Mindfulness and Ethos

Compatibility, Challenges and Opportunities in the Irish Catholic Primary School

Religion, Education and Values

Volume 19

PETER LANG
Oxford · Berlin · Bruxelles · Chennai · Lausanne · New York

Mindfulness and Ethos

Compatibility, Challenges and Opportunities in the Irish Catholic Primary School

Thomas Carroll

PETER LANG
Oxford · Berlin · Bruxelles · Chennai · Lausanne · New York

Bibliographic Information published by the Deutsche Nationalbibliothek
The Deutsche Nationalbibliothek lists this publication in the Deutsche Nationalbibliografie; detailed bibliographic data is available online at http://dnb.d-nb.de.

Library of Congress Cataloging-in-Publication Data
Names: Carroll, Thomas, 1991- author
Title: Mindfulness and ethos : compatibility, challenges and opportunities in the Irish Catholic primary school / Thomas Carroll.
Other titles: Evaluation of the compatibility of mindfulness and ethos in the Irish Catholic primary school
Description: Oxford ; New York : Peter Lang, [2025] | Series: Religion, education and values, 2235-4638 ; volume 19 | Revision of the author's thesis (PhD, University of Limerick, 2021) under the title: An evaluation of the compatibility of mindfulness and ethos in the Irish Catholic primary school. | Includes bibliographical references.
Identifiers: LCCN 2025000629 (print) | LCCN 2025000630 (ebook) | ISBN 9781803740362 paperback | ISBN 9781803740379 ebook | ISBN 9781803740386 epub
Subjects: LCSH: Catholic Church--Education--Ireland--History | Education, Primary--Ireland--History | Mindfulness (Psychology)--Religious aspects | Catholic elementary schools--Ireland--History
Classification: LCC LC506.I7 C366 2025 (print) | LCC LC506.I7 (ebook)
LC record available at https://lccn.loc.gov/2025000629
LC ebook record available at https://lccn.loc.gov/2025000630

A catalogue record for this book is available at the British Library.

The cover image:
Students practicing mindfulness with a Christian symbol in the background
© iStock-1463488020.jpg

ISSN 2235-4638
ISBN 978-1-80374-036-2 (Print)
ISBN 978-1-80374-037-9 (EPDF)
ISBN 978-1-80374-038-6 (EPUB)
DOI 10.3726/b20326

Published by Peter Lang Ltd, Oxford (United Kingdom)

info@peterlang.com www.peterlang.com

This publication has been peer reviewed.

To my wife Emma and Henry, the king of the doggos

Contents

List of Figures

Abbreviations

ASA	A Secular Age
CCE	Congregation for Catholic Education
CES	Catholic Education Service
CS	The Catholic School
CSO	Central Statistics Office
CSP	Catholic Schools Partnership
DES	Department for Education and Skills
EFH	Educating to Fraternal Humanism: Building a 'Civilisation of Love' 50 Years after Popolorum Progressio (2017)
EIDCS	Educating to Intercultural Dialogue in Catholic Schools: Living in Harmony for a Civilisation of Love (2013)
GE	Gravissimum Educationis (1965)
MBCT	Mindfulness-Based Cognitive Therapy
MBI	Mindfulness-Based Interventions
MBSR	Mindfulness-Based Stress Reduction
NA	Nostra Aetate (1965)
PPI	Positive Psychology Interventions
RDECS	The Religious Dimension of Education in a Catholic School (1988)
SSE	School Self-Evaluation

Preface

Ireland has undergone seismic cultural and societal transformations in recent decades. The most recent census found that 69% of citizens in the Irish Republic identify as Catholic, a drop of 10% from the previous statistics. Concurrently, the number of nonreligious has grown to the second largest demographic in the state, solidifying the reality that Ireland is becoming less religious in terms of belief and practice. The Catholic Church has lost its hitherto status as a monopoly religion due to secularisation, accelerated by clerical abuse scandals and cover-ups. As Crawford Gribben concluded in his 2023 book *The Rise and Fall of Christian Ireland*, 'What has passed as Christian Ireland is dead.' Yet over 88% of Irish primary schools are under Catholic patronage, a visible expression of the tension between Ireland's historical Catholic hegemony and the post-Catholic society of today.

Within this milieu, the contemporary phenomenon of mindfulness has emerged, surging in popularity and visibility in many sectors of society, including education, and by extension, Catholic primary schools. Deriving from forms of Buddhist meditation, mindfulness is associated with positive outcomes such as improved mental well-being and reduced stress among a myriad of other claims. As a Catholic primary school teacher, a researcher in Catholic education, and a person with an interest in forms of mindfulness practice, I have wondered about the intersection point of these schools with their distinctive educational and theological vision and the popularity of mindfulness practice, a phenomenon originating from Eastern wisdom traditions. This book is the result of that wonderment, drawing upon insights from scholars including Charles Taylor, Lieven Boeve, Tomáš Halík and Michael Paul Gallagher to first outline a coherent narrative of how religious belief is experienced in our contemporary Western context and by extension, Ireland.

The ubiquity of mindfulness in contemporary life means that the term is often used loosely to convey a variety of meanings and values, leading to the risk of opacity in what exactly mindfulness means. The concept, origin, etymology, history and recontextualisations of mindfulness are presented here to offer the reader an overview of the term. The role of mindfulness in Irish education is also explored, situating the practice within an evolving framework of curricular reform and policy development, with particular reference to the relationship between mindfulness and well-being. In doing so, the reader receives a snapshot of changing educational terrain in Ireland, as novel conceptions of the intentions and purposes of education and flourishing emerge, suggesting turns to contemplative and holistic visions of education.

This book provides a comprehensive overview of a coherent and robust vision of Catholic education, drawing upon various voices in the field, particularly those in Ireland and the United Kingdom, such as Stephen McKinney, Patricia Kieran and John Sullivan. For those interested in the purpose, themes and Church publications on Catholic education, this book provides an accessible resource to make sense of these areas.

Ultimately, this book seeks to establish if mindfulness is compatible with the Catholic primary school ethos in Ireland. It establishes moments of both compatibility and incompatibility, outlining the consequences for both in the life of Catholic schools. It is a dialogue between mindfulness and Catholic education, seeking fruits that can be life-giving to those who work in Catholic schools. Areas of discussion include mindfulness as pre-evangelisation, the relationship between mindfulness and prayer, and mindfulness as other and other-centred. For those interested, enthused, or concerned by mindfulness practice in Catholic schools, this book is a resource to meet such needs and motivations. Its findings and recommendations are important to all those interested in contemporary developments in Catholic education, policy and practice.

Originally a doctoral thesis, the book fills the lacuna of knowledge originally identified with updated research to demonstrate the current state of play regarding mindfulness and Catholic education. Building from that work, I extend my thanks to my supervisors and guides, Rev. Prof. Eamonn Conway (University of Notre Dame) and Dr. Daniel O' Connell (Mary Immaculate College), for giving me the confidence to take the thesis and do something more with it. My thanks also to the insights and advice of my colleagues and fellow academics as I charted this journey. Finally, I thank Tony Mason, Commissioning Editor at Peter Lang, and his team for their professionalism and support during this process.

Introduction

We are witnessing what writer and mindfulness coach Barry Boyce has termed the 'mindfulness revolution'.[1] Mindfulness has exploded in popularity in recent decades across many areas of society, including healthcare, commerce and education. This phenomenon has become increasingly common in Irish schools. Mindfulness practice is supported by a growing body of literature, promoting benefits such a physical and mental wellbeing, improved socialisation and enhanced academic performance.

Given that a significant majority of Irish primary schools have a Catholic ethos,[2] it is important to consider what the implications are for mindfulness practice in these schools. This was exemplified in 2019, when Dr. Alphonsus Cullinan, Bishop of Waterford and Lismore, claimed in a letter to the diocesan schools that mindfulness and yoga were not Christian activities and not suitable for practice during religious education.[3] For some media outlets, such comments were deemed a controversial and unhelpful input, despite the Bishop's correct assertion that Buddhist mindfulness did not have a Christian origin, and as such, the Catholic school was not a suitable site for such a practice. Such demarcations are of paramount importance as schools with a Catholic ethos have a right and a responsibility to provide religious

1 Barry Boyce, ed., *The Mindfulness Revolution: Leading Psychologists, Scientists, Artists, and Spiritual Teachers on the Power of Mindfulness in Daily Life* (Boston, MA: Shambala, 2011).

2 'Catholic schools still comprise the vast majority of primary schools, with 88.4 per cent of schools having a Catholic ethos in 2023/2024.' Department of Education and Skills, *Statistical Bulletin, August 2024: Overview of Education: 2003/04–2023/24* (Dublin: Rialtas na hÉireann, 2024). <https://www.gov.ie/en/collection/annual-statistical-reports/>. Accessed on 31st August 2024.

3 Darren Skelton, 'Bishop of Waterford Warns Against Yoga and Mindfulness in Schools', *The Journal.ie*, 18 October 2019. <https://www.thejournal.ie/waterford-bishop-alphonsus-cullinan-yoga-mindfulness-4857160-Oct2019/>. Accessed on 5 August 2020.

education in the Christian tradition, available to all, using appropriate teaching methods and pedagogies.[4]

This raises questions as to whether mindfulness is compatible with the Catholic ethos, but also on a more general level, what does mindfulness mean, and how can it be understood in our contemporary context? Are some forms of mindfulness compatible with the Catholic ethos, and if so, how so? Conversely, how are those other forms of mindfulness incompatible with the Catholic ethos? The 2018 publication by the Irish Bishops' Conference's Council for Catechetics, *A Reflection on Mindfulness: Rediscovering the Christian Tradition of Meditation and Contemplation,*[5] attempted to address some of these questions and offered guidance to schools on mindfulness in Catholic schools. This included recognising that meditation was an activity seen across many different wisdom traditions, and contemplative prayer was also to be found in the Christian tradition. It also made reference to some of the spiritual riches of Christian contemplative prayer and meditation as practiced by several of the great mystics of the Church.[6,7]

4 Irish Catholic Bishops' Conference, *Guidelines for the Faith Formation and Development of Catholic Students* (Dublin: Veritas, 1999).

5 Council for Catechetics, Irish Catholic Bishops' Conference, *A Reflection on Mindfulness: Rediscovering the Christian Tradition of Meditation and Contemplation* (Dublin: Veritas, 2018).

6 Ibid, 16. 'Among those who promoted attentiveness to the present moment, we can think of Meister Eckhart (thirteenth/fourteenth century), the anonymous author of "The Cloud of Unknowing," St Catherine of Siena (fourteenth century), Julian of Norwich (late fourteenth, early fifteenth century), St Teresa of Ávila (sixteenth century) and Jean-Pierre de Caussade (eighteenth century). In modern times, saints and teachers such as St Thérèse of Lisieux, Dom John Main, Thomas Merton, Abbot Thomas Keating, Pope St John Paul II, Chiara Lubich and St Mother Teresa have all insisted that this contemplative attentiveness to the present moment must be taught once again and so preached and taught the importance of the practising attentiveness to the present moment as a presence of God.'

7 The work of Dr Noel Keating is significant here. Keating has sought to introduce children in Irish primary schools to the practice of Christian meditation, a traditional form of Christian contemplative prayer which was rediscovered and popularised by the Benedictine monk John Main. <http://www.christianmeditation.ie/?q=meditationwithchildren>.

However, research remains at an early stage on the relationship between Christian spirituality and mindfulness,[8] with few articles exploring the relationship between Catholic schools and mindfulness.[9] In this sense, this book makes a meaningful contribution to Catholic educational research, particularly within the Irish Catholic educational context. It fills a lacuna of knowledge in relation to how mindfulness is to be understood today and how it is operative in Irish Catholic primary schools. Given the legacy of debilitating effects of the COVID-19 lockdown on the wellbeing of so many Irish children, this research provides an opportunity to address the implications of mindfulness practice in Irish education, its possible benefits and how there are many riches in a Catholic educational vision that can contribute to each child being enabled to flourish and reach their full potential.

The conclusions, findings and recommendations are of interest to patrons and managerial bodies who may see mindfulness as incompatible with the ethos of Catholic schools, or who understand contemporary mindfulness practice as a spiritual practice belonging to Buddhism. It may prompt them to consider what mindfulness may contribute to the Catholic educational vision of these schools, and likewise, what resources in the Catholic faith tradition could also be drawn upon to promote Christian contemplative or silent prayer. For Catholic educational practitioners, it may encourage them to explore how mindfulness practice contributes to the holistic development of the child and how it would contribute to their distinctive Catholic school ethos. This work thus seeks to marry theological research with the practical implications of mindfulness practice in Irish Catholic primary schools.

8 See Stefan G. Reynolds, *Living with the Mind of Christ: Mindfulness in Christian Spirituality* (London: Darton, Longman & Todd, 2016) and Peter Tyler, *Christian Mindfulness: Theology and Practice* (London: SCM Press, 2018).

9 Stefan G. Reynolds, 'Mindfulness, Yoga and Schools: An Opportunity or a Problem?', *The Furrow* (December 2019); Thomas Carroll, 'Mindfulness as *Praeparatio Evangelica* in the Irish Catholic School', *Irish Theological Quarterly 88*(4) (2023), 323–39 and Thomas Carroll, 'Mindfulness in Catholic Primary Schools: An Irish Perspective', *Religions 14*(11) (2023), 1348.

Book Structure

The book is divided into six chapters.

Chapter 1 contextualises this research by exploring the conditions of religious belief and experience operative today. Five significant thinkers are brought into conversation with each other in this regard. First, the work of moral philosopher Charles Taylor is examined, with particular reference to his seminal work, *A Secular Age*. Second, the work of theologian Lieven Boeve, who argues that our contemporary context is both post-Christian and post-secular, is explored. Third, the thought of Irish theologian Michael Paul Gallagher on the crisis of the imagination and the rise of cultural unbelief is investigated. Fourth, Czech philosopher, sociologist and theologian Tomáš Halík's work is examined. Halík proposes a seeker-dweller paradigm to best understand the mission of the Church today. Finally, Grace Davie's thought is explored, with reference to her analytical tools of appraising religious beliefs and practice from a religious sociological perspective. From this interdisciplinary interaction between interlocutors, several themes emerge that shape the parameters of this book.

Chapter 2 is an examination of the contemporary phenomenon of mindfulness. It explores the origins, development and scientific benefits of mindfulness, recognising the importance it plays in the Buddhist wisdom tradition. It also charts the evolution of mindfulness from Eastern religious practice to Western secular phenomenon through the socio-historical processes of Buddhist modernism. Moreover, this chapter explores and critiques the three distinctive strands of mindfulness operative in the West today. Mindfulness 1 represents the secularised, psychologised mode of practice made famous by molecular biologist Jon Kabat-Zinn. Mindfulness 2 relates to the privatised, commodified version of mindfulness, exemplified in the many books, apps and products with the mindfulness brand. Finally, Mindfulness 3 signifies the post-secular spirituality model. This form, while deracinated from Buddhism, offers many people who do not identify as religious a practice that answers some desire for fulfilment or spiritual need.

Chapter 3 considers how mindfulness is increasingly influential in the Irish education system today, with particular reference to the concept of wellbeing. This includes investigating the growing presence of mindfulness, through the vehicle of wellbeing, in educational policy and curricular reform at Irish primary and post-primary levels. Current research on mindfulness in education is also investigated to ascertain whether the benefits of mindfulness to children have been conclusively proven or whether further, more rigorous study is needed. This chapter also explores two programmes operative in Irish primary schools that use mindfulness to promote positive wellbeing: Paws b and Weaving Wellbeing.

Chapter 4 develops criteria for a Catholic educational vision that will be used to evaluate the compatibility of mindfulness with Irish Catholic primary school ethos. First, it surveys the landscape of Church literature on Catholic education since the Second Vatican Council. This involves examining several influential documents to ascertain what key themes are present in Catholic education, including *Gravissimum Educationis (1965)*, *The Catholic School (1977)* and *The Religious Dimension of Education in a Catholic School (1988)*, as well as the more recent *Educating to Intercultural Dialogue in Catholic Schools: Living in Harmony for a Civilisation of Love (2013)* and *Educating to Fraternal Humanism: Building a 'Civilisation of Love' 50 Years after Populorum Progressio (2017)*. This also involves how Catholic education in Ireland is envisioned, with reference to important documents within the Irish Church over recent decades. Following this, the framework for the distinctiveness of Catholic education offered by theologian Thomas Groome will be investigated in dialogue with other significant thinkers in this area, such as John Sullivan, Patricia Kieran and Stephen McKinney. From this, key themes for a Catholic educational vision emerge, which will serve as the evaluative criteria to evaluate the compatibility of mindfulness with Irish Catholic primary school ethos.

Chapter 5 is the evaluative chapter, these criteria of a Catholic educational vision: (1) Theological Anthropology; (2) Christocentricity; (3) Sacramentality; (4) Evangelisation; (5) Academic Integrity and Autonomy of Subjects; (6) Dialogue between Faith and Culture and (7) Social Justice, are utilised to judge how and when mindfulness is congruent with Catholic ethos. Several opportunities emerge here, such as the benefits of mindfulness to the holistic development of the child, mindfulness as a contemplative practice and mindfulness as a means of pre-evangelisation. However, challenges also emerge, such as the dangers of mindfulness being utilised solely for academic performance, or as an individualist means of soothing rather than subverting sources of suffering in society and in those around them.

Finally, Chapter 6 presents the conclusions, findings and recommendations of the book. It charts out how mindfulness is not only compatible with the ethos of Irish Catholic primary schools but is, in fact, a potentially invaluable resource to a Catholic educational vision lived out in these schools.

CHAPTER 1

The Conditions of Religious Belief and Experience in the Contemporary European Context

In order to evaluate the relationship between mindfulness and ethos in Irish Catholic primary schools, it is imperative first to understand and appreciate the current conditions of religious belief and experience operative within the contemporary European context. While this work focuses on the Irish context, it is important to include the European context in the framework. While Ireland maintains comparatively higher levels of religious belief and practice than many other European countries, irreligiosity has emerged as the second largest belief category in Ireland's 2022 Census.[10] The causes of this shift in religious belief merit reflection from a theological perspective, as argued by theologian Stephen Bullivant.[11]

What will now be presented are the perspectives of prominent thinkers who have researched religious belief and experience in the

10 The 2022 Census data indicated that 69% of the population in the Republic of Ireland self-identified as Catholic, a 10% decrease from the previous Census results six years earlier, while irreligion simultaneously solidified its place as the next largest grouping at 14%, an increase of 4%. See Central Statistics Office (CSO), *Census of Population 2022—Summary Results*. Available online: <https://www.cso.ie/en/releasesandpublications/ep/p-cpsr/censusofpopulation2022-summaryresults/migrationanddiversity/ (accessed on 21 September 2024)>.

11 Stephen Bullivant notes the findings of the 2008 International Social Survey Programme (ISSP) which outlines the huge variance in people identifying as atheist or agnostic. 'Cyprus had the lowest incidence with a combined total of 5% ... closely followed by Portugal (8%) and Poland and Ireland (both 9%) At the opposite end of the spectrum were the Czech Republic (52%), Sweden (39%), France (37% ... The sheer existence of unbelief on this scale poses Christianity and its followers with a large number of important and uncomfortable questions'. Stephen Bullivant, *Faith and Unbelief: Faith Going Deeper* (London: Canterbury Press Norwich, 2013), xiv–xv.

contemporary European context, encompassing the Irish experience. These interlocutors come from different academic backgrounds, but each provide a unique and pertinent reading of the times. Moreover, in order to present a more comprehensive outline of the contemporary spiritual climate, an interdisciplinary approach is necessary to address this phenomenon from perspectives including theology, sociology of religion and moral philosophy.

The first is Canadian moral philosopher Charles Taylor, whose seminal text *A Secular Age* has had a profound impact on research into religious belief and experience in an age increasingly characterised as postmodern. Described as '... one of the finest intellectual commentators on Western culture and religion',[12] Taylor's work focuses on the concept of the modern social imaginary and the search for authenticity of the self.

Belgian theologian Lieven Boeve is credited with characterising our current context as post-Christian and post-secular, as well as exploring how to maintain the particularity of the Christian narrative in an increasingly pluralist society. Boeve has been particularly influential in the establishment of Catholic Dialogue Schools in his native Belgium[13], attempting to enable Catholic education to flourish within a detraditionalised, postmodern context, and, as such, his insights are extremely important in contextualising this work.

The late Irish theologian Michael Paul Gallagher's work provides a theological perspective on the relationship between faith and culture, articulating a creative reading of the contemporary crisis of belief and imagination. Gallagher's prophetic insights are relevant as they identify shifts from belief to unbelief in the Irish context, recognising that high mass attendance and self-identification as Catholic do not necessarily equate to a rich spiritual life.

Czech philosopher, sociologist and theologian Tomáš Halík offers a unique perspective of the believer living in an overwhelmingly secular

12 Richard Kearney and Jens Zimmerman, *Reimagining the Sacred: Richard Kearney Debates God* (NY: Columbia University Press, 2016), 76.

13 Lieven Boeve, 'Faith in Dialogue: The Christian Voice in the Catholic Dialogue School', *International Studies in Catholic Education 11*(1) (2019), 37–50.

society. Halík advocates a patient faith that bears the doubts of atheism and a Church that reaches out to those seeking meaning in their lives on the margins of faith. A former atheist, Halík is helpful here in recognising the need to further explore that grey area between belief and unbelief, and the contemporary hunger for meaning felt by many.

Finally, sociologist of religion Grace Davie provides sociological resources in exploring the prevailing role of religion in society. Davie is credited with the terms 'believing without belonging' and 'vicarious religion' to diagnose how religious belief and experience have changed and evolved in modern times. Davie stresses the importance of the social sciences not being limited by secular assumptions, as a detached, neutral viewpoint will not adequately address the prevalence of religion in people's lives. Davie's insights are particularly relevant here, given her position as an Anglican vicar as well as a prominent sociologist of religion.

By bringing these interlocutors into dialogue with each other, it will be illustrated that there are sometimes striking differences as well as similarities in interpreting the religious signs of the times. In this way, essential criteria will emerge that will provide a theological framework for this project, contextualising the question at the heart of this work, the compatibility of mindfulness and ethos of Irish Catholic primary schools. The first interlocutor to be explored is Charles Taylor.

Charles Taylor

In his seminal work, *A Secular Age*, Charles Taylor explores the interaction between religion and modernity and its implications for how people construct identity and discover meaning. Taylor maps out how the conditions of religious belief and experience have altered over time from a hitherto undoubted assumption of theistic belief to one where the very plausibility of such belief is in question. As such, Taylor asks:

> How did we move from a condition where, in Christendom, people lived naïvely within a theistic construal, to one where we all shunt between two stances, in which

> everyone's construal shows up as such; and in which, moreover, unbelief has become the major default option?[14]

Taylor identifies 'us' in his question as those in Western nations, where unbelief has become the norm, rather than the exception. While some countries, including Ireland still possess a relatively high (albeit decreasing) rate of religious belief, an elite intellectual class in society can influence and transmit secular enlightenment views, changing the conditions of the plausibility of theistic belief. This trend has been noticed by sociologist of religion Peter Berger.[15]

Before outlining Taylor's approach to secularity, it is important to describe what Taylor means by religion. Taylor understands religion as any worldview that allows for the possibility of an experience of transcendence, stating that '… a reading of "religion" in terms of the distinction transcendent/immanent is going to serve our purposes here.'[16] Such an approach enables religion to be understood as more than theism, as that represents just one option of an openness to transformation that goes beyond human flourishing in an immanent sense. For this reason, Taylor includes non-theistic wisdom traditions such as Buddhism, which can present both an immanent

14 Charles Taylor, *A Secular Age* (Cambridge: Harvard University Press, Belknap Press, 2007), 14. Hereafter, this text will be referred to as *ASA*, unless otherwise stated. Taylor's question on how Western society has undergone such a radical change in religious belief and experience can be asked in blunter terms: 'Why was it virtually impossible not to believe in God in, say 1500 in our Western society, while in 2000 many of us find this not only easy, but even inescapable?' Ibid, 19.

15 Peter Berger, *The Desecularization of the World: Resurgent Religion and World Politics* (Grand Rapids: Eerdmans, 1999), 10. 'There exists an international subculture composed of people with Western-type higher education, especially in the humanities and social sciences, that is indeed secularized. This subculture is the principal "carrier" of progressive, Enlightened beliefs and values. While its members are relatively thin on the ground, they are very influential, as they control the institutions that provide the "official" definitions of reality, notably the education system, the media of mass communication, and the higher reaches of the legal system.'

16 *ASA*, 15.

and transcendent axis.[17] In this sense, Taylor offers an inclusive definition of religion in exploring how people experience the sacred in a secular age.

Taylor adopts three classifications of the term 'secular' in mapping out the altered circumstances surrounding the rise of widespread unbelief. For Secular 1, following medieval or classical accounts, 'secular' was the realm of the temporal and profane, existing on a different plane to the sacred. Philosopher James Smith proposes:

> This is the "secular" of the purported sacred/secular divide. The priest for instance, pursues a "sacred" vocation, while the butcher, baker and candlestick maker are engaged in "secular" pursuits.[18]

These were planes of reality with porous borders, where the mundane realm of the temporal could be penetrated and upended by the sacred. Secular 1 highlights the premodern imaginary, where belief in God was taken to be axiomatic, and that objects and things were imbued with spiritual or sacred power, which was beyond human perception or understanding. Such examples include the spiritual power attributed to relics or cathedrals. Secular 1 signifies the permeable boundary between the ordinary, earthly aspects of reality and the enchanted, otherworldly realm of the sacred.

Secular 2 corresponds to the decline in the number of people who identify with religious affiliation, particularly the Christian faith, '... people turning away from God, and no longer going to Church'.[19] This understanding of secularity can be seen most clearly in contemporary debates on the place of religion in public life. Such a definition of secularity is common in arguments

17 Ruth Abbey elaborates on Taylor's broad definition of religion. 'Any orientation toward the transcendent where the understanding of transcendence feeds back into a conception of human flourishing and fullness, counts as religion for the purposes of Taylor's analysis of the secular age. He offers Buddhism as an example of this- it has a transcendent axis that informs its conception of human flourishing, but it is not a traditional form of theism.' Ruth Abbey, 'The Missing Question Mark', in Ian Leask, ed., *The Taylor Effect: Responding to a Secular Age* (Newcastle: Cambridge Scholars Publishing, 2010), 11.

18 James K.A. Smith, *How (Not) to Be Secular: Reading Charles Taylor* (Grand Rapids: Eerdmans, 2014), 20–21.

19 *ASA*, 2.

for religious belief to be sidelined into private life and that the public square should be governed by political institutions underpinned by a neutral, rational viewpoint. As Smith puts it, 'Secularism is always secularism 2'.[20]

Secular 2 represents a shift from Secular 1 in that the previously porous boundary between the sacred and secular realms hardens, both realms becoming distinctive locations within institutions and society. The plausibility of belief in an independent eternal reality is challenged as Secular 2 generates an areligious space where life for many is buffered from the intrusions of transcendental experience. In this way, Secular 2 represents the modern phenomenon of the contest between religion and secularism in the public square.

In marking the shift from Secular 1 to Secular 2, Taylor is critical of previous sociological theories, such as the secularisation thesis, which suggests that the narrative of modernity and freedom from superstition gradually eclipses religious belief and experience. He outlines the various arguments proposing the secularisation thesis:

> ... that religion must decline either (a) because it is false, and science shows this to be so; or (b) because it is increasingly irrelevant now that we can cure ringworm by drenches (the 'artificial-fertilizers-make-atheists' argument); or (c) because religion is based on authority, and modern societies give an increasingly important place to individual autonomy; or some combination of the above.[21]

For Taylor, the secularisation thesis has some value in that it rightly identifies cultural forces that influenced secularisation, such as industrialisation, urbanisation and fragmentation of the religious community.[22] However, it fails to account for the conditions of religion and unbelief today, how people feel or sense the sacred in this secular age. Thus, Taylor's most original contribution to this discussion is found in his articulation of a third definition of secularity, unique from the social theories of the previous secular categories. Taylor focuses on the conditions of belief,[23] on what the experience of a religious believer or a non-believer is like in contemporary

20 James K.A. Smith, *How (Not) to Be Secular: Reading Charles Taylor* (Grand Rapids: Eerdmans, 2014), 21.

21 *ASA*, 428–9.

22 Ibid, 436.

23 Ibid, 2–3.

Western societies, rather than on expressions of belief. Smith points out the philosophical perspectives that undergird Taylor's Secular 3:

> It is important to appreciate that, philosophically, Taylor is working from the tradition of hermeneutic phenomenology, an heir to Heidegger and Merleau-Ponty. So he equates the 'conditions' of belief with the "background" we bring to our perception of reality.[24]

Taylor is thus less concerned with data on how religious affiliation is practiced and more concerned with how the individual's very experience of reality interacts with some form of religious or transcendental experience. In Secular 3, the shift in the conditions of the plausibility of religious belief is '... a move from a society where belief in God was unchallenged and indeed, unproblematic, to one in which it is understood to be one option among others and frequently not the easiest to embrace'.[25]

Taylor presents a radically transformed context for religion in a secular age, where the essential change lies on the level of the social imaginary, the ways people perceive or sense their social surroundings, which operates on a deeper and broader level that is different to intellectual frameworks.[26] In this sense, Taylor seeks to shift the debate about secularisation from visible and quantifiable changes in social practice to deeper movements of spiritual imagination and sensibility. Secular 3 highlights how the background of how we imagine our social existence has radically shifted, particularly in terms of being aware of a transcendental level to reality. For Taylor, people now possess an altered social imaginary, which is expressed through images, symbols and stories rather than by interpretations of data and theories.

24 James K. A. Smith, *How (Not) to Be Secular: Reading Charles Taylor* (Grand Rapids: Eerdmans, 2014), 18.

25 *ASA*, 3.

26 Taylor defines social imaginary as '... something much broader and deeper than the intellectual schemes people may entertain when they think about social reality in a disengaged mode. I am thinking, rather, of the ways people imagine their social existence, how they fit together with others, how things go on between them and their fellows, the expectations that are normally met, and the deeper normative notions and images that underlie these expectations.' Charles Taylor, *Modern Social Imaginaries* (Durham, Duke University Press, 2004), 23.

Secular 3 highlights the conditions of religion and unbelief that have made possible '… new ways of existing both in and out of relation with God' via the modern social imaginary'.[27] For Taylor, this is manifested in the unprecedented phenomenon that humans can now live without any link or interest in transcendence or form of religion, where '… a purely self-sufficient humanism came to be a widely available option … a humanism accepting no final goals beyond human flourishing; nor any allegiance to anything beyond this flourishing. Of no previous society was this true'.[28]

This is in stark contrast to the porous self of premodern times, where the medieval social imaginary allowed for openness and vulnerability to an enchanted world where meaning and significance could be derived from. Human agents were not understood to be the sole possessors of power and agency in the face of spirits, demons and magic. Moreover, the belief in an eternal realm independent of the secular world was seen as axiomatic, providing a transcendent backdrop to the mundane experiences of people.

Smith highlights the significance Taylor places on the porous self's openness to experience of some external spiritual realm or from transcendence, noting that '… the self is essentially vulnerable (and hence also 'healable'). To be human is to essentially be open to an outside (whether benevolent or malevolent), open to blessing or curse, possession or grace'.[29] This highlights an understanding of the human person as connected and open to the experience of the transcendent. However, this porous self is shattered by the contemporary growth of the buffered self and the immanent frame.

As the premodern imaginary moved to the modern imaginary, so did the porous self develop into the buffered self. This was '… a new sense of the self and its place in the cosmos: not open and vulnerable to a world of spirits and powers'.[30] The magic of the premodern world was disenchanted, and the vulnerability or openness to transformation through transcendence receded as Secular 2 advanced. For Taylor, the buffered self is operative in

27 *ASA*, 437.
28 Ibid, 18.
29 James K. A. Smith, *How (Not) to Be Secular: Reading Charles Taylor* (Grand Rapids: Eerdmans, 2014), 29.
30 *ASA*, 27.

Secular 3, making possible a perception of the world where transcendence or the experience of the transcendent is deemed irrelevant or implausible.

This buffered self is not open to normative demands from any agency external to itself. The transcendent realm is eclipsed by the immanent, creating a mode of existence devoid of any connection to a supernatural reality or experience of transcendence. Sacred time and space become increasingly sidelined in favour of a secular realm where human flourishing is seen as being independent of the sacred or transcendent. Taylor refers to this modern social imaginary as being operative within the immanent frame.

> So the buffered identity of the disciplined individual moves in a constructed social space, where instrumental rationality is a key value, and time is pervasively secular. All of this makes up what I call 'the immanent frame'.[31]

The immanent frame is '... common to all of us in the modern West'.[32] It is a mode of living within each person operates within, where cosmic, ethical and social orders do not need explanation or meaning from any transcendent or supernatural reality. Such a self-sufficient way of living allows for the possibility of exclusive humanism, where human flourishing is understood as a goal without a transcendent aspect. This reading does not occur from intellectual enquiry, rather, it is a part of our social imaginary, a deeper sensibility towards the backdrop of how we perceive reality.[33]

Taylor is critical of a closed reading or 'closed spin' of the immanent frame. An open reading allows at least for the possibility of believing in transcendence, whereas a closed spin rejects it outright. This inflexibility signifies the assumed implausibility of belief in anything beyond a secular, rational frame of reference. Given the conditions of Secular 3, belief in God or a sacred realm is seen at best irrelevant and at worst hostile and dangerous to a place in the public square. These views are pervasive among many figures in the academic world, where secular enlightenment values are

31 *ASA*, 542.

32 Ibid, 543.

33 How you inhabit the immanent frame is less a fruit of deduction and more a "vibe". It is less a reasoned position or articulated worldview and more a Wittgensteinian 'picture' that holds is captively precisely because it's not conscious.' James K. A. Smith, *How (Not) to Be Secular: Reading Charles Taylor* (Grand Rapids: Eerdmans, 2014), 95.

disseminated and confidently assumed in the plausibility of their worldview while equally dismissive of the possibility of the sacred realm or experience of the transcendent.

Taylor challenges this '… spin of closure which is hegemonic in the Academy'[34] and questions the confidence of such a position, arguing that the closed spin assumes a viewpoint that goes beyond mere rationality.[35] Taylor's critique of the closed spin is that it takes as obvious and self-evident that any experience of transcendence is implausible. It does this despite having no evidence or reason to draw such a certain conclusion. Moreover, the closed spin highlights the way questions of the transcendent are dealt within the immanent frame.

However, the predictions of secularisation theories that religion would be eclipsed by rationality have not necessarily been proven. Religion remains a potent force of meaning for many, and a desire for living fully and authentically is pervasive. Rather than arriving at a stage of comfortable unbelief, a search for authenticity and a spiritual hunger generates unrest in a secular age.

This lack of contentment culminates in what Taylor calls the 'nova effect'. This concept indicates the explosion of multiple options for seeking authenticity, meaning and fullness in life. In Secular 3, the individual operating the immanent frame is '… living in a spiritual supernova, a kind of galloping pluralism on the spiritual plane'.[36] The rise of the possibility of exclusive humanism does not do away with experiencing the transcendence; rather, it leads to a pluralisation and fragilisation of positions on searching for meaning and significance in our lives, an explosion of religious and non-religious spiritual options.

For Taylor, many initially will retain a comfortable distance from this gamut of worldviews as they appear so other as being inaccessible or irrelevant

34 Ibid, 549.

35 Educational Pádraig Hogan summarises Taylor's challenge to this type of reading which '… makes its own leap of faith in the non-existence of a "beyond". But it remains unaware of the element of credulity in this stance due to its own domestication in privative accounts of secularisation.' Pádraig Hogan, 'Inheritances of Learning and the "Unquiet Frontiers of Modernity"', in Ian Leask, ed., *The Taylor Effect: Responding to a Secular Age* (Newcastle: Cambridge Scholars Publishing, 2010), 140.

36 *ASA*, 300.

to how the individual engages in the world. Moreover, a closed spin approach is not challenged by these options, as there is an assumption that questions of spirituality or narratives that call for personal transformation will not break the protective shell of the buffered self. However, given the continued pluralisation and fragmentation of positions and exposure to people with different perspectives, many individuals are eventually confronted by this novel effect and an awareness of alternatives to their position.[37]

Thus, everyone inhabiting the immanent frame is faced with 'cross-pressures'. Rather than the subtraction theories of secularisation, the explosion of options means that there is a constant fragilisation of viewpoints that can seem strange and contestable. People are constantly exposed to various beliefs and worldviews that challenge their own perceptions of reality. This means that they have a heightened sense of awareness of spiritual options and positions different from theirs. Moreover, cross-pressures are experienced by people across the spectrum of belief and unbelief on the level of the social imaginary in Secular 3, where the conditions of belief have changed.

Even those who live with a 'closed spin reading' of the immanent frame can feel the loss of transcendent experience as part of their implicit background. Any sense of the sacred or the depth of mystery seems to be flattened by the superficial nature of much of contemporary living. Taylor notes how this loss can be felt in the mundaneness of everyday life.

> ... some people feel a terrible flatness in the everyday, and this experience has been identified particularly with commercial, industrial, or consumer society. They feel emptiness of the repeated, accelerating cycle of desire and fulfilment, in consumer culture; the cardboard quality of bright supermarkets, or neat row housing in a clean suburb.[38]

Our consumerist culture seems to be shorn of any orientation towards the sacred, any significance or meaning beyond the flatness of a disenchanted world. This malaise of immanence means that many people may question whether their life has ultimate meaning and whether sources for flourishing

37 'Then the issue posed by the difference becomes more insistent: why my way, and why not hers? There is no other difference left to make the shift preposterous and unimaginable'. Ibid, 304.

38 Ibid, 309.

or living authentically can be found.[39] This does not necessarily mean that a return to an openness to transcendence is inevitable. Rather, many seek satiety or fullness within the immanent world through a variety of means, which in turn leads to the nova effect.

Taylor argues that '... life is fuller, richer, deeper, and more worthwhile, more admirable, more what it should be'.[40] For Taylor, fullness takes us beyond human flourishing in an immanent sense and into the sacred or transcendent. These experiences of fullness can be moments of intense joy and fulfilment, but also traumatic and bewildering. There is a depth of meaning in these moments of transcendence that strike at the heart of our modern social imaginary. The buffered self is confronted with a sense of something mysterious that is beyond our secular language and frames of reference.

> They can orient us because they offer some sense of what they are of: the presence of God, or the voice of nature, or the force which drives through everything, or the alignment in us of desire and the drive to form. But they are also often unsettling and enigmatic. Our sense of where they come from may also be unclear, confused ... We are deeply loved, but also puzzled and shaken. We struggle to articulate what we have been through.[41]

Taylor questions how we can then speak of fullness without some transcendental aspect in this secular age with its altered conditions of belief. Taylor sees fullness as the condition we aspire to that exists beyond the malaise of immanence, but also beyond human flourishing. It transcends our human vocabulary and cannot be controlled or mastered through rational means or human will. Within the Christian tradition, such an ideal of fullness is teleological, which Taylor calls 'final goals'.[42] For Taylor, fullness from a theological perspective is '... a condition in which our highest spiritual and

39 Costello cites three modes of malaises which Taylor explores. '(1) the fragility of meaning, the loosening of a sense of or search for an over-arching significance. (2) the felt flatness of attempts to solemnise important moments of our lives and (3) the emptiness of the ordinary'. Stephen Costello, "Beyond Flourishing: 'Fullness' and 'Conversion' in Taylor and Lonergan", in Ian Leask, ed., *The Taylor Effect: Responding to a Secular Age* (Newcastle: Cambridge Scholars Publishing, 2010), 140.

40 *ASA*, 5.

41 Ibid, 6.

42 Ibid, 16.

moral aspirations point us inescapably to God, one might say, make no sense without God'.[43] This idea of God as rooting a sense of human flourishing will be explored in greater detail in later chapters, which explore the theological anthropology within Catholic education. At this time, however, it is enough to note the theological perspective of human life made for a relationship with God.

In Secular 3, fullness or ultimate meaning is understood within an immanent framework, thus providing a take on meaning that closes the window on any transcendental dimension. However, the prevailing cross-pressures mean that the individual is confronted with a gamut of spiritual options that cause them to ask questions of their own position. This does not mean a return to seeing the world through a sacred lens. However, the possibility of transcendent experience continues to exist and be encountered in life, despite the malaise of modernity. For Taylor, ultimate fulfilment is found through an encounter with God, through an experience of the transcendent that pushes oneself beyond mere human flourishing and transforms us in a way that exclusive humanism cannot. In this way, the confident predictions of secularisation theses have failed to account for the continued search for ultimate meaning and fullness in life that many still seek.

Taylor's taxonomy of secularity, most notably his designation of Secular 3, provides a useful framing of the contemporary conditions of religious belief and experience. His discussion of the buffered self and the immanent frame highlights the secularised imagination of many people today who live with no reference or connection to any sense of the sacred or transcendent. Taylor's exploration of the nova effect and the subsequent cross-pressures demonstrates that the pluralisation and fragilisation of spiritual and non-spiritual options cause individuals to confront what is life-giving and authentic about their worldview. Moreover, despite the secular conditions of our age, many are haunted by a loss of depth or authenticity in their lives and search for fullness or ultimate meaning in their lives. Thus, spiritual hunger remains pervasive in a secular age.

43 Ibid, 26.

Lieven Boeve

Belgian theologian Lieven Boeve offers a cultural analysis of the transformation of the Christian narrative in the European context. Boeve is concerned with how Christian faith can be conceptualised '… as being both distinctive and maintaining an intrinsic relation between tradition and context at the same time'.[44] This presents a tension between maintaining the particularity and continuity of the Christian faith while also being responsive to the increasingly pluralised, detraditionalised context of contemporary Europe.

For Boeve, this contemporary context can be categorised as postmodern, his perspective influenced by French philosopher Jean-François Lyotard's interpretation of postmodernism as a suspicion of grand narratives.[45] In this regard, the transmission of the Christian faith passed down through the generations has lost its axiomatic character. There is an increased awareness of the diversity of worldviews and religious beliefs that challenge the previously unassumed plausibility of the Christian narrative. Boeve proposes a theoretical framework to diagnose the contemporary conditions of religious belief and experience in this context.

Boeve's most significant contribution to this conversation is his thesis that the European context is both post-Christian and post-secular.[46] Boeve argues that such a perspective is vital in exploring the current context as it does not suffer the same limitations found in secularisation theories predicting the disappearance of religion from Europe. Like Taylor, Boeve feels

44 Lieven Boeve, *God Interrupts History: Theology in a Time of Upheaval* (New York: Continuum, 2007), 81.

45 'In Lyotard's view, we entered postmodernity at the point when the modern master narratives of knowledge and emancipation (which received their social form in the great ideologies) lost their legitimacy and plausibility.' Lieven Boeve, *Interrupting Tradition: An Essay on Christian Faith in a Postmodern Context* (Louvain: Peeters Press, 2003), 51. For further reading on Boeve's exploration of the relationship between the postmodern thought of Lyotard and theology, see Lieven Boeve, *Lyotard and Theology* (London: Bloomsbury, 2014).

46 See Lieven Boeve, *God Interrupts History: Theology in a Time of Upheaval* (New York: Continuum, 2007).

that there is more to be said about how people believe than is predicted by secularisation theses.

The term 'post' is not to be understood as something that has occurred after an event, nor have both the realities and embodiments of Christianity or secularity vanished.[47] Rather, it highlights how the ways we interact with both the Christian narrative and the processes of secularisation have changed, in the same way that postmodernity does not mean the end of modernity, but rather its transformation.[48] Boeve proposes:

> The term post-Christian then indicates that, although the traces of Christian faith in our society and in our culture, in our collective and individual identity formation, are still in abundance, at the same time the Christian faith is no longer the obvious, accepted background that grants meaning.[49]

Christian faith still offers a fundamental life-option into a loving relationship with the God who saves through Jesus Christ. However, the implicit understanding of the Christian narrative as dominant within society has passed. There are echoes here of Taylor's observation that the premodern social imaginary, which assumed Christianity as the source of meaning and fullness, has gone. It is now possible to perceive human flourishing with no connection to any sense of the sacred or transcendent.

Moreover, there may be a significant group within society that feels some vague connection to a Christian identity due to a formal catechesis in schooling, but any living expression of that faith is tenuous at best and

47 Lieven Boeve, 'Interrupting Christian Identity Construction: Catholic Dialogue Schools and Negative Theology', *Religions 13*(2) (2022), 170.

48 Dermot Lane expresses some theological reservations with the term 'post secular'; '… in that it seems to imply that religion can bypass the secular' and that such a reading 'misunderstands the intrinsic value of the secular for religion'. However, despite these misgivings, Lane is sympathetic towards the term as it '… does try to convey, however inadequately, a shift surrounding religion and secularism'. Dermot A. Lane, *Religion and Education: Reimagining the Relationship* (Dublin: Veritas, 2013) 8.

49 Lieven Boeve, 'Religious Education in a Post-secular and Post-Christian Context', *Journal of Beliefs and Values: Studies in Religion and Education 33*(2) (2012), 145.

non-existent at worst.[50] This highlights the perceived lack of a faith community or any sense of the Christian faith as a source of overarching significance in life. The Christian language and practice of faith become less relevant or meaningful to this cohort.

Boeve draws upon the work of sociologist Yves Lambert to highlight the change in religiosity in younger generations in Europe, borrowing Grace Davie's descriptive term 'believing without belonging'. Lambert defines this development as an '… autonomous, diffused 'off-piste' religiosity (which) is illustrated mainly through variables which are typically less Christian.'[51] The previously commonplace institutional affiliation to a religious belief system is replaced by a more independent search for meaning, values, and identity. This shift to spirituality over adherence to an established religious tradition includes characteristics such as interest in meditation, other wisdom traditions and transcendent beliefs such as life after death.[52] In this sense, the term 'post-Christian' highlights the contemporary interest in fullness that goes beyond a merely secular viewpoint. There remains a hunger for spiritual fullness and authenticity, albeit increasingly outside the Christian narrative.

For Boeve, defining the current European context as post-secular relates to the social processes of secularisation associated with conventional sociology of religion; the gradual receding of Christian faith and practice on a cultural and personal level as a result of modernisation, urbanisation and

50 'Here attention is given to the fact that although still a great deal of them are baptised and received religious education in school, most often they are only partially initiated and possess merely a fragmentary involvement with faith and faith communities'. Lieven Boeve, 'Religion after Detraditionalization: Christian Faith in a Post-Secular Europe', *Studies: Irish Theological Quarterly 70*(2) (2005), 104.

51 Yves Lambert, 'A Turning Point in Religious Evolution in Europe', *Journal of Contemporary Religion 19* (2004), 38.

52 Boeve identifies some of the variables in religiosity for those in the category of 'believing without belonging' as '… importance of meditation and contemplation; belief in a higher power, spirit, or force, rather than a personal God; belief in life after death (including reincarnation); an interest in different religious traditions rather than one particular tradition'. Lieven Boeve, *God Interrupts History: Theology in a Time of Upheaval* (New York: Continuum, 2007), 18.

secularisation.[53] Like Taylor, Boeve disputes the so-called zero-sum theories of secularisation, which propose that the growing influence of modernisation on society equates to the lessening of the role religion plays in the public sphere.[54]

Boeve refers to prominent proponents of the secularisation thesis, such as Peter Berger and Harvey Cox, who have since recanted their position as religion has not dissipated from modern society as predicted.[55] Moreover, the prominence of religion in public discourse globally as well as in Europe highlights that modernisation has not relegated religion as a means of individual and social identity construction, with Boeve claiming 'Modernisation in Europe has caused a transformation of religion, not its disappearance'.[56] This statement is congruent with Charles Taylor's designation of Secular 3, in that the conditions of religious belief and experience of the contemporary context have been altered and not annihilated.

Boeve analyses this change through the perspectives of detraditionalisation and individualisation, which are not limited by the implicit assumptions of the secularisation thesis. 'Detraditionalisation as a term hints at the socio-cultural interruptions of traditions (religious as well as class, gender … traditions), which are no longer able to pass themselves from one generation to the next'.[57] Detraditionalisation affects all religious and non-religious

53 Boeve cites the work of sociologist Steve Bruce who offers a contemporary defence of the secularisation thesis. See Steve Bruce, *God is Dead: Secularization in the West, Religion in the Modern World* (Malden, MA: Blackwell, 2002).

54 'Once the secularization process is completed, a secular Europe will be realized, a Europe in which religion no longer plays a role in the construction and legitimation of individual and social identities. It would now appear, however, that this thesis has ultimately been falsified by the facts, and that many have come to recognize this reality.' Lieven Boeve, *God Interrupts History: Theology in a Time of Upheaval* (New York: Continuum, 2007), 14.

55 Boeve references Harvey Cox, 'The Myth of the Twentieth Century: The Rise and Fall of Secularization', in Gregory Baum and Harvey Cox, eds, *The Twentieth Century: A Theological Overview* (New York: Orbis, 1999), 135–43 and Peter Berger, *The Desecularization of the World: Resurgent Religion and Global Politics* (Grand Rapids: Eerdmans, 1999), 1–18.

56 Lieven Boeve, 'Religion After Detraditionalization: Christian Faith in a Post-Secular Europe', *Irish Theological Quarterly* 70(2) (2005), 104.

57 Ibid.

beliefs and ideologies. From a Christian perspective, the Christian tradition can no longer be passed down to the next generation as the unchallenged and axiomatic basis for identity development and source of overarching meaning. Moreover, the individual must now construct their own identity rather than simply inherit a set of narratives and traditions. Boeve thus treats detraditionalisation and individualisation as inextricably linked within this new socio-cultural context.

Individualisation refers to the individual constructing their own identity from the broad range of possibilities available. Previous resources for such construction are still available, such as the Christian narrative, but the quasi-unquestioned transmission of those traditions, customs and values is no longer self-evident.[58] Boeve's idea of individualisation here echoes that of Taylor, where the porous self is replaced by the buffered self. In the past, Christians inherited their rituals, traditions and practices as a 'package deal' as Taylor calls it. This 'package deal' was based on a perspective that saw the world as created, sustained and redeemed by God. The human person was understood as being made in the likeness and image of God, a reflection of a transcendent reality. Now, this buffered self is not open to normative demands from any agency external to itself. The individual must construct their identity, where religious belief is an optional extra rather than a central meaning-making tenet in how they perceive reality.

Boeve argues that pluralisation is operative parallel to individualisation. The gamut of different perspectives and fundamental life options available to the individual is one of the defining characteristics of our contemporary

58 Boeve argues that 'The roots causes of the process of individualization are to be found in the centuries-old process of modernisation. Accompanying aspects ... include: (1) Increased education and educational level, resulting in the relativization of the family as the primary context of socialisation; (2) increased economic capital that guarantees both material independence- thus facilitating individual choice- and the material potential to realise individual options; (3) urbanisation via the process of migration from traditional village and neighbourhood contexts; (4) significantly increased mental and geographical mobility; (5) massively expanded leisure possibilities and to conclude, (6) the persistent rationalisation of the lifeworld via, for example, the infiltration of scientific, medical and psychological insights that undermine traditional conceptualisations and practices'. See Lieven Boeve, *Interrupting Tradition: An Essay on Christian Faith in a Postmodern Context* (Louvain: Peeters Press, 2003), 52.

context, which is synonymous with Taylor's nova effect thesis. Boeve outlines some of the most prominent developments from the plethora of religious views available:

> ... the vague religiosity of many of our contemporaries, referred to ironically be some as 'something-ism'... the widespread search for spirituality (instead of "ethics,") ... replacement of the term 'religion' with 'spirituality'... the tendency to religious indifference and relativism, and to practical agnosticism and atheism instead of theoretical agnosticism and atheism ... etc.[59]

Analysing the religious situation in Europe as post-Christian and post-secular corresponds to a present reality where a plurality of religious and non-religious beliefs and fundamental world views co-exist and compete. The predictions of secularisation theories have not accounted for this post-modern transformation of religion in continuing to shape individual and social identity. A secularist Europe has not emerged; rather, there is a diversity of views, much more complex than a simplistic religious/secular binary.[60] Rather, a competitive and diverse marketplace of religious and non-religious options has emerged.

Due to the processes of individualisation, detraditionalisation and pluralisation, Christian identity has become more reflexive. The marketplace of beliefs requires the Christian to choose to be a Christian. For those with a vague, dissociated relationship with Christianity, this can be accompanied by individuals constructing self-identity from fragments of different religions in their search for meaning, rather than Christianity.[61] Given these processes, we have no choice other than to seek meaning in the uncertainty and multitude of narratives present in postmodernity. Boeve's argument

59 Ibid, 14–15.

60 Boeve highlights some of these perspectives: 'Besides Christians (divided into different denominations), there are atheists, agnostics, Muslims, Jews, Buddhists, ex-Christians (or post-Christians), the indifferent, individualists, people belonging to neo-religious movements (such as New Age), etc. This diversity is becoming increasingly visible and poses new and different challenges for Christian believers, over and above those of the "de-christianisation" of society'. Lieven Boeve, 'The Shortest Definition of Religion: Interruption', *Communio Viatorum 46* (2004), 303.

61 Lieven Boeve, *God Interrupts History: Theology in a Time of Upheaval* (New York: Continuum, 2007), 18–24.

here is akin to the situation people face in Taylor's nova effect, where they must confront the vast array of options on the spiritual plane in an effort to find experiences of authenticity or fullness.

Boeve illustrates the 'culture of the kick' as one of the primary reactions to this new postmodern situation. 'Kicks imply sensation, stimulus and intensified thrill, and postmodern people seem to be addicted to them. In their hunger for experience, they look for more, for quicker and more intense experiences'.[62] In a post-secular and post-Christian context, the individual faces the challenge of searching for meaningful experience through having to choose from fragments of narratives in order to construct a basis for values, meaning and identity. However, the culture of the kick treats the intensity of an experience as the metric for its meaningfulness.

The culture of the kick is thus a protest to the supposed contingency and meaningless of postmodern life by forcing the subject to experience something other than one's own narrative. For Boeve, this meaningful experience is to be found in a boundary experience, where the ego is confronted with otherness. Such experiences are not in self-realisation. Rather, they are to be found in radical events that dramatically cause us to question the self-assuredness of our own narratives, such as death, illness and despair. They can also be moments of joy and beauty that push us beyond the limitations of our constructed identity.

> All such experiences are rooted in an incomprehensible sense of fullness that has the capacity to extend our boundaries. Time and time again, such boundary experiences, both positive and negative, challenge our ongoing narratives to turn outwards, to become open narratives.[63]

Boeve's reading of the culture of the kick bears a strong correlation with Taylor's work on the immanent frame. The boundary experience is the person breaking out of the immanent frame and experiencing something deeper and mysterious than a secular, materialist viewpoint. There is a hunger for meaningful experience or human flourishing that transcends the arbitrary meaninglessness felt by many in the post-secular and post-Christian age.

62 Ibid, 86.
63 Ibid, 89.

Boeve cites 'something-ism', the term coined by Dutch atheists to illustrate the vague religiosity felt by many in Europe now, despite the modernising effects of secularisation. Boeve notes, 'It would seem that the demythologisation of the world has left people unsatisfied, leading them to search for 'something more'.[64] Such something-ism represents a religious longing for meaning beyond the secular, materialist world. This demythologisation also occurs on the level of what Taylor calls the social imaginary, the implicit background to how people interact and make sense of the world. The secularisation of images, stories and symbols has cut off the roots to meaning-making for many in a post-secular post-Christian age.

In this search for an experience of otherness, Boeve proposes drawing upon the Christian tradition of negative or apophatic theology. This theology proposes that the assumed images and language of God are inadequate and limited, as our human experience and language always fall short of the incomprehensible. Otherness of God. Boeve cites the work of theologian Denys Turner in critiquing the modern scientific understanding of the experience of God, which can lead to a theological positivism that falls short of what constitutes negative theology or mysticism.[65]

In the post-Christian, post-secular age, the Christian narrative must then cultivate a contemplative orientation open to God's grace. This interruption of God in our lives cannot be compartmentalised by language, symbols, narratives or stories, which are always partial and contextually determined. 'Which such determinations can never describe God, let alone attain him—they can point to, or better still, testify to God—they remain our only means to refer to God, "our means", "our narrative"'.[66]

64 Lieven Boeve, *God Interrupts History: Theology in a Time of Upheaval* (New York: Continuum, 2007), 139.

65 The modern scientific understanding of the experience of God, '... when applied in theology, leads to a theological positivism: by analogy with the (natural sciences), mystical experience is supposed to serve as positive proof of the truth claims of religion. Thus, mysticism is for theology what sensory experience is for the sciences. Such a vision does not do justice to mysticism and negative theology'. Ibid, 158. See Denys Turner, *The Darkness of God: Negativity in Christian Mysticism* (Cambridge: CUP, 1995).

66 Ibid, 160.

A hermeneutic of apophatic theology enables the Christian in the post-Christian and post-secular age to re-discover the particularity of their own faith as well as religious experience. Such a hermeneutic is a resource for recontextualisation, presenting the Christian tradition as an open narrative that creates the possibility for dialogue in a postmodern world by virtue of the particularity of its own truth claims, while challenging the closed narratives of relativisation and fundamentalism. This Christian narrative with its own particular teachings, traditions and images enables the fostering of a religious experience that interrupts our perceptions and is a condition of the possibility of an encounter with the incomprehensible mystery of God.

> The Christian narrative which has become conscious of its own particularity and contingency can only adequately relate to the transcendent when it (1) opens itself up, cultivating a sort of contemplative openness into which the transcendent as interruptive event can enter, and (2) bears witness in a non-hegemonic way to the transcendent with the help of its own, always fragmentary words, images, stories, symbols and rituals.[67]

A contemplative openness thus becomes a necessary capacity for the Christian today. The turn to apophatic theology provides an instructive approach to nourishing religious experience in the Christian narrative. It is then central to representing the authenticity of the Christian faith in a post-secular and post-Christian context while maintaining an openness to dialogue with other narratives. This possibility of a contemplative disposition echoes theologian Karl Rahner's famous claim that 'The Christian of the future will be a mystic, or he will not exist at all'. Moreover, it offers a theological resource in conceptualising the Christian narrative as being both distinctive and keeping an intrinsic relation between tradition and context at the same time.

67 Lieven Boeve, 'Thinking Sacramental Presence in a Postmodern Context: A Playground for Theological Renewal', in Lieven Boeve and Lambert Leijssen, eds, *Sacramental Presence in a Postmodern Context* (Leuven: Leuven University Press, 2001), 21.

Boeve in conversation with Taylor

Several of Boeve's ideas correlate with those of Charles Taylor. First, both Boeve and Taylor share scepticism of secularisation theses, as while secular rationality is prevalent today, it must still co-exist with the influential role religion plays in contemporary society. Moreover, Taylor's designation of Secular 3 finds an ally in Boeve's assertion that postmodernity has meant the transformation of the conditions of how we experience religion today, not the death of religion as predicted by secularisation theses.

Second, what Boeve designates as post-secular and post-Christian, Taylor terms Secular 3, the altered conditions of belief. These are broadly compatible as both thinkers acknowledge the pluriformity of worldviews and truth claims operative today. For Boeve and Taylor, Christianity has lost its previously held position as the dominant, unquestioned narrative and signifier of meaning for individuals. It is now one view among many. Taylor develops this idea with his usage of the 'nova effect', where there is an explosion of views that the individual has to contend with and investigate. Boeve would argue that the processes of detraditionalisation, pluralisation and individualisation have all contributed to this in terms of identity formation today.

Both thinkers address the continuing spiritual hunger of individuals seeking meaning and fullness in their lives. Taylor calls these cross-pressures, while Boeve examines the culture of the kick, which shares several similarities. Central to their argument is the fact that people still desire meaning that transcends the borders of their experience, a hunger for fullness or authenticity that goes beyond human flourishing in the immanent sense.

Finally, while broadly in agreement, Boeve and Taylor offer different theories on how this spiritual searching may develop. For Boeve, a contemplative outlook developed through Christian apophatic theology offers hope. Such an approach enables the Christian narrative to contextualise to the postmodern setting while retaining the particularity of its truth claims. However, Taylor speaks of religion as any approach that enables encounter with the transcendence, including non-theistic traditions like Buddhism. From this perspective, Taylor sees people's search for fullness continuing in a Secular 3 age. In this sense, Boeve's work has a more fixed position as he is writing exclusively on the Christian narrative, while Taylor's broader definition of religion allows him to make broader claims on how the hunger for transcendence will continue to be operative in our current context.

Michael Paul Gallagher

The work of the late Irish theologian Michael Paul Gallagher explores the significance of unbelief and imagination through an analysis of the interaction between faith and culture in the contemporary Western context. Gallagher often draws upon literary perspectives to enrich his surveying of how religious experience is felt, particularly in an Irish context which has undergone profound secularisation in recent decades, citing, among others, T. S. Eliot.[68]

This change in spiritual sensibility was identified by Gallagher at a time when the Irish Church commanded extremely high mass attendance and Irish citizens overwhelmingly self-identified as Catholic. Gallagher recognised that high Mass attendance did not necessarily correspond to a rich and lived faith experience. Gallagher's prophetic observation generated a new conversation on how the authentic experience of the Catholic faith was being stymied by an institution that was failing to address the spiritual needs of a new generation of Catholics.[69] For Gallagher, there were deeper

68 'The problem of the modern age is not merely the inability to believe certain things about God and man which our forefathers believed, but the inability to feel towards God and man as they did' T.S. Eliot, *On Poetry and Poets* (London: Faber & Faber, 1957), 25.

69 'At that time, huge emphasis was placed on attendance at Mass as a sign of a healthy Church, whereas in Michael Paul's analysis, this practice was spiritually impoverished, having little prayerfulness, no sense of living worship and no real attempt to create a human community.' Thomas G. Casey, *Wisdom at the Crossroads: The Life and Thought of Michael Paul Gallagher SJ* (New Jersey: Paulist Press, 2018), 53.

questions to be asked about how people felt towards God in the contemporary context, which could not be answered solely by metrics.

Gallagher does not romanticise Catholic Ireland of the 1950s but recognises that the religious foundations of that time allowed more space for religious imagination and experience.[70] Social changes such as detraditionalisation and secularisation have had a profound effect on how religious beliefs and practices are transmitted to the next generation. Gallagher summarises: 'In short, such rapid social change has spelt the death of conventional religion in so far as it remains merely conventional'.[71] The connection to religious faith, which was previously inherited by people, is interrupted by these social forces, effectively ending the hitherto unquestioned status of Christianity as the definitive foundation for identity construction and authenticity in life. In this sense, Gallagher is referring to the same sociological processes as Boeve, in transforming the contemporary conditions of religious belief and experience. Moreover, Taylor's categorisation of Secular 3 is an appropriate synonym for Gallagher's diagnosis in that Gallagher is speaking of the altered conditions of religious belief and experience in the Irish context.

In light of these social changes, Gallagher is concerned with the orientation towards religious experience being undernourished, leading to a distancing from the reality of Christian faith, eventually rendering religious faith implausible. Gallagher recognises this indifference towards faith as a crisis of religious consciousness. Indifference represents a form of atheism in that the existence of God is not so much as challenged as considered irrelevant, occurring on the imaginative level rather than the cognitive.

> The term not only covers the strong meaning of closedness to any horizon of transcendence, but also a whole spectrum of what the French would call distanciation; where

70 'In short, a simpler world, a more ordered or obedient world … You might describe it more critically as too protected, ruled by fear and very conformist. Yes, perhaps, but there was a certain rootedness and security in spite of the warts'. Michael Paul Gallagher, *Questions of Faith* (Dublin: Veritas, 1996), 37.

71 Michael Paul Gallagher, *Struggles of Faith: Essays by Michael Paul Gallagher* (Dublin: Columba Press, 1990), 45.

> the meaning or value of some component of religion becomes dulled and one finds oneself consciously or unconsciously 'distanced' from any contact with it.[72]

Gallagher's approach is robustly compatible with Taylor's writing on the modern social imaginary, which grounds the immanent frame. The window to the transcendental horizon of meaning is closed off, rendering spiritual consciousness and awareness meaningless. Spiritual imagination and religious language become secularised and ineffective, leaving the indifferent person without an openness or awareness of a transcendent horizon of existence.[73] It is now possible to envision a conception of human flourishing with no reference to the sacred, where God is no longer thought of as the ultimate source of meaning and fullness of life. Unbelief rather than belief becomes a more plausible and coherent outlook.

Central to Gallagher's approach to unbelief is his analysis of the interaction between faith and contemporary culture. The possibility of religious faith has become trivialised in the public sphere through a secularisation of attitudes rather than ideas or concepts.

> Our receptivity for revelation is more shaped by culture than by philosophical clarities. We seldom live by ideologies but rather by images of life communicated by our surrounding worlds. Hence the cultural wavelength is central for understanding the shifting currents within religious commitment now.[74]

Gallagher offers numerous interpretations of what culture can be understood as, including a lens, an ever-present horizon, an ocean or a prison.[75] Culture includes values, images and meanings which are not equivalent to the external structures that we exist within. Similar to Taylor's social

72 Ibid, 43.

73 See Michael Paul Gallagher, *Help My Unbelief* (Chicago: Loyola University Press, 1988). Gallagher devotes this text to exploring the psychological roots of unbelief, identifying three main forms; alienation, anger and apathy.

74 Michael Paul Gallagher, *Clashing Symbols: An Introduction to Faith and Culture* (New York: Paulist Press, 2003), 7.

75 For a full account of Gallagher's understanding of culture, see Michael Paul Gallagher, *Clashing Symbols: An Introduction to Faith and Culture* (New York: Paulist Press, 2003), 1–26.

imaginary, Gallagher's cultural wavelength is a deeper orientation towards meaning that occurs on the symbolic or imaginative level rather than through cognition. Due to processes of secularisation, pluralisation and detraditionalisation, our contemporary cultural wavelength can shift our religious consciousness away from an openness to transcendence and religious experience. This change occurs on a deeper level of symbols and imagination, '... a shift in personal paradigms of meaning, and when those horizons are in flux, images may often embody the transition better than ideas'.[76]

Gallagher is influenced by fellow Jesuit theologian Bernard Lonergan in gauging the place of faith in a more secular time, that the present moment is less a crisis of faith as a crisis of culture. Because of this crisis, the Christian faith cannot be transmitted to the next generation as it was in the past, due to new and alternative frameworks of meaning and values. The symbols, images and stories of contemporary culture mean that not only is Christian faith a choice today, but it is also often a choice that is increasingly counter-cultural. The radical message of self-giving love in the Gospels is in tension with the consumerist, materialist tendencies found in modern culture, meaning that faith is not as easily translated to others as in past decades.

The receptivity to religious experience is lessened predominantly through apathy, a form of cultural unbelief that deadens the imagination to the possibility of belief in God. While many younger baptised generations in Ireland receive faith formation and the sacraments as rites of initiation, their experience of religion or the Church is extremely weak. The question of God becomes irrelevant as basic attitudes and assumptions have become less attuned to the wavelength of an experience of the transcendent. This has significant implications for Catholic education but also the Church

76 Michael Paul Gallagher, 'Secularization and New Forms of Faith', *Studies, An Irish Quarterly Review, Spring* (1985) 12.

more generally,[77] where younger generations inherit a deracinated faith; a cultural unbelief with only a tenuous, vague connection to the Christian faith.[78] In particular, there exists for many younger Catholics a profound religious illiteracy which renders the language and ritual of Christian faith strange and alien.

Gallagher identifies four operative types of cultural unbelief. Firstly, religious anaemia refers to the weakening of identification with the traditional roots of Church experience. A lack of vibrancy in education, formation and evangelisation leads to the language of faith losing meaning to the next generation. Such staleness disenchants and distances the receiver from a meaningful faith experience. 'In short, religious anaemia is produced when the receiver encounters only the conventional or complacent externals of an institution, and when the communication of faith fails to enter imaginatively into the culture of the receiver'.[79] This would link with Gallagher's earlier warning of perceiving the Irish Church as in good health by virtue of high Mass attendance. It does not account for whether the spiritual needs

77 Gallagher's fellow Jesuit Karl Rahner offers a considered opinion on the challenges of living the Christian faith in a culture often at odds with the Gospel message. Moreover, Rahner also identifies the transformation of faith from family inheritance to personal choice. '… (1) faith is constantly threatened from without and received no support from institutional morality, custom, civil law, tradition, or public opinion. It is no longer a matter of family inheritance, but of conscious, personal choice; (2) a considerable part of the riches of culture is no longer specifically Christian and may even exert a negative influence on a Christian's moral life; (3) the Church will be a Church of the laity, where they will assume increasingly important roles and will take over many of the duties previously reserved to the clergy; (4) the clergy will no longer belong to the upper privileged levels of society (5) the conflict will occur not so much between the Church and the State but in the conscience of the individual who is asked to make a choice between the values of the gospel and the dominant cultural mores'. See Karl Rahner, Cecily Hastings (Trans.), 'The Present Situation of Christians' in *The Christian Commitment; Essays in Pastoral Theology* (New York: Sheed & Ward, 1963), 23–6.

78 What emerges is that, especially in younger generations, unbelief has become an inherited confusion, a distance from roots, an unaggressive puzzlement about religious practices and their language. As a result, they experience unbelief as a cultural by-product.' Michael Paul Gallagher, *Clashing Symbols: An Introduction to Faith and Culture* (New York: Paulist Press, 2003), 131.

79 Ibid, 132.

of Catholics are being met or a life-giving capacity for encounter with Jesus Christ is being cultivated.

The second grouping, secular marginalisation, relates to the increasing preconception that democracy equates to a secular liberal viewpoint. Faith is implicitly treated as unimportant and more suited to the individual's private life. Powerful social influencers such as the academy, media and politicians can marginalise the plausibility structures of belief, rendering it less important and less believable.[80] The images and language of faith recede in the face of an ever more influential secular viewpoint, leading to religion being less visible in public discourse and gradually less relevant in everyday life. This would bear a resemblance to Charles Taylor's designation of Secular 2.

The third grouping, anchorless spirituality, is a reaction to the religious anaemia found in Church experience. People drift from the roots of Christian faith in search of fundamental meaning in other places. These searchers have an awareness of a hunger for spiritual nourishment, but can end up falling into a range of belief systems that lack any roots.

> It is that drifting that constitutes a danger: the hunger is good but insofar as the lived culture weakens people's Christian roots ... In the context of religious malnutrition, such lonely spirituality easily becomes another form of deChristianisation. Without community and contemplation, it risks becoming a narcissism without Christ.[81]

While spiritual hunger remains fundamentally important for many, the lonely spirituality that Gallagher warns of is superficial, in theologian Nicholas Lash's words, a means of soothing rather than subverting our well-heeled complacencies.[82] Any spirituality that rejects personal transformation for

80 Gallagher references the work of law professor Stephen Carter on this form of interaction between faith and the public sphere and the tensions that follow. For further reading, see Stephen L. Carter, *The Culture of Disbelief: How American Law and Politics Trivialize Religious Devotion* (New York: Basic Books, 1993).

81 Michael Paul Gallagher, *Clashing Symbols: An Introduction to Faith and Culture* (New York: Paulist Press, 2003), 132.

82 See Nicholas Lash, *The Beginning and End of Religion* (Cambridge, Cambridge University Press, 1996), 174.

comforting the ego can lead spiritual seekers to a self-centred and unfulfilling outlook.

Cultural desolation is the fourth type of cultural unbelief, one which represents both a challenge and an opportunity to an openness to a transcendent horizon of religious experience. 'The key idea is that the pressures of the dominant culture leave many people blocked in a cultural desolation on the level of disposition and readiness for faith'.[83] Among these, pressures are contemporary phenomena such as globalisation, consumerism and pluralisation. These can inculcate this desolation in terms of generating attitudes that interrupt a transcendental or religious outlook. These also include an excessive anthropocentrism, materialism and moral relativism, which deaden the search for fullness or authenticity in life that transcends the boundaries of everyday experience.

Gallagher identifies the breakdown in religious imagination as the key blockage for those facing cultural desolation. This deeper sensibility is the *a priori* awareness of the mystery of God which transcends our words, thoughts and actions. This is the most fundamental change that secularisation has brought into the interaction between faith and culture. The fading of one's religious imagination entails an anthropological concern with how we discern ultimate meaning and our place in the world. Our spiritual imagination exists on a deeper level of images and symbols, which provide us with values and meaning. To lose this represents a seismic shift in self-identity.

> If our spiritual imagination is the battleground of our self-meanings, we need to reflect on this deeper secularisation of the sensibility, as going beyond the crisis of religious structures in a more plural Ireland. It involves not just a measurable problem of belonging and believing but a crisis of ultimate identity.[84]

In discerning how Christian faith is to respond to this secularisation of feeling in contemporary culture, withdrawing to a fundamentalist, reactionary viewpoint risks Christianity being reduced to a militant, unreasonable voice in public discourse. However, there is also a danger in thoughtlessly buying

83 Michael Paul Gallagher, *Clashing Symbols: An Introduction to Faith and Culture* (New York: Paulist Press, 2003), 133.

84 Michael Paul Gallagher, 'Imagination Gone Secular?', *The Furrow*, 57(11) (Nov 2006), 592.

into the values of a dominant culture, devoid of attempting to influence or challenge certain values. Moreover, some interpretations of pluralism can lead to a vague disposition of all images and symbols in culture having equivalent value, without any metric for discerning truth in a cultural context. This relativist position leaves all narratives flattened of their distinctiveness and particularity.

Gallagher advocates an open disposition to those in cultural desolation, and from a pastoral perspective, draws on the work of theologian Karl Rahner on 'mystagogy', to be led onto mystery. Gallagher biographer Thomas Casey outlines this term in both Rahner's and Gallagher's theology. 'His (Rahner's) idea is simple: it is necessary to find and name some signs of God's presence in a person's experience before telling that person about the Good News'.[85] Such an approach is strongly influenced by the Ignatian spirituality of 'seeing God in all things'. Moreover, this approach strongly correlates with the notion of pre-evangelisation, the removal of barriers to belief and nurturing of a religious literacy. Such a development is a prerequisite for evangelisation to flourish.[86]

Gallagher sees language as sacramental and reality as graced, in that creation contained images and signs of God. These images have the potential to enable people to have an awareness of the sacred in everyday life. Rahner's quote that the Christian of the future being a mystic is then instructive in understanding Gallagher's approach. It does not mean that each person must have a profound religious experience. Rather, it means the possibility of an experience of mystery, seeing God mediated through experience of the world and having the capacity to transcend the shallow surface of profane reality.[87] For Gallagher, this enflaming of the imagination is a vital step in

85 Thomas G. Casey, *Wisdom at the Crossroads: The Life and Thought of Michael Paul Gallagher SJ* (New Jersey: Paulist Press, 2018), 56.

86 Michael Paul Gallagher, 'What Are We Doing When We Do Theology?', *Landas: Journal of Loyola School of Theology* 28 (2024) 1–12.

87 Gallagher would explain this theological concept as; '… discerning and disclosing the mysteries within each person's life-story; as such it would communicate the indifferent, not primarily in terms of God and faith, but in terms of their own experiences of self-transcendence and struggle, with the confidence that within these experiences the presence of God can be unveiled'. Michael Paul Gallagher, *Struggles of Faith: Essays by Michael Paul Gallagher* (Dublin, Columba Press, 1990), 49.

bridging the gap between cultural desolation and learning into the Christian faith for young Catholics and spiritual seekers. This means asking questions, becoming mindful of their inner feelings, thoughts and sources of meaning before being open to the Christian life.[88]

The fragmentation of culture means that many people, both believers and non-believers, are searching aimlessly to satisfy their spiritual hunger without any roots or anchors to support them. Gallagher recognises spirituality as a constituent of the human person and this openness to spiritual depths is in danger of being blocked by modern social processes and influences. Gallagher advocates silent prayer as one such anchor, which offers a means of awakening in our depths to mystery, to an experience of God.

> Silent prayer enables an entering into a more profound experience of mystery without the distractions of the ego, and this transition is a vital step towards a more contemplative level of prayer. It means an emergence from self-strength to a trust that God is 'there' in all his strange shyness.[89]

This approach to prayer can help engender a contemplative outlook, discerning the presence of the Holy Mystery that transcends our partial language, signs and symbols. For the generations experiencing different categories of unbelief, such a transition offers an opening to a sense of religious imagination and wonder. Gallagher recognises that we have moved from a 'culture of obedience to a culture of experience'.[90] Such a turn to silent prayer allows for the possibility of making religious experience more meaningful and vibrant to those seeking spiritual nourishment. Such prayer allows for a greater sense of awareness of one's own deep hungers. Moreover, for those who have a vague,

88 Casey recalls one incident or Gallagher offering advice to a fellow priest trying to reach out to young parishioners: 'They needed help to find their own questions before they would be open to the wisdom emanating from the Christian tradition. They needed to pay attention to their own experience and discover their own depth before they would be ready to appreciate the depth of their faith'. Thomas G. Casey, *Wisdom at the Crossroads: The Life and Thought of Michael Paul Gallagher SJ* (New Jersey: Paulist Press, 2018), 114.

89 Michael Paul Gallagher, *Struggles of Faith: Essays by Michael Paul Gallagher* (Dublin, Columba Press, 1990), 135.

90 Ibid, 81.

anchorless connection to the Christian faith, being present in moments of silence allows the person to become consciously aware of mystery, a sense of otherness that transcends their everyday experience and social imaginary.

Gallagher in conversation with Taylor and Boeve

Several themes emerge from Gallagher's writings that resonate with those of Taylor and Boeve. First, all three acknowledge the effects of pluralisation, secularisation and detraditionalisation on the contemporary conditions of religious belief and experience, albeit in different ways. Taylor speaks of the immanent frame, whereas Gallagher speaks of these changed conditions as a crisis of culture and a secularisation of the imagination, both thinkers referring to a sensibility or implicit background deeper than intellect or cognition, where the manner we make meaning or engage with the possibility of the transcendent is buffered by a secular rationality. Moreover, Boeve's post-secular and post-Christian designation can apply to Gallagher's surveying of the religious landscape. The Christian faith is no longer the pre-eminent locus of meaning for many, and individuals are challenged to construct their identity in light of a gamut of contested and contesting truth claims and worldviews.

Second, Gallagher's exploration of unbelief correlates with Taylor's Secular 3, in that in each there is a sense that the question of God or the possibility of transcendent experience is deemed irrelevant due to a deadening of a spiritual orientation or awareness. In this sense, Taylor's idea of the buffered self-correlates with Gallagher's work on forms of unbelief, highlighting the manner in which contemporary cultural forces contribute to eclipsing the possibility for conceptions of human flourishing that transcend our everyday experience.

Finally, Boeve, Taylor and Gallagher share the belief that this culture is haunted by a desire for meaningful experience, be that the culture of the kick, cross-pressures or Gallagher's reference to this being an age of experience over authority. Moreover, Boeve and Gallagher agree that a significant opportunity may be contemplative prayer. Such a prayer does not undercut religious symbols and teachings, rather, it is an opportunity for those searching for the Other to encounter in the silence a mystery beyond the experience of the world. In engaging in such silent prayer, those seeking may find an anchor for their spirituality and the possibility of falling in love with the Christian story.

Tomáš Halík

Czech philosopher and theologian Tomáš Halík offers a unique perspective on the dynamics of faith and religious experience in a secularised culture.[91] This is shaped by his own experience of living under totalitarian atheist Communist rule, which included a clandestine ordination and theological studies in secret.[92] Even after the collapse of the regime, the Czech Republic has a significantly higher level of citizens who identify as atheist than most European countries. In this sense, Halík writes from the perspective of a Catholic who belongs to a section of society outnumbered by secular counterparts, which can be instructive for the Irish context, where changes in the conditions of religious belief and experience are being felt.[93]

91 Halík's unique approach to examining the relationship between theology and secularity has led to Aden Cotterill labelling Halík's work a theology for the post-secular. See Aden Cotterill, 'Tomáš Halík: A Theology for the Post-Secular', *Theological Studies* *85*(1) (2024), 78–95.

92 Tomáš Halík, *From the Underground Church to Freedom* (Notre Dame, Indiana: University of Notre Dame Press, 2019).

93 'Czechs generally speaking feel an *a priori* distrust towards institutionalized and organized religion. Czech believers are therefore in a unique situation. They are a small minority, surrounded by a secular majority. So their experience with the effective (and also ineffective) ways of evangelization and reaching out to contemporary seekers may perhaps be useful for other Christians, facing similar conditions or struggling with gradual changes of general attitudes towards the Church similar to those typical of the Czech situation'. Pavel Hošek, 'Introduction: Towards a Kenotic Hermeneutics of Contemporary Czech Culture', in Tomáš Halík and Pavel Hošek, eds, *A Czech Perspective on Faith in a Secular Age* (Washington: Council for Research and Values in Philosophy, 2015), 2.

In the wider European context, the traditional role of Christianity as a common language or the integrative influence in society[94] has been transformed by secularisation and the pluralisation of ideas and narratives. Halík differentiates between secularisation and secularism. Secularisation is a historical process that represents a change in the forms of religious belief.[95] On the other hand, secularism '... describes an ideology that interprets this (secularisation process) as necessary, irreversible progress from "religious superstition" to a bright future under the aegis of reason and science.'[96] Secularism advocates a modern positivist rationale of neutral objectivity. This ideology includes categories of militant atheism that can turn secularism into a form of religion with intolerant and oppressive aspects.[97]

Halík thus interprets secularisation as a necessary burning away of false certainties of Christian faith.[98] In this vein, Halík wonders whether secularisation could be understood as a particular form of Christianity, suggesting that the secular age we live in is, in fact, the reality of Christ's kenosis (self-emptying).[99] For Halík, Christianity must articulate the particularity of the Good News in an age where the Church is no longer the

94 Halík understands religion here in terms sociological functionalism. '... religion as an integrating social force, as a "common language"- whatever holds society together is its religion (*religo*)'. Tomáš Halík, 'Europe between Laicity and Christianity', in Tomáš Halík and Pavel Hošek, eds, *A Czech Perspective on Faith in a Secular Age* (Czech Philosophical Studies V, Christian Philosophical Studies X, 2015), 55.

95 Tomáš Halík, 'Europe between Laicity and Christianity', in Tomáš Halík and Pavel Hošek, eds, *A Czech Perspective on Faith in a Secular Age* (Washington: Council for Research and Values in Philosophy, 2015), 56.

96 Ibid, 57.

97 Halík differentiates between 'soft secularism' and 'hard secularism'. The hard form is reminiscent of the totalitarian atheism of Communist regimes that Halík endured, where believers are subject to religious persecution. Soft secularism represents 'attempts to marginalising Christianity in the name of the ideology of multiculturalism and political correctness'. Ibid, 57.

98 See Tomáš Halík, *The Afternoon of Christianity: The Courage to Change* (Notre Dame, Indiana: University of Notre Dame Press, 2024), 50–1.

99 Halík shares this kenotic interpretation with philosopher Gianni Vattimo. For further reading see Gianni Vattimo, *Belief* (Cambridge: Polity Press, 1996) and Gianni Vattimo, *After Christianity* (New York: Columbia University Press, 2002).

assumed common language of society. It is a transformation rather than the extinction of religion.

> Yes the form of religion that we are accustomed to is truly 'dying off'. The history of religion and of Christianity consists of periods of crisis and periods of renewal; the only religion that is truly dead is one that does not undergo change, the one that has to be dropped out of that rhythm of life.[100]

Halík's perspective here echoes that of Boeve, who argues that postmodernity has transformed rather than killed religion. This purgative change represents the end of one form of Christianity and simultaneously a recontextualisation of the Christian narrative. Martin Koči and Pavel Roubík summarise Halík's view that 'The disappearance of Christianity from European culture does not turn Europe into an atheistic or non-religious entity. Rather, Europe has become "religious" in a different way when compared with the classical understanding'.[101,102] This perspective is congruent with those offered by Taylor and Gallagher, in that the conditions of religious belief and experience have changed. Being religious today feels different due to the effects of secularisation and pluralisation.

Despite the high rates of atheism in the Czech context as well as a secularising European context, Halík argues that the hitherto dichotomy of believers and unbelievers is no longer adequate in addressing the question of religious belief and experience. Western culture no longer accommodates this demarcation and instead a seeker-dweller paradigm offers a more appropriate construal.

> If we want to understand the spiritual situation of contemporary Western post secular society, we have to move from the traditional believers-nonbelievers paradigm to the

100 Tomáš Halík, *Night of the Confessor: Christian Faith in an Age of Uncertainty* (New York: Image Books, 2012), 8.

101 Martin Koči and Pavel Roubík, 'Searching the Altar of an Unknown God: Tomáš Halík on Faith in a Secular Age', in Tomáš Halík and Pavel Hošek, eds, *A Czech Perspective on Faith in a Secular Age* (Washington: Council for Research and Values in Philosophy, 2015), 103.

102 For further reading, see Tomáš Halík, 'Embracing Atheism' in Anselm Grün, Tomáš Halík and Winfried Nonhoff, eds, *Is God Absent? Faith, Atheism and Our Search for Meaning* (NJ: Paulist Press, 2016), 12–32.

> new seekers-dwellers paradigm. Believers and non-believers are not two strictly separated groups. The contemporary Western person is often 'simul fidelis et infidelis'.[103]

Dwellers are those who belong and form identity in the Christian faith. Their worldview is permeated by the belief in God and in the mission of the Church, discerning ultimate meaning in their lives from their faith. However, Halík is particularly concerned with the seekers, those who are seeking meaning but experience Christ from a distance for whatever reason, in that undefined or grey area between religious conviction and affirmed atheism.[104] These seekers experience doubt and uncertainty, living in the midst of a postmodern world that does not offer answers.[105] In this sense, seekers are people of questions, searching for fullness or authenticity in life.

This grey zone is a diverse and growing category, including those who would identify as being 'spiritual but not religious' and those who are apathetic towards the claims of religious narratives. This is a reference to the growing populace of Europeans that seek spiritual experience in forms derived from Eastern religions, meditations and alternative spiritualties. For Halík, the seekers are on a spiritual journey, much like Christian dwellers, searching for authenticity beyond the materialistic realm of secular culture. This longing disposition creates an opportunity for dialogue between the two factions, as Halík, they are both on a spiritual journey, seeking something that transcends their construal of the world.

Halík is sympathetic to the doubts and questions that seekers may have on the God of Christian faith, even if from a distance, such that Koči and Roubík argue '*Den Fremden verstehen* – understanding the stranger is the

103 Tomáš Halík, Church for the Seekers, Tomáš Halík and Pavel Hošek, eds, *A Czech Perspective on Faith in a Secular Age* (Washington: Council for Research and Values in Philosophy, 2015), 127.

104 See Alister E. McGrath, 'On the Threshold of Mystery: Tomáš Halík on Cultural Witness in an Age of Uncertainty and Change', *Religions 14* (2023), 399.

105 For further reading, see Tomáš Halík, 'Religion and the Spiritual Seeker' in Anselm Grün, Tomáš Halík and Winfried Nonhoff, eds, *Is God Absent? Faith, Atheism and Our Search for Meaning* (NJ: Paulist Press, 2016), 72–84.

hermeneutical principle of Halík's theology'.[106] For Halík, true faith is not unwavering, rather, it needs to be dynamic and alive to critical questions. Faith is kept from stagnant complacency by being shaken into discernment and reflection.[107] This self-questioning does not reduce faith to a half-hearted commitment but instead recognises that unshakeable faith is one in danger of complacency. Faith is then a journey of searching, which must remain animated and self-questioning and able to interact with paradox and mystery.

Halík is thus particularly interested in understanding the perspectives of the seekers in the grey area, those with questions who prefer to stay at a distance from the institutional Church they have no connection with and look at with suspicion. As part of its mission, the Church needs to be open to engagement with these seekers in a spirit of seeking itself, providing a space for questions to be asked, which is necessary for faith to be nurtured and deepened. Moreover, it is necessary for dwellers to engage in such dialogue to enable being shaken out of a complacent, buffered faith. This spirit of dialogue echoes Gallagher's outlook, which suggests that the next generation needed help to find their own questions before engaging with the Christian tradition. In this sense, both Halík and Gallagher argue that seekers must discover their own depths and questions as part of their spiritual journey.

Halík cites the tax collector Zacchaeus from Luke's Gospel (Lk: 19: 1–10) as an example of the principled seeker who watches Christ from a distance. Zacchaeus responded quickly when Jesus called him by name. Zacchaeus' watchfulness has its genesis in God '... the foundation and fount of our seeking, our watchfulness, our openness, our self-transcendence'.[108]

106 Martin Koči and Pavel Roubík, 'Searching the Altar of an Unknown God: Tomáš Halík on Faith in a Secular Age', in Tomáš Halík and Pavel Hošek, eds, *A Czech Perspective on Faith in a Secular Age* (Washington: Council for Research and Values in Philosophy, 2015), 102.

107 Halík argues that this doubt and questioning is fundamental to what a theologian does. 'Theologians are professional doubters. Even when they are fully anchored by God in sincere and ardent faith, it is their duty to be a part of the band of seekers by exploring questions in the light of their own way of living, understanding, and expressing their faith'. Tomáš Halík, *I Want You to Be: On the God of Love* (Indiana: Notre Dame Press, 2016), 6.

108 Tomáš Halík, *Patience with God: The Story of Zacchaeus Continuing in Us* (New York: Doubleday, 2009), 53.

Halík is sympathetic to the challenges faced by the contemporary examples of Zacchaeus. Rather than ostracise those in the liminal area between faith and atheism, Halík argues that they are on their own journey, perhaps wary of the confident claims of some Christians or wary of the institutional Church. Moreover, Luke's Gospel does not tell the reader whether Zacchaeus became a disciple of Christ or underwent some form of spiritual transformation. Halík's Zacchaeus analogy is powerful and one that could apply far beyond his own Czech context.

The grey area that the modern Zacchaeuses inhabit is central to the future of the Church. By accepting that doubt and searching are constituents to faith, the Church can follow Christ's example in standing with those on the margins of society as well as those on the margins of faith. Halík seeks to understand the stranger's perspective on Christian faith and uses this perspectivism to advocate a fresh and dynamic approach to deepening our own faith. Halík argues the atheist perspective can provide an opportunity for Christians to reflect on their faith and shake any false certainties they hold. While there are various atheistic perspectives,[109] Halík focuses on atheists who take religion and the question of God seriously as opposed to New Atheism advocates such as Richard Dawkins who dismiss religion as pernicious and cancerous. The atheists Halík refers to are critics of false images and understandings of God that hamper the need for constant searching and questioning of faith.[110] Halík advocates the interface between this enquiring form of atheism and Christian faith insofar as it enables the purging of overconfidence and false representations of God. This leads to the dweller constantly appraising and reflecting upon their faith in God as transcendent Holy Mystery.

109 For further reading, see John Gray, *Seven Types of Atheism* (London: Penguin Books, 2019).

110 As Cotterill puts it, '… atheism as critical unbelief is where Halík finds an ally: the sharp and thoughtful atheism of someone like a Nietzsche or Feuerbach'. Aden Cotterill, 'Tomáš Halík: A Theology for the Post-Secular', *Theological Studies 85*(1) (2024), 84.

Halík emphasises that there are some questions so fundamentally profound that they eclipse the importance of any forthcoming answer.[111] Mystery cannot be mastered like an academic subject or compartmentalised into a formula or equation. Halík quotes Augustine's mantra that '*Si comprehendis, non est Deus*—if you think you know something, then you can be sure it is not God'.[112] The reality of God transcends all our conceptions and language; the eternal Mystery is hidden from human reality insofar as God is not human reality.

Halík turns to apophatic theology for theological reflection on the mystery of God. By removing affirmative statements about what God is, we remove any false idolising of a transcendent reality beyond our language and concepts. This path of negation stresses that God transcends the scope of our cognition, imagination, and language which is always partial, fragmented and contextually determined. Halík is following a rich Christian contemplative tradition here, including early Church Fathers such as Clement of Alexandria and Psuedo-Dionysius as well as the medieval mystics Meister Eckhart and the *Cloud of Unknowing* author. Moreover, this approach mirrors that of Boeve, who argues that the transcendent mystery of God interrupts our narratives and human experiences. In a post-secular, post-Christian age, the turn to apophatic theology provides an instructive approach to nourishing religious experience within the Christian narrative.

Apophatic theology can help the believer and atheist alike remove false images of God as well as incoherent interpretations of encountering and experiencing God. As the Mystery of God is infinite, seekers must continue to search and question deeper into this Mystery. Negative theology reduces the threat of false anthropocentric understandings of God as some Zeus-like figure. It conveys to us that the Divine Mystery is so radically Other that to experience God's presence in the world is only through God's absence or hiddenness.

111 Halík recalls seeing the phrase 'Jesus is the answer' graffitied on a Prague subway station wall, only to note that underneath someone else had responded with 'But what was the question?' Tomáš Halík, *Patience with God: The Story of Zacchaeus Continuing in Us* (New York: Doubleday, 2009), 6.

112 Tomáš Halík, *I Want You to Be: On the God of Love* (Indiana: Notre Dame Press, 2016), 19.

> God cannot be the object of love because God is not an object; objective perception of God leads to idolatry. I cannot love God in the same way that I love another human being, my city, my parish, or my work. God is not in front of me, just as light is not in front of me: I cannot see light; I can only see things in light. Likewise, I cannot see and visualise God. Even faith does not show him ... With faith, all I can do is see the world in God.[113]

Halík's appeal to apophatic theology highlights how the Christian can be oriented to transcendent experience in their lives. Seeing the world in God is possible through an openness to mystery that Taylor's immanent frame and Gallagher's secularised imagination treat as implausible. However, apophatic theology represents a valuable resource in this endeavour to experience the transcendent. First, it purges false certainties and images of God in the Christian faith, shaking it out of complacency. Second, and more importantly, it challenges the immanent frame's perception that everything can be explained, and that human knowledge is limitless. In this sense, apophatic theology makes possible a contemplative outlook.

In the face of a growing vague religiosity, Christianity is challenged to recontextualise itself while maintaining the particularity of its narrative. While Halík is keen to engage with seekers, he critiques modern spiritualties emphasising an experience of self-fulfilment without the prospect of personal transformation. Contemporary forms of spirituality that improve personal wellbeing can positively contribute to society. These exist in an age with altered conditions of religious belief and experience, where it is now possible to conceive of human flourishing in a totally immanent sense.

However, in a post-secular and post-Christian context, the individual faces must search for meaningful experience by choosing fragments of narratives in order to construct values, meaning and identity. But this spiritual search can treat the intensity of an experience as the metric for its meaningfulness. 'Many people continue to confuse authenticity with emotional spontaneity, and regard the intensity of an emotional experience as the main criterion for assessing an event in their own lives'.[114] In this way, Halík agrees with Gallagher on this being an age of experience over authority. Moreover,

113 Ibid, 24.
114 Ibid, 73.

Halík's analysis is synonymous with Boeve's 'culture of the kick'. This desire for spiritual meaning is a protest against the proposed meaninglessness and arbitrariness of postmodernism. There is a desire for experience that transcends the mundaneness of everyday life. For the dweller, God is that condition which makes possible a religious or transcendent experience.

Halík argues that we must continue to search the endless depths of mystery that transcend our language and concepts, as that is where God dwells. God's hiddenness is the opportunity to seek further into the deep with questions and reflection, and Halík challenges Christians to relearn true prayer by vanquishing false images and language of God to go deeper into the depths of God's mystery. The altered conditions of belief call Christians to reinterpret their faith anew in the face of contrasting narratives. Through contemplation, Christians can become attentive to the transcendent reality of God, encountering God's closeness in His hiddenness, His presence through His absence. 'It is necessary for us Christians to learn contemplation once more: the art of inner silence, in which God will be able to speak to us through our own lives and His unique events'.[115] In this sense, Halík shares Gallagher's conviction that a contemplative orientation is necessary for Christians today, seeing God in the world and feeling God's presence break into our lives.

Halík in conversation with Taylor, Boeve and Gallagher

Halík offers several insights that correspond to themes identified in the work of the other interlocutors so far. Among these are the transformative effects of postmodernism on the conditions of religious belief and experience, apophatic theology as an important resource and the call for a renewal in contemplative outlook.

First, Halík agrees with Taylor, Boeve and Gallagher that secularisation has remade the contemporary conditions of how religion is felt and

115 Ibid, 212.

experienced today. Secularisation has broken the tradition of Christianity as the common language for discerning values, meaning and identity. However, Halík strikes a decidedly optimistic tone that such a crisis for faith represents an opportunity for renewal, as secularisation can help to shake faith out of complacency and purge Christian faith of false and anthropocentric projections of God.

Second, like Boeve, Halík argues that apophatic theology is a necessary companion to Christian life today. At a time of pluralisation and fragmentation of grand narratives, negative theology recognises the limitations of language, images and conceptions of the Otherness of God. In order to orient an openness to the transcendent, we must shed our partial, contextually determined projections of God to go deeper in seeing God in the world.

Finally, in light of the gamut of new worldviews and positions, Halík offers a pastoral reflection similar to Gallagher, in that he sees a spiritual renewal of the imagination possible through a re-learning of silent prayer and a contemplative outlook. In this sense, both theologians see our present context as an opportunity to cultivate the pre-religious awareness that can open the individual up to the experience of the Holy Mystery of God in their lives. Moreover, this also means a spirit of openness with those who are seeking spiritual meaning, entering into dialogue with their questions, doubts and uncertainties as both dweller and seeker are on a spiritual journey.

Grace Davie

Sociologist of religion Grace Davie provides a detailed analysis of belief in contemporary Western society, offering several methodological tools to map the religious climate of today. A lay Anglican canon, Davie is keen to stress that sociology and theology can complement each other in exploring the relationship between religion, the human person and society. Davie argues that sociologists of religion must treat theology and religious studies more seriously, especially considering the continuing tenacity of religion in the modern world. A more collaborative approach between the social sciences and theology can lead to fruitful research due to shared interests and concerns surrounding fundamental questions of what it means to be human and what the conditions of religious belief and experience are today.

Davie is aware of the secular presuppositions of the social sciences and the challenges this presents to a more intellectually robust sociology of religion. She notes that within contemporary sociology '... there remains ... a deep-seated resistance to the notion that it is entirely normal in most parts of the world to be fully modern and fully religious'.[116] This secular outlook affects contemporary sociology insofar as it views religion as a subjective, private matter that is in tension with modern society and culture. This secular/religious dichotomy echoes Taylor's view that the academy can be highly influential in promoting a concept of modernity that relegates religion to belonging to the private sphere, and that the closed spin of the immanent frame neglects the transcendent as a source of meaning and identity for people.

Citing the continued prevalence of religion in public discourse, Davie stresses that in isolation, the secularisation thesis which has influenced modern sociology of religion, cannot account for the current conditions of belief. Europe has become increasingly secular in terms of societal functions such as healthcare and educational provision, which were previously controlled by the Church. Moreover, the institutional Church is no longer the dominant influence or common language for the transmission of morals and values in society. For Davie, however, the challenges faced by religious institutions are not based on the secularisation thesis, as political institutions and groups like trade unions are also under pressure from decreasing numbers of committed adherents.[117] In this sense, Davie shares Taylor and Boeve's scepticism of the predictions of secularisation theses.

Davie notes that a shift from a culture of obligation to one of consumption represents a key change in the conditions of belief in Europe. In the past, a more explicit social pressure was operative, which expected adherence to

116 Grace Davie, *The Sociology of Religion: A Critical Agenda* (London: SAGE Publications, 2013), xxi.

117 Ibid, 5. 'The reasons for these shifts lie primarily in the changing nature of economic and social life, the subject matter of mainstream sociology. Religious indifference is less important; it is, in fact, more likely to be the result than the cause of the institutional changes that are so clearly occurring'.

traditional teachings and regular attendance at church worship, which is no longer the case today. To be religious today is a personal option rather than a societal expectation. This leads to greater variety in religious adherence, where Christian self-identity is more detached from active participation in liturgies or communal rituals.

> Religiously active Europeans now go to church or to another religious organisation because they choose to, sometimes for a short period or sometimes for longer, sometimes regularly and sometimes less so, but they feel no obligation either to attend that church in the first place or to continue if they no longer want to.[118]

This increased autonomy and flexibility in religiosity adds to a pluralised context with a gamut of spiritual and non-spiritual outlooks. Moreover, increased immigration in Europe has led to even more religious narratives present in a Western context previously characterised by Christendom. Rather than religion fading away with the tides of rational progress, religiosity has fragmented and diversified into a plethora of spiritual outlooks in a contesting and contested marketplace. Economic and social changes have led to this transformation in religious experience, where personal choice becomes the decisive element. Davie's thesis here mirrors that of Boeve, who views the social processes of pluralisation and individualisation as significant in mapping out how the religious landscape has changed so drastically.

The marketplace has expanded further through spiritual practices '... guided by internal motivations rather than external constraints'.[119] These innovations are extremely varied in their beliefs and tenets and free from the perceived limitations of institutional religion, and have seen exponential growth in mainstream society.[120] These 'new' spiritualties are often ill-defined and diverse but commonly centred on the self and connectedness. These includes

118 Grace Davie, 'Religion in 21st Century Europe: Framing the Debate', *Irish Theological Quarterly* 78(3) (2013), 283.

119 Grace Davie, *Religion in Britain: A Persistent Paradox, 2nd Edition* (Oxford: Blackwell Press, 2015), 159.

120 Grace Davie, *Religion in Modern Europe: A Memory Mutates* (New York: Oxford University Press, 2000), 139. '... the New Age movement itself produces a mountain of published material, a fact that can be ascertained across Europe in any general bookshop with a section on religion'.

aspects of self-spirituality like '... the God in me, reaching fulfilment, realising my potential ... and the interconnected person (mind, body and spirit) and the interconnected universe (each individual is part of a cosmic whole)'.[121] The emergence of these new beliefs and outlooks are highlighted by Boeve's insights on 'something-ism', the growing demographic of those who identify as spiritual but not religious. Moreover, the popularity of these new spiritualties highlights a contemporary hunger for spiritual experiences that transcend the mundaneness of everyday experience, which gives life a sense of fullness or authenticity, as has been highlighted by each of the interlocutors.

Davie proposes two conceptual tools to aid the sociologist in analysing the current conditions of religiosity in the European context, believing without belonging and vicarious religion. Davie offers the term 'believing without belonging' as an analytical tool for the specific conventions of religious belief in Europe, which have developed from a complex historical and sociological past. Late-modern Europe '... is a part of the world characterised by unusually low levels of active religiousness, but with relatively high levels of nominal belief: or to put this into a convenient shorthand, Europe believes but it does not belong'.[122]

Believing without belonging is operative beyond the religious context, as traditional activities focused on regular social gatherings, such as membership of trade unions and leisure activities have also declined. Thus, the decrease in church attendance should not be interpreted as being indicative of an increasingly rational people disentangling themselves from the binds of superstitious religion. Instead, believing without belonging is a pervasive characteristic of contemporary society. The phrase denotes the discrepancies between indicators of religiousness. There is a clear reduction in 'hard' forms of religious life, such as a decrease in attending regular worship and adhering to the orthodoxy of credal statements.

This religious category has significantly declined in contemporary Europe, not least in the Irish context. However, Davie argues that despite this change, a significant number of Europeans express a belief in God and

121 Grace Davie, *The Sociology of Religion: A Critical Agenda* (London: SAGE Publications, 2013), 167.

122 Grace Davie, *Religion in Modern Europe: A Memory Mutates* (New York: Oxford University Press, 2000), 33.

an interest or belief in categories of experience that could be classed as religious or spiritual. This lessening of doctrinal and orthodox belief and forms of worship present both opportunities and challenges. Davie argues that '… the situation described as believing without belonging is neither better nor worse than a more straightforwardly (if one may use that term) secular society. It is simply different'.[123] Boeve and Halík make a similar point on this new climate of belief, stating that the conditions of religious belief and experience have changed, not ended.

Davie cites data from the European Values Survey to highlight how a significant number of young people have a sensibility towards the more heterodox forms of belief, such as belief in life after death, a vague belief in God or a higher spiritual power and an interest in supernatural dimensions of reality.[124] Davie proposes a changed religious landscape of the future where belief of some sort will go on existing alongside more secular understandings of life, contrary to the claims of secularisation theses.[125] This prediction that religion and secularity will continue to interact mirrors the perspectives of Taylor and Boeve.

However, Davie warns against treating 'believing without belonging' as a thesis to fully explain the religious situation in contemporary Europe. Rather, it is but one conceptual tool that the sociologist can draw upon, as this view is reflected in contemporary sociological research.[126] Davie notes the pitfalls of applying 'believing without belonging' in isolation, suggesting that too rigid an application can distort the sociologist's attempt to map out the persistence of the sacred in contemporary society, despite the decline in church attendance.[127]

123 Grace Davie, *Religion in Britain: A Persistent Paradox, 2nd Edition* (Oxford: Blackwell Press, 2015), 80.

124 Grace Davie, *The Sociology of Religion: A Critical Agenda* (London: SAGE Publications, 2013), 142.

125 Ibid.

126 See David Voas and Alasdair Crockett, 'Religion in Britain. Neither Believing nor Belonging', *Sociology, 39*(1) (2005), 11–28, Tony Glendenning and Steve Bruce, 'New Ways of Believing or Belonging: Is Religion Giving Way to Spirituality?' *The British Journal of Sociology, 57*(3) (2006), 399–414.

127 Grace Davie, *Religion in Britain: A Persistent Paradox, 1st Edition* (Oxford: Blackwell Press, 1994), 93–4.

Davie recognises that without scrutiny, 'believing without belonging' can present a misleading dichotomy between hard and soft forms of belief, oversimplifying the complexity of contemporary religiosity.[128] In order to alleviate such conceptual challenges, Davie proposes vicarious religion as a second analytical tool to diagnose the current religious climate as it may be more accurate and perceptive.

> By vicarious is meant the notion of religion performed by an active minority but on behalf of a much larger number, who (implicitly at least) not only understand, but appear to approve of what the minority is doing ... The second half is best explored by means of examples. It captures better than 'believing without belonging' the legacy of a historically dominant church.[129]

Vicarious religion is operative in a more implicit way than believing without belonging and is difficult to quantify with traditional sociological metrics. However, it offers an important conceptual resource in mapping how people retain a vague connection to religiosity and identification with a faith perspective, despite little adherence to communal worship. Moreover, it highlights the change in conditions of religious belief and experience, where religious practice becomes a personal choice rather than an explicit societal expectation. Davie's work on this phrase is influenced by research on the highly secular Nordic countries, which scholars have characterised as

128 Davie surmises this point at the 2005 Faith Angle Conference; 'In some ways I think that the phrase "believing without belonging" is a little misleading, because it isn't that belonging is hard and belief is soft. Both of them can be hard and soft. For example, if you ask European populations- and here I'm generalizing- do you believe in God, and you're not terribly specific about the God in question, you'll get about 70 percent saying yes, depending where you are. If you say, do you believe that Jesus Christ is the Son of God, you'll get a much lower number. In other words, your question into a credal statement, the percentages go down. The looser your definition of belief, the higher the percentage of believers.' <www.pewforum.org/2015/12/05/believing-without-belonging-just-how-secular-is-europe/>. Accessed 8 August 2019.

129 Grace Davie, *Religion in Britain: A Persistent Paradox, 2nd Edition* (Oxford: Blackwell Press, 2015), 6.

belonging without believing.[130] Davie highlights the prevalence of religion in Nordic society despite high levels of belief and low levels of religious institutional worship, where many retain religious identity with Lutheran churches, connecting with national identity and an important cultural component.[131]

Despite a growing secular population, there is still a significant demand for religious rituals which mark significant moments in life be performed by religious leaders. In particular, there remains a significant demand for Christian funerals which highlight the resilience of vicarious religion.[132] Significant sectors of the population would take great offence to such pastoral care or services not being offered to the bereaved as it would rupture deeply held assumptions about the role of these religious institutions. Davie notes the death of reality television star Jade Goody who having received a terminal cancer diagnosis turned to the Anglican church. Having been baptised, along with her children, she chose to have a traditional church funeral and passed away aged 28. Davie elaborates on the importance of treating this kind of religious experience seriously from a sociological perspective.

> These are moments when the 'secular' routines of life are suspended, when- to put the same point in a different way- the abnormal (the articulation of religion in words and actions) becomes at least for a short time normal. For this reason alone they merit careful sociological attention.[133]

130 See Anders Bäckström, Nina Edgardh and Per Pettersson, *Religious Change in Northern Europe: The Case of Sweden* (Stockholm: Verbum, 2004) and Andrew Greeley, *Religion in Europe at the End of the Second Millennium: A Sociological Profile* (London: Transaction, 2003) for further reading on this Nordic concept of belonging without believing.

131 Grace Davie, *The Sociology of Religion: A Critical Agenda* (London: SAGE Publications, 2013), 143.

132 Davie cites statistics from the Church of England, citing how in 2009, 43 percent of adults attended a religious ceremony for someone who had died. According to the latest data available: There were 81,000 Church of England baptisms and services of thanksgiving for the gift of a child during 2022. There were 31,400 Church of England marriages and services of prayer and dedication after civil marriages during 2022 and there were 103,500 Church of England-led funerals during 2022, 64% of which took place in churches. See <https://www.churchofengland.org/sites/default/files/2023-11/statisticsformission2022.pdf>. Accessed on 31 October 2024.

133 Grace Davie, *Religion in Britain: A Persistent Paradox, 2nd Edition* (Oxford: Blackwell Press, 2015), 87.

Davie is articulating here what Boeve refers to as boundary experiences, those moments of otherness and profound meaning which can be found in moments of joy and grief that break through the mundaneness of everyday life. Moreover, the persistence of moments such as the funeral of Jade Goody signifies the persistence of the sacred in contemporary life, contrary to the predictions of the secularisation thesis. Despite the changed conditions of religious belief and experience, such moments of otherness are possible, taking people beyond the boundary of Taylor's immanent frame.

Davie argues that vicarious religion requires sociologists of religion to be more imaginative in analysing the implicit and explicit ways in which people experience religion in the contemporary European context. Rather than an interpretation of data detached from an awareness of religious culture, Davie advocates greater creativity in appreciating the implicit backgrounds and assumptions of people towards belief and culture, which hitherto have been downplayed. 'This approach may vary from place to place, but it requires above all a developed sociological imagination and an awareness of culture as well as religion'.[134]

This appeal to the imagination echoes Gallagher's work on the secularised imagination. The modern social imaginary treats belief in the transcendent as implausible, meaning that sociological approaches to the study of religion risks neglecting those deeper spiritual wavelengths of faith perspectives. To better understand how religion and the sacred is operative in contemporary culture, an open spirit of enquiry and imagination is needed in contemporary sociology of religion. Davie's observation that sociologists must appreciate the implicit assumptions and dispositions of religion in human life seriously highlights the importance of inter-disciplinary research in these areas. The social sciences are concerned with the human person in the world, as are theology, religious studies and philosophy. In this sense, Davie is reinforcing the motivation of this opening chapter, that in order to get a better picture of the contemporary conditions of religious belief and experience, a variety of perspectives and academic lenses is required.

134 Ibid, 84.

Davie in conversation with interlocutors

Grace Davie's sociological perspective offers several themes that interact with those of the other interlocutors. First, Davie agrees with Taylor and Boeve on the failures of the secularisation thesis. Rather than the death of religion, they agree that a dynamic and complex interaction between religion and secularity has emerged rather than a monolithic master narrative operative. This is in broad agreement with Boeve's classification of the post-Christian and post-secular era, as well as Taylor's Secular 3 designation.

Second, Davie's illustration of Christian funerals as observable and common moments where the sacred interrupts the secular norms of everyday life mirrors Boeve's boundary experiences. Transcendent experience remains a possibility in contemporary life, which can give people a sense of otherness or meaning that gives life a fullness beyond immanent conceptions of flourishing. This would also support Taylor's work on the cross-pressures people feel as a response to the flatness of life, as well as Boeve's writing on the culture of the kick.

Finally, Davie's observation of contemporary interest in spirituality echoes the spiritual hunger identified by the other interlocutors. These phenomena, which jettison religious doctrines and social teaching for more vague connections to God and intense experience, mirror Halík and Gallagher's view that experience rather than authority is the paradigm for discovering and constructing meaning for many today. In this sense, religious adherence is now a choice rather than an inherited worldview or societal expectation, echoing Boeve's claim of the reflexivity of Christian identity.

A synthesis of ideas

Having provided an overview of various interpretations of the current conditions of religious belief and experience by some contemporary thinkers, certain key themes emerge. These key themes will now be categorised, contextualising the question of the compatibility of mindfulness and ethos in Irish Catholic primary schools, which is at the heart of this work.

The secularisation thesis has failed to come to pass

Despite the predictions of various sociologists of religion, the modern narrative of the progress of rationality, science and technological advancement at the cost of religion has not happened. Religious attitudes, beliefs and identity remain prominent in many parts of Europe. There have been decreases in certain forms of religious practice and communal worship, but the prophecy of the widespread receding place of religious believers has not occurred. This is not to overstate the place of religion in the contemporary European context. Religion does not hold the same prominence as the unassumed source of meaning and the common language of Western people. While the secularisation thesis has not wholly succeeded, the conditions of religious belief and experience have changed due to the processes of modernity. As Yves Lambert puts it, 'In Europe, God is neither as dead nor as alive as some now maintain'.[135]

Institutional religion is challenged by new narratives

Virtually all countries in Europe are seeing a continuing decrease in numbers attending Mass and participating in the liturgical life of the Church. This recession in Church attendance is also observable in other traditional social groupings and memberships in the political sphere. These social and economic changes have played at least some part in this decline. There is a widespread apathy or suspicion towards previously respected pillars of society, including political, financial and religious institutions. The claims and authority of modern narratives are increasingly challenged by postmodern perspectives that are wary of any position that makes universal truth claims.

135 Yves Lambert, 'A Turning Point in Religious Evolution in Europe', *Journal of Contemporary Religion 19* (2004), 44.

A new and growing marketplace of religions is operative

Through the modern processes of pluralisation, secularisation and detraditionalisation, there has been an explosion of religious and non-religious worldviews present in contemporary Europe. This gamut of worldviews become products to be consumed, as individuals can choose to become involved or members of groups that promote an alternative spirituality or religious experience. While many people are still born into a particular Christian tradition, they may now opt for another religious faith or no faith at all with far greater frequency than in previous decades. New Age spiritualities and westernised forms of oriental beliefs, such as Buddhism, have grown, and the promotion of meditation and mindfulness are now a common practice in mainstream society.

Many now identify as spiritual but not religious

As greater numbers of the European population leave conventional Christian churches, softer forms of religiosity remain high. A relatively large demographic is born into the Christian faith but retain a tenuous connection to this faith community outside of ceremonies such as baptism, weddings and funerals. Despite the decrease in 'hard forms' of religiosity, such as adherence to religious doctrines and attendance at communal worship, they retain vague beliefs in an afterlife and God. This demographic identifies as spiritual in that they believe there is something more or deeper to reality than the life around them, transcending the mundaneness of everyday life.

Meditation and silent practice remain sources of spiritual nourishment

Despite the modernising processes of secularisation, pluralisation and detraditionalisation, many people are invariably drawn to experiences beyond the immanent and material influences of modern life. From a theological anthropological perspective, many people feel a restlessness or hunger within their lives for something that goes beyond their everyday lives and experiences, transcending immanent conceptions of human flourishing.

The increased plurality of religious and non-religious outlooks means that there is a contemporary interest in forms of spirituality which include silent reflection, meditation and mindfulness practices derived from Vedic religions such as Buddhism. These practices have grown in popularity, especially observed in the explosion in interest in mindfulness. This contemporary practice demonstrates the need for silent practices that address a dissatisfaction felt by many in their lives.

In the Christian context, there remains an interest in silent prayer and reflection, as according to St John of the Cross, silence is God's first language. In this sense, silent prayer and meditation remain an important theological resource for Christians today, as for faith to thrive today, Karl Rahner argues that the Christian of the future must be a mystic. This means that an orientation to the transcendent horizon of meaning must be cultivated and nurtured for the Christian faith to engage in the contemporary world.

Theology faces a contextual challenge in addressing this changing culture

Faith does not occur in a vacuum; it is operative within a particular culture and tradition. Many people now live their lives without any explicit awareness of the transcendent and can conceive of human flourishing in a immanent sense. Theology faces the challenge of translating the spiritual fruits of Christian faith in this fragmented and detraditionalised context. Theology is challenged to transmit religious language into a medium applicable and relevant to the lives of those seeking authenticity and meaning in their lives. Abstract and cerebral notions of God must be distilled into the language of an experience of the Holy Mystery that transcends all words and concepts. Creative solutions such as apophatic theology can attend to this deadening of the religious imagination and present Christianity as life-giving to seekers of faith. A renewal of experiential spirituality, such as meditation and silent prayer needs to be recontextualised to address the waning religious imagination and experience of today.

This chapter outlined the contemporary conditions of religious belief and experience in the contemporary European context. In order to contextualise our question on the compatibility of mindfulness with ethos in Irish

Catholic primary schools, the theological, philosophical and sociological insights of several imminent interlocuters were drawn upon.

The shared interdisciplinary conversation between Charles Taylor, Lieven Boeve, Michael Paul Gallagher, Tomáš Halík and Grace Davie provides a map of the terrain of how belief is operative, felt and experienced today. This enabled the distillation of several consistent themes, which will frame the rest of this work. Having contextualised our question in terms of religious belief and experience, we now turn to the contemporary phenomenon of mindfulness.

CHAPTER 2

The Contemporary Phenomenon of Mindfulness

Having framed the conditions of religious belief and experience in the Irish context in the previous chapter, we will explore the term 'mindfulness' and how it is operative within this context. In relation to Irish Catholic primary schools, there has been a growing interest in mindfulness practices to bring about stress reduction, greater concentration and academic improvement in students.[136] Thus to answer the question at the heart of this book, it is imperative to understand the origins, development and contemporary applications of the concept of mindfulness.

The first half of the chapter will investigate the concept and etymology of mindfulness as understood in contemporary discourse. This will include the role of mindfulness in Buddhist teachings and precepts, with particular reference to the Pāli term '*sati*'. This will also include mapping the evolution of mindfulness as an aspect of Buddhist wisdom traditions to a Western phenomenon through the paradigm of Buddhist modernism.

The second half will then examine the contemporary strands of mindfulness operative within the Western context, as identified by Buddhist scholar Rupert Gethin will be examined and critiqued. By offering a detailed insight into what mindfulness is and how it is operative in contemporary life, we

136 Michelle McBride, 'Bells and Mind Jars: Mindfulness comes to School', *Irish Times*, 17 January 2017 <https://www.irishtimes.com/news/education/breathing-bells-and-mind-jars-mindfulness-comes-to-school-1.2933176> and Celine Naughton, How Mindfulness is Teaching Children to Cope in School, *Irish Independent*, 12 April 2016. <https://www.independent.ie/life/health-wellbeing/how-mindfulness-is-teaching-children-to-cope-in-school-34618690.html>. This has also included the Professional Development Service for Teachers (PDST) offering a dedicated page to Irish educators on mindfulness practice in schools. <https://pdst.ie/MSP2016> (all resources accessed on 3 February 2024).

are better equipped to evaluate the compatibility of mindfulness and ethos in Irish Catholic primary schools.

Mindfulness: definitions, origins and developments

We are witnessing what writer and mindfulness coach Barry Boyce has termed the 'mindfulness revolution'.[137] This phenomenon has swept into the mainstream lexicon and has interacted with many areas of society including education, commerce and healthcare. Moreover, personal use of mindfulness techniques for therapeutic and wellbeing purposes has exploded through the use of mindfulness apps, courses and websites. Such has been the exponential growth of mindfulness that in 2014, *TIME* magazine ran a cover titled '*The Mindful Revolution*' along with a piece discussing the ever-rising influence of mindfulness meditation in a wide variety of sectors of Western society.[138] Since that publication, there has been no indication that this phenomenon is set to fade from contemporary life, adding credence to Wong's claim that '... in the early twenty-first century, mindfulness will be regarded as one of the major cultural icons'.[139]

The most common definition of the term in contemporary discourse is offered by molecular biologist and founder of the Mindfulness-Based Stress Reduction program (MSBR), Jon Kabat-Zinn. He defines mindfulness as '... paying attention in a particular way: on purpose, in the present

137 Barry Boyce, ed., *The Mindfulness Revolution: Leading Psychologists, Scientists, Artists, and Spiritual Teachers on the Power of Mindfulness in Daily Life* (Boston, MA: Shambala, 2011).

138 Kate Pickert, 'The Mindful Revolution'. *TIME Magazine*, 3 February 2014. <http://content.time.com/time/subscriber/article/0,33009,2163560,00.html> (accessed 4 November 2019). In the same year the *Huffington Post*, a popular American news site which has its own Mindfulness news section, declared 2014 the 'Year of Mindful Living'.

139 Penelope Wong, 'Dissenting Voices of and About Mindfulness: What Can We Learn?' *Journal for the Liberal Arts and Sciences* 24(2) (2021), 65.

moment, and nonjudgmentally'.[140] Bishop et al. offer a more detailed definition, stating 'Broadly conceptualised, mindfulness has been described as a kind of non-elaborative, non-judgmental, present-centred awareness in which each thought, feeling or sensation that arises in the attentional field is acknowledged and accepted as it is'.[141] This definition presents mindfulness as a human faculty, encompassing a non-evaluative awareness and acceptance of the present moment. Langer and Piper's thesis mirrors this, arguing that mindfulness is a basic human capacity which can be achieved without religious or prayerful practices.[142]

This raises the question of how the relationship between mindfulness and meditation can be understood. Moreover, it is important to differentiate between mindfulness and meditation as these terms are often used somewhat interchangeably in mindfulness discourse. Poirier offers an instructive means of distinguishing between the terms, proposing that meditation represents a more concentrated, ritualised practice of attention whereas mindfulness is an extension of that cultivated attention into everyday life.[143] This does not deny the possibility of a symbiosis between mindfulness and meditation. If mindfulness is an innate human faculty, then meditation can be understood as a method or practice that focuses and attunes the person to full attention or mindfulness to the present moment. In this sense, mindfulness will be presented within this work as the non-judgemental awareness and acceptance of the present moment, with meditation understood as a ritualised method to cultivate a mindful state.

140 Jon Kabat-Zinn, *Wherever You Go, There You Are: Mindfulness Meditation for Everyday Life* (London: Piatkus, 1994), 4.

141 Scott Bishop, Mark Lau, Shauna Shapiro, Linda Carlson, Nicole D. Anderson, James Carmody, Zindel V. Sega, Susan Abbey, Michael Speca, Drew Velting and Gerald Devins, 'Mindfulness: A Proposed Operational Definition,' *Clinical Psychology: Science and Practice 11* (2004), 3.

142 Ellen Langer and Alison I. Piper, 'The Prevention of Mindlessness', *Journal of Personality and Social Psychology 53* (1987), 280–7.

143 Marc R. Poirier, 'Mischief in the Marketplace for Mindfulness'. In Robert Meikyo Rosenbaum and Barry Magid, eds, *What's Wrong with Mindfulness (And What Isn't): Zen Perspectives* (Somerville, MA: Wisdom Publications, 2016), 14.

The contemporary phenomenon of mindfulness practice is commonly understood as being extracted or inherited from Buddhism.[144] In the context of this book, this means that to evaluate the relationship between mindfulness and ethos in Irish Catholic primary schools, the connection between mindfulness and Buddhism must be investigated. This means applying a critical socio-cultural overview to gain a fuller understanding of the meanings mindfulness has held and the implications this has on contemporary forms and applications of mindfulness.

In exploring the Buddhist understandings of mindfulness, it is first important to note that Buddhism itself is a pluralist tradition, consisting of many distinct schools of thought, otherwise known as vehicles. The three most common vehicles are Theravada, Mahayana and Vajrayana.[145] As such, conceptions and practices of mindfulness differ between these respective Buddhist vehicles.[146] Harrington and Dunne stress that the investigator must be cognisant of these distinctions when exploring themes within Buddhism, including mindfulness:

> Many participants in today's conversations tend to talk about an entity called 'Buddhism' as if we had here to do with a monolithic and unchanging ancient tradition that speaks in a single voice. Buddhism in fact is a dynamic, pluralistic and even quarrelsome set of cultural traditions, and every researcher or clinician implicitly or explicitly engages, not with the whole but with a part.[147]

144 Elizabeth Landeau, 'Can Mindfulness Help Manage Pain and Mental Illness?', *CNN Edition*, 16 November 2010). 'Mindfulness as a concept comes from Buddhism and is key to meditation in that tradition'. <https://edition.cnn.com/2010/HEALTH/11/16/mindfulness.therapy.meditation/index.html> (accessed on 24 March 2021) and Kate Pickert, 'The Mindful Revolution', *TIME Magazine*, 3 February 2014. 'Mindfulness is rooted in Eastern philosophy, specifically Buddhism'. <http://content.time.com/time/subscriber/article/0,33009,2163560,00.html> (accessed 4 November 2019).

145 Peter Harvey, *An Introduction to Buddhism: Teachings, History and Practices* (2nd Edition) (Cambridge: Cambridge University Press, 2013), 4–5.

146 Georges Dreyfus, 'Is Mindfulness Present-centred and Non-judgmental? A Discussion of the Cognitive Dimensions of Mindfulness', *Contemporary Buddhism 12*(1) (2011), 42.

147 Anne Harrington and John Dunne, 'Mindfulness Meditation: Frames and Choices', *American Psychologist*, 2. <http://nrs.harvard.edu/urn-3:HUL.InstRepos:10718406>. Accessed 6 November 2019.

While these three main schools of Buddhist teaching have evolved differently over time, Peter Harvey argues that despite the variance in some teachings and practices, mindfulness and meditation retain huge significance across the complex network of Buddhism, with mindfulness being '... a crucial aspect to any Buddhist meditation'.[148] The two qualities most associated with achieving enlightenment in Buddhist meditation are *samatha* and *vipassanā*.[149] *Samatha* relates to the calming of the mind through focus on a particular object of concentration. By focusing one's attention on the object, the practitioner is enabled to empty their minds of other thoughts and distractions. Thus, the practitioner is focused upon the present moment in concentration.[150]

Once this state of calm concentration has been achieved, *vipassanā* may be initiated. This centres on practising clear insight; rather than focusing on a sole object, the practitioner observes feelings and experiences come and go. An awareness of breath is typically used in order to aid freedom from distractions as one explores the nature of reality as they experience it. Influential Buddhist monk Thich Nhat Hanh explains this process as following the calm state of mind cultivated through *samatha*:

> Because you are calm and concentrated, you are really there for deep looking. You shine the light of mindfulness on the object of your attention, and at the same time you shine the light of mindfulness on yourself. You observe the object of your attention and you also see your own storehouse full of precious gems.[151]

148 Peter Harvey, *An Introduction to Buddhism: Teachings, History and Practices* (1st Edition) (Cambridge: Cambridge University Press, 1990), 70.

149 Peter Harvey, *An Introduction to Buddhism: Teachings, History and Practices* (2nd Edition) (Cambridge: Cambridge University Press, 2013), 324.

150 'Calm-abiding is a settled one-pointedness of mind, not a sleepy or blank state. One rests in the experience of the present moment, neither distracted by thoughts of past or future nor anxiously grasping and whatever is arising right now. It is a state that is stable, open and clear, in which thoughts are neither suppressed nor cultivated'. Lama Jampa Thaye, *Wisdom in Exile: Buddhism and Modern Times* (Bristol: Ganesha Press, 2017), 72.

151 Thich Nhat Hanh, *The Heart of the Buddha's Teaching: Transforming Suffering into Peace, Joy and Liberation* (New York: Harmony Books, 2015), 66.

These two facets of Buddhist meditation aid the practitioner in achieving Nirvana, the ultimate state of liberation from suffering which is at the heart of the Buddha's teaching. Meditation is then an important aspect of key teachings such as the Noble Eightfold Path,[152] which traverse the Buddhist landscape. These factors represent guidelines for the transition from the endless cycle of rebirth (*samsara*) to the soteriological freedom of Nirvana and the final dissolution of the illusion of the self. These eight factors can be divided into three categories: Morality (*sīla*), which relates to the perfection of ethical and moral virtues; Wisdom (*paññā*), which is the cultivation of intellectual virtues; and Meditation (*samādhi*), concentrative states that attune the mind on the path towards Nirvana.[153] The three factors associated with Meditation (*samādhi*) are Right Effort, Right Mindfulness and Right Concentration.

These three categories of the Noble Eightfold Path are 'three sides of a triangle'.[154] The calmness of meditation and intellectual investigation cultivates an ethical benevolence towards others in the pursuit of Nirvana and liberation of all beings from suffering, which is fundamental to the Buddha's teaching on the Four Noble Truths.[155] Thus, meditation occupies a central role in practically all forms of Buddhism and is inseparable from the categories

152 Damien Keown, *Buddhism: A Very Short Introduction* (Oxford: Oxford University Press, 2013), 58–59. The Noble Eightfold Path represents a key tenet of Buddhism, offering the factors necessary for a way of life that leads the practitioner closer to Nirvana. Keown quotes The Buddha's teaching on the Truth of the Eightfold Path: 'This, O Monks, is the Truth of the Path which leads to the cessation of suffering. It is this Noble Eightfold Path, which consists of (1) Right View, (2) Right Resolve, (3) Right Speech, (4) Right Action, (5) Right Livelihood, (6) Right Effort, (7) Right Mindfulness, (8) Right Meditation.'

153 Ibid, 59–60.

154 Ibid, 111.

155 For further reading, see Robert Scharf, 'Epilogue', in Robert Meikyo Rosenbaum and Barry Magid, eds, *What's Wrong with Mindfulness (And What Isn't): Zen Perspectives* (Somerville, MA: Wisdom Publications, 2016), 140. Scharf outlines the Four Noble Truths of the Buddha. '(1) to live is to suffer, (2) the only genuine remedy to suffering is escape from samsara (the phenomenal world) altogether, and (3) escape requires, among other things, abandoning hope that happiness in this world is possible.' The Fourth Noble Truth relates to the Noble Eightfold Path as the way towards enlightenment and liberation.

of morality and wisdom. While the various schools of thought may vary in emphasis and approaches to this trio of concepts, they are operative precepts across the Buddhist landscape.

Keown warns against meditation being understood as a detachable utility to success in the other two categories, citing the practice of the Buddha himself who continued to meditate after having achieved enlightenment. In the Buddhist tradition, the triumvirate of *sīla, paññā* and *samādhi* are interdependent upon one another and cannot be fully applied or appreciated in isolation. 'Meditation, however, is not just a *means* to virtue and wisdom: if it were, it would be merely a technique which can be discarded once they had been attained'.[156]

Despite the variety of Buddhist schools of thought, meditation that cultivates a mindful state is integral to key Buddhist teachings such as the Noble Eightfold Path. In this regard, it is an interrelated and reciprocal aspect of the development of the ethical, moral, and intellectual virtues towards the ultimate goal of Nirvana. This means that mindfulness meditation is not a technique or tool but rather an essential component of following the path of the Buddha.

As has been highlighted, many contemporary forms of mindfulness are overwhelmingly associated with Buddhist origins. A key concept in this regard is the Pāli word *sati*. It was not until 1881 that mindfulness as related to the Buddhist tradition first emerged in Western thought, through scholar Thomas William Rhys Davids' translation of the Pāli word *sati* as mindfulness.[157] Tyler highlights the equivalent term in the Sanskrit canon (of *sati*) is *smṛti,* which literally means 'that which is remembered'[158] and elaborates on the important connection between these terms in respect of Buddhist teaching on mindfulness:

156 Damien Keown, *Buddhism: A Very Short Introduction* (Oxford: Oxford University Press, 2013), 111.

157 '*Sati* is literally memory but is used with reference to the constantly repeated phrase 'mindful and thoughtful'... that activity of mind and constant presence of mind which is one of the duties most frequently inculcated on the good Buddhist'. Thomas William Rhys Davids, *Buddhist Suttas* (Oxford: Clarendon, 1881), 145.

158 Peter Tyler, *Christian Mindfulness: Theology and Practice* (London: SCM Press, 2018), 8.

> As many commentators have noted, the cognate resonance of sati with the Sanskrit smṛti reminds us to recall our fundamental orientation to the precepts and the path of the Buddha as we engage in observation of the self- thus implying that there is such a thing as wrong mindfulness: the mindfulness of, say, a terrorist preparing to detonate a bomb or attack civilians.[159]

This is an important point as it implies that far from being a morally neutral practice, *sati* involves self-awareness informed by other Buddhist precepts such as the Eightfold Path, entailing rules such as Right Action and Right Speech. This understanding of *sati* can differ from contemporary iterations of mindfulness such as the forms promoted by prominent mindfulness practitioner Jon Kabat-Zinn, which emphasise non-evaluative attention to the present moment, representing a shift from traditional Buddhist approaches to mindfulness.[160]

Reynolds details how traditionally, mindfulness was a more active practice rather than the passive form seen in the contemporary mindfulness practice often associated with Kabat-Zinn, arguing '... in early Buddhist understandings of mindfulness, awareness is not just a passive acceptance of what is, but active vigilance against what is unhelpful and cultivation of positive states of mind'.[161] This again highlights the interplay between *sati* and the precepts of the Noble Eightfold Path and the Four Noble Truths. In order to achieve liberation from suffering (Nirvana), the Buddhist attempts to live in accordance with these precepts.

159 Ibid, 9.

160 A helpful analogy of early Buddhist understandings of *sati* is offered by Hwang and Kearney. '*Sati* as memory does not refer to memory in the ordinary sense of remembering the past; rather, *sati* remembers the present, by keeping the present in mind. We find the same concept presented in the exhortations at railway stations to "mind the gap" when stepping between a train and the platform. Minding the gap here means remembering the act of entering and exiting a train during the actual moment of transit. Mindfulness practice is remembering to stay present. It is the art of not forgetting, and entails tracking both awareness and the object of awareness over time'. Yoon Suk Hwang and Patrick Kearney, *A Mindfulness Intervention for Children with Autism Spectrum Disorder: Mindfulness in Behavioural Health* (Cham: Springer International Publishing, 2015), 6.

161 Stefan G. Reynolds, *Living with the Mind of Christ: Mindfulness in Christian Spirituality* (London: Darton, Longman & Todd, 2016), 47.

When faced with social structures that perpetuate suffering or injustice, the Buddhist challenges these sources of suffering rather than observing them in a non-evaluative manner. In this regard, traditional understandings of mindfulness are interdependent upon other precepts such as Right Action and Right Intention. This means that there is an intrinsic link between the Buddhists' efforts to be mindful of sources of suffering and their efforts in actively reducing and challenging them. As such, Buddhist mindfulness is not a passive or neutral technique.

Wallace argues that those seeking to deepen their understanding and experience of Buddhist meditation need to understand the nuances and subtleties of terms such as *sati*. Otherwise, they are in danger of a shallow, anchorless experience that provides no true insight:

> Sati has a much richer connotation, so those wishing to practice Buddhist meditation are well advised to gain as clear an understanding of this and other related terms as they can … Otherwise Buddhist meditation quickly devolves into a vague kind of 'be here now' mentality, in which the extraordinary depth and richness of Buddhist meditation traditions are lost.[162]

Wallace's warning here raises an interesting question: Are those who engage in contemporary mindfulness practices self-identifying as Buddhist practitioners, or do they interpret mindfulness as a secular activity outside of Buddhism? In the context of this work, it is important to ascertain whether mindfulness practices in Irish Catholic primary schools are to be understood as Buddhist meditation or a secular method inspired by Buddhism. In order to answer this question, it is thus necessary to examine how mindfulness meditation has evolved from a Buddhist precept in the East to a contemporary phenomenon in the West.

As stated previously, mindfulness across practically all of the Buddhist spectrum of practice is underpinned by the Buddha's teaching on the Noble Eightfold Path. One of these factors is Right Mindfulness, which is itself interdependent on the other seven elements of the Path. In this sense, there is a clear distinction between mindfulness in foundational Buddhist teachings and contemporary forms of mindfulness which promote non-evaluative

162 B. Alan Wallace, 'A Mindful Balance', *Tricycle, XVII, (3)*, Spring (2008), 62.

attention to the present moment, including those operative in Irish Catholic primary schools, which will be explored in the next chapter.[163]

This evolution of mindfulness can be framed as a complex intellectual interaction between Eastern wisdom traditions and Western Enlightenment over the past 150 years which has resulted in what has been termed 'Buddhist modernism'.[164] This multifaceted process relates to the ways that different Buddhist schools of thought, beliefs and practices including mindfulness have interacted with the prevailing narratives of modernity in the West. This had led to emergent understandings of Buddhism as a result of the interplay between aspects of Buddhist teaching and a Western context typically characterised by rationality and secularism.[165]

However, McMahan points out that these contemporary developments of Buddhist modernism are '… the result of a process of modernisation, westernisation, reinterpretation, image-making, revitalisation and reform that has been taking place not only in the West but also in Asian countries for over a century'.[166] Modern forms of Buddhism are seen as compatible with a scientific, rationalist Western worldview as they are perceived as non-theistic modes of spirituality rooted in empirical investigation. Early Buddhist religious teachings, such as reincarnation and karma, are demythologised. Religious rituals such as prayer wheels and chants to invoke protection and prayerful devotion towards images of the Buddha[167] are generally replaced by meditative practices that can be decontextualised from teachings such as the Noble Eightfold Path.

163 Mindfulness programmes available for Irish Catholic primary schools such as Paws b and Weaving Wellbeing will be explored in Chapter 3 to further examine the distinction between Buddhist precepts and nonevaluative attention to the present moment.

164 For further reading, see David L. McMahan, *The Making of Modern Buddhism* (Oxford: Oxford University Press, 2008) and Robert Scharf, 'Buddhist Modernism and the Rhetoric of Meditative Experience', *Numen 42*(3) (1995), 228–83.

165 Donald Lopez, 'Foreward', in Paul Carus, ed., *The Gospel of Buddha: According to Old Records* (LaSalle, Illinois: Open Court Publications, 2004), vii–ix.

166 David L. McMahan, *The Making of Modern Buddhism* (Oxford: Oxford University Press, 2008), 5.

167 See Harvey's chapter on the role of devotion in Buddhist practice in Peter Harvey, *An Introduction to Buddhism: Teachings, History and Practices* (2nd Edition) (Cambridge: Cambridge University Press, 2013), 237–63.

Tensions can arise between adherents of traditional Buddhist schools and more modern forms,[168] where proponents of a modernist school remove the explicitly religious elements of older forms of Buddhism. As a result of the processes of Buddhist modernism, spiritual approaches that focus less on doctrine and metaphysical presuppositions have become more popular and widespread. This was observed in the previous chapter with the growing contemporary interest in Eastern meditation as well as the growth in those who identify as spiritual but not religious. One of the emergent developments from this process is how for some, modern Buddhism is seen as a practice that does necessarily require adherence to teachings or rituals previously seen as important in Buddhist wisdom traditions.[169]

Consequently, modern Buddhism has brought about a significant, contemporary reinterpretation of *sati* as a non-judgemental, non-reactive awareness also known as 'bare-attention'. This development of 'bare-attention' mindfulness is seen in the writings of influential Buddhist teachers such as Mahāsī Sayādaw[170] and Nyanaponika

168 For further reading, see Robert Meikyo Rosenbaum, '"I" Doesn't Mind', in Robert Meikyo Rosenbaum and Barry Magid (Eds.), *What's Wrong with Mindfulness (And What Isn't): Zen Perspectives* (Somerville, MA: Wisdom Publications, 2016) and James Mark Shields, 'The Scope and Limits of Secular Buddhism: Watanabe Kaikyoku and the Japanese New Buddhist "Discovery of Society"', in Hanna Havnevik, Ute Hüsken, Mark Teeuwen, Vladimir Tikhonov, and Koen Wellens, eds, *Buddhist Modernities: Re-Inventing Tradition in the Globalizing World* (New York: Routledge, 2017), 15–32.

169 Stephen Batchelor, 'A Secular Buddhist' (2012) 2. A Secular Buddhist (gaiahouse.co.uk). Accessed on 18 December 2019.

170 Scharf argues Sayādaw; '... developed the technique that is best known today, in which the practitioner is trained to focus on whatever sensory object arises in the moment-to-moment flow of consciousness. Mahāsī designed this method with laypersons in mind, including those with little or no prior exposure to Buddhist doctrine or liturgical practice. Perhaps most radical was Mahāsī's claim that the cultivation of liberating insight did not require advanced skill in concentration (*samatha*) or the experience of absorption *(jhāna)*. Instead, Mahāsī placed emphasis on the notion of *sati*, understood as the moment-to-moment, lucid, non-reactive, non-judgmental awareness of whatever appears to consciousness'.

See Robert Scharf, 'Is Mindfulness Buddhist? (and Why it Matters)', *Transcultural Psychiatry* 52(4) (2015), 472.

Thera[171], who promoted this type of moment-to-moment awareness, which did not require prior experience of Buddhist meditation or any connection to Buddhist teachings or philosophy.[172] One reason for this was the emergence of forms of meditation movements from traditional Buddhist contexts such as Myanmar, Thailand and Sri Lanka, which understood meditation as the cornerstone of achieving liberation over ritual and liturgy. McMahan points to examples of the disembedding of Zen meditation (*zazen*) from traditional institutional contexts of the Japanese, Chinese, Korean, Tibetan and Vietnamese monasteries.

> The idea that the goal of meditation is not specifically Buddhist, and that "Zen" itself is common to all religions, has encouraged the understanding of zazen (meditation) as detachable from the complex traditions of ritual, liturgy, priesthood, and hierarchy common in institutional Zen settings.[173]

This represents broader processes of detraditionalisation and individualisation within Buddhist practices on a global scale in the past century. This echoes Boeve and Taylor's observations in Chapter 1 of similar cultural and sociological processes as in the Western religious context, which changed the way religious belief was felt by many. Moreover, Western society has proven to be a particularly fertile ground for these contemporary detraditionalised forms of Buddhist meditation free from religious language and concepts.[174]

171 See Nyanponika Thera, *The Heart of Buddhist Meditation: The Buddha's Way of Mindfulness* (San Francisco, CA: Weiser Books, 2014). The text was originally published, and such has been its influence, that on the front cover of the 2014 edition, Jon Kabat-Zinn's endorsement reads simply; 'The book that started it all'.

172 It is worth noting that long-term student of Nyanponika Thera, Bhikku Bodhi claims his teacher's interpretation of bare attention differed from that seen in contemporary Western mindfulness. See Bhikku Bodhi, 'What Does Mindfulness Really Mean? A Canonical Perspective', *Contemporary Buddhism: An Interdisciplinary Journal 12* (2011).

173 David L. McMahan, *The Making of Modern Buddhism* (Oxford: Oxford University Press, 2008), 187.

174 Ibid, 188–208. McMahan offers several reasons why Western culture has been so receptive to mindfulness meditation, including the subjective turn associated with modernity, where the individual enjoys the self-determination and autonomy to develop their own privatised religious imaginary, rather than be bound to a single tradition for meaning. Moreover, other conditions include the rise of meditation being seen as an object of science, as well as a phenomenon that could share common ground and psychoanalysis.

The contemporary practice of mindfulness in the Western context can be seen as a decontextualisation of Buddhist teaching in that there is a consistent de-emphasis of the explicitly religious and supernatural elements associated with Buddhist teachings such as karma, samsara, ghosts and demons. Moreover, as McMahan argues, this decoupling of meditation from tenets of Buddhist tradition can be so radical that meditation practice for many is no longer understood as a Buddhist tenet at all.

> Paradoxically, while meditation is often considered the heart of Buddhism, it is also deemed the element most detachable from the tradition itself. It has in some sectors become disembedded from the Buddhist tradition and rearticulated as a technique of self-investigation, awareness, personal satisfaction, and ethical reflection, taking on a life of its own, in some cases altogether outside of Buddhist communities.[175]

Buddhist modernism has led to the development of new trends and forms of Buddhism globally. However, in the Western context, mindfulness meditation has interacted with a setting underpinned by a pluralisation of worldviews and a reduction in people who identify as religious, as was observed in the previous chapter. This interplay of mindfulness with a secularised West has been helped by the popular perception of Buddhism being a non-theistic tradition that is compatible with a secular or rationalist viewpoint.[176]

Contemporary Western culture has inherited mindfulness through the processes of Buddhist modernism and shows no signs of abating. Unlike mainstream religions, mindfulness is accepted by secular society as an activity independent of religious dogma and any commitment or affiliation to a faith tradition. As it is seen as outside of religion, it has been able to enter areas of civic and commercial life that religion would often find inaccessible.

175 Ibid, 185.
176 See Caroline Starkey, 'British Buddhism, Secular Mindfulness and the Politics of Sustainability,' *Religion* 2023.

Contemporary forms of mindfulness

Having mapped the migration of mindfulness from Eastern wisdom tradition to Western phenomenon, the idea that mindfulness is itself a static, monolithic activity in twenty-first-century secular culture is challenged. To this end, Peter Tyler summarises authoritative Buddhist scholar Rupert Gethin's position on the contemporary iterations of mindfulness, arguing that there are three distinctive strands currently operative:

> … first, clinically mindfulness as developed by practitioners such as Kabat-Zinn and (Mark) Williams in their MBSR (Mindfulness-Based Stress Reduction) and MBCT (Mindfulness-Based Cognitive Therapy) courses. Second, mindfulness as a commercial phenomenon, promulgated by apps for making you a better worker, businessman, lover, etc.- what is sometimes called 'McMindfulness'. And finally, mindfulness as a new Western phenomenon that… 'eschews the traditional framework of karma and rebirth, where the goal of nirvana is understood as liberation from the round of rebirth, and replaces these with a more therapeutic framework where nirvana is understood as a kind of equilibrium and state of well-being achieved by mindfulness meditation'. Such practitioners will still claim the title of being 'Buddhist' and hold that 'mindfulness', is as they see it, the essence of Buddhism.[177]

These three strands offered by Gethin will be critiqued in order to discern similarities and differences between the respective approaches. By critiquing these forms of mindfulness, conclusions about the contextualisation of mindfulness as Buddhist and/or secular will emerge. The critique in this instance is not meant to undermine the efficacy of mindfulness; rather, it is a creative process of questioning the underlying assumptions and conventions of the contemporary mindfulness movement.

In the context of this work, such a critique is necessary, as in order to evaluate the compatibility of mindfulness and ethos in Irish Catholic primary schools, we first need to interrogate what kinds of mindfulness are operative today, as well as their relative strengths and weaknesses. In doing so, we are better equipped to discern how mindfulness interacts in Irish primary schools and its implications for the ethos of the Catholic school.

177 Peter Tyler, *Christian Mindfulness: Theology and Practice* (London, SCM Press, 2018), 15.

For the purposes of clarity, these forms of mindfulness will be classified as Mindfulness 1, Mindfulness 2 and Mindfulness 3 unless otherwise stated.

Mindfulness 1

Mindfulness has been absorbed into several therapeutic interventions in recent decades. The academic interest in Mindfulness 1 as it relates to psychological and psychiatric treatments and interventions has grown exponentially in recent years. As of July 2021, there have been over 17,500 scholarly articles featuring the word 'mindfulness' since 2010 on *PsychInfo*, the online database for the American Psychological Association.[178]

Hayes has referred to these therapies, which integrate Buddhist mindfulness meditation, as third-generation cognitive-behavioural approaches, following behavioural therapy and cognitive behavioural therapy (CBT).[179] Farias and Wikholm posit that where CBT tries to challenge and alter negative or problematic behaviours, third-wave therapies (or mindfulness-based interventions) see thoughts as impermanent and cultivate a non-evaluative outlook towards them:

> So, with mindfulness-based interventions, the aim is not to change your thoughts, but your global beliefs about thoughts- essentially, you're expected to stop believing that your thoughts are necessarily true or important. This is where the Buddhist philosophy really kicks in: your thoughts are mere 'mental events'- just thoughts, nothing more- and they don't necessarily warrant any action. All you're aiming to do is to be aware.[180]

178 A search in October 2024 found over 24,600 articles on mindfulness, double that of the 11,700 results found in November 2019. APA PsycNet Search Results. Accessed on 29 October 2024.

179 Stephen C. Hayes, 'Acceptance and Commitment Therapy, Relational Frame Theory and the Third Wave of Behavioural Therapies', *Behaviour Therapy*, *35*(4), *Autumn* (2004), 639.

180 Migel Farias and Catherine Wikholm, *The Buddha Pill: Can Meditation Change You?* (London: Watkins, 2015), 104.

Moreover, while Mindfulness 1 integrates aspects of Buddhist philosophy into a therapeutic approach, the therapist ensures that any connections to religious language or concepts are removed in order to make the therapy available to anyone that is not Buddhist. In this way, Mindfulness 1 can be framed as a secular psychological therapeutic approach.[181]

A growing body of research indicates that mindfulness practice has identifiable physical and mental health benefits ranging from an increase in alertness and wellbeing of older people[182] to effectiveness in reducing alcohol and cigarette addiction.[183] Meta-analyses of clinical trials provide evidence of positive impacts of mindfulness-based interventions on a wide variety of ailments and conditions.[184] Outside of mental health and psychology, mindfulness techniques have provided evidence of increased effectiveness in cognitive functioning, performance, stress-resilience, and wellbeing in educational settings[185] and the workplace.[186]

While there has been a significant quantity of research on the benefits of mindfulness, some have voiced concerns over the quality of research methods involved in a section of these studies. One significant systematic

181 Stefan G. Reynolds, *Living with the Mind of Christ: Mindfulness in Christian Spirituality* (London: Darton, Longman & Todd, 2016), 50–1. 'Behaviour therapists try to use strictly secular language in Mindfulness theories. Stripping mindfulness from any religious connotations makes it available to non-Buddhists. Mindfulness is used strictly as a therapeutic tool, instrumental to mental health, stability and cognitive clarity'.

182 Ellen Langer, 'A Mindful Education', *Educational Psychologist* (2003), 43–50.

183 J. Mark G. Williams and Jon Kabat-Zinn, eds, *Mindfulness: Diverse Perspectives on its Meaning, Origins and Applications* (Abingdon: Routledge, 2013).

184 For further reading, see Alberto Chiesa and Alessandro Serretti, 'Mindfulness Based Cognitive Therapy for Psychiatric Disorders: A Systematic Review and Meta-analysis', *Psychiatry Research, 187*(3), (2011), 441–53, and Shian-Ling Keng, Moria J. Smoski and Clive J. Robins, 'Effects of Mindfulness on Psychological Health: A Review of Empirical Studies', *Clinical Psychology Review*, *31*(6) (2011), 1041–56.

185 See Chiesa and Serretti (ibid), and Richard Burnett, 'Mindfulness in Schools: Learning Lessons from the Adults, Secular and Buddhist', *Buddhist Studies Review*, *28*(1) (2011), 79–120.

186 Ute R. Hülsheger, Hugo J. E. M. Alberts, Alina Feinholdt, and J. W. B. Lang, 'Benefits of Mindfulness at Work: The Role of Mindfulness in Emotion Regulation, Emotional Exhaustion, and Job Satisfaction', *Journal of Applied Psychology*, *98*(2) (2013), 310–25.

review has argued for more robust research to be conducted in the area.[187] Further, Thompson argues that some studies on mindfulness can be affected by poor-quality research at times, which renders some results meaningless.[188] Another study found significant publication bias, which could overstate results.[189] Dobkin and Zhao urge caution in the perceived universal benefits of MBIs, as there has not been extensive evidence that meditation is the definitive catalyst for effective therapeutic treatment in these programs.[190] It is evident from the current research that while mindfulness is shown to provide benefits in therapeutic, educational and occupational contexts, further research and more rigorous meta-analyses are necessary to prevent overstating the efficacy and outcomes of mindfulness.[191]

Several major therapies of the third generation of cognitive behavioural approaches have been identified,[192] with each of these having connections

187 Madhav Goyal, Sonal Singh, Erica Sibinga, Neda F. Gould, Anastasia Rowland-Seymour, Ritu Sharma, Zackary Berger, Dana Sleicher, David D. Maron, Hasan M. Shihab, Padmini Ranasinghe, Shauna Linn, Shonali Saha, Eric B. Bass and Jennifer Haythornthwaite, 'Meditation Programs for Psychological Stress and Well-being: A Systematic Review and Meta-analysis', *JAMA Internal Medicine, 174*(3) (2014), 357.

188 Katherine Thompson, *Christ-Centred Mindfulness: Connections to Self and God* (Sydney: Acorn Press, 2018), 36. Thompson stresses potential pitfalls such as not adequately matching groups in cross-sectional studies, which can lead to confounding variables which can influence and nullify results.

189 Stephanie Coronado-Montoya, Alexander W. Levis, Linda Kwakkenbos, Russell J. Steele, Erick H. Turner, and Brett D. Thombs, 'Reporting of Positive Results in Randomized Controlled Trials of Mindfulness-based Mental Health Interventions', *PLOS ONE, 11*(4) (2016).

190 Patricia Lynn Dobkin and Qinki Zhao, 'Increased Mindfulness – The Active Component of the Mindfulness–based Stress Reduction Program?', *Complementary Therapies in Clinical Practice, 17*(1) (2011), 22–7.

191 Moloney critiques other limitations and methodological weaknesses in MBIs as well as scrutinising the 'Mindful Nation' report promoted by MPs in Westminster. See Paul Moloney, 'Mindfulness: The Bottled Water of the Therapy Industry,' in Ronald E. Purser, David Forbes and Adam Burke, eds, *Handbook of Mindfulness: Culture, Context and Social Engagement* (Basel: Springer Publishing, 2016), 269–92.

192 Thompson lists these as Mindfulness-Based Stress Reduction (MBSR), Mindfulness-Based Cognitive Therapy (MBCT), Dialectical Behaviour Therapy (DBT) and Acceptance and Commitment Therapy. (ACT). See Katherine Thompson, *Christ-Centred Mindfulness: Connections to Self and God* (Sydney: Acorn Press, 2018), 26–43.

to meditation derived from Buddhist schools.[193] Mindfulness-Based Stress Reduction (MBSR) will be the central focus of this evaluation of Mindfulness 1, as it is the approach that has most successfully moved beyond clinical and healthcare settings other sectors of society, such as education and commerce.

MBSR was developed by molecular biologist Jon Kabat-Zinn at the University of Massachusetts in the late 1970s as a participant-centred behavioural medicine program initially designed to empower patients to engage proactively in their own healing and pain reduction.[194] The original targets for this program were those patients with chronic pain who found conventional medical treatment inadequate.[195] Moloney outlines the basic tenets of this program that now form the pillars for the official eight-week MBSR program:

> Participants were asked to commit to daily practice of mindfulness exercises, mostly in the form of sitting or vipassana meditation (in which attention is focused upon your breath) and also in regular movement awareness and 'body scanning' exercises, taught in a series of weekly sessions. These exercises were intended to dispel physical and mental tension and to foster the relaxed state conducive to the pursuit of meditation.[196]

Kabat-Zinn proposed a robust training program that would ultimately focus on radically changing how the patient viewed their illness and their lives more generally. By transforming a patient's attitude to their momentary experience through non-judgemental awareness and acceptance, this could reduce suffering and symptoms such as depression and anxiety. Mindfulness-based programs such as MBSR have yielded positive

193 Kirmayer offers a useful table outlining the cognitive therapies and their respective links to Buddhist meditation techniques. See Laurence J. Kirmayer, 'Mindfulness in Cultural Context', *Transcultural Psychiatry 52*(4) (2015), 454–6.

194 Jon Kabat-Zinn, *Full Catastrophe Living: Using the Wisdom of Your Body and Mind to Face Stress, Pain and Illness* (New York: Bantam Dell, 2000).

195 Gavin Ivey, 'The Mindfulness Status of Psychoanalytic Psychotherapy', *Psychoanalytic Psychotherapy 29*(4) (2015), 382–98.

196 Paul Moloney, 'Mindfulness: The Bottled Water of the Therapy Industry'. In Ronald E. Purser, David Forbes and Adam Burke, eds, *Handbook of Mindfulness: Culture, Context and Social Engagement* (Basel: Springer Publishing, 2016), 269–70.

results in these areas.[197] This experiential approach uses mindfulness, which while inspired by Buddhism,[198] is reframed as a secular psychological practice. Harrington and Dunne identify the Buddhist vehicles and practices that influenced Kabat-Zinn's original development of MBSR, including '… the mindfulness-based practices of Zen, Theravada Buddhism and yoga practice, along with significant influences from Tibetan and Vietnamese Buddhism'.[199]

While MBSR techniques stem from Buddhist meditative practices, Kabat-Zinn consistently stresses that mindfulness can be practiced by anyone as it is a universal capacity outside the realms of a religious worldview or belief system. Kabat-Zinn states his aim as such, is to provide '… the wisdom

197 See Jon Kabat-Zinn, *Full Catastrophe Living: Using the Wisdom of Your Body and Mind to Face Stress, Pain and Illness* (New York, NY: Delacorte Press, 1990) and Jon Kabat-Zinn, 'An Outpatient Program in Behavioral Medicine for Chronic Pain Patients Based on the Practice of Mindfulness Meditation: Theoretical Considerations and Preliminary Results', *General Hospital Psychiatry 4*(1) (1982), 33–47. Also, see Jon Kabat-Zinn, Leslie Lipworth, and Robert Burney, 'The Clinical Use of Mindfulness Meditation for the Self-regulation of Chronic Pain,' *Journal of Behavioural Medicine 8*(2) (1985), 163–90; Aleksandra Zgierska, David Rabago, David, Neharika Chawla, Kenneth Kushner, Robert Koehler and Allan Marlatt, 'Mindfulness Meditation for Substance Use Disorders: A Systematic Review', *Substance Abuse 30* (2009), 266–94 and Philippe R. Goldin and James J. Gross, 'Effects of Mindfulness-Based Stress Reduction (MBSR) on Emotion Regulation in Social Anxiety Disorder', *Emotion, 10*(1) (2010), 83–91.

198 Jon Kabat-Zinn, *Full Catastrophe Living: Using the Wisdom of Your Body and Mind to Face Stress, Pain, and Illness* (New York: Delacorte, 1990), 11. 'This "work" involves above all the regular, disciplined practice of moment-to-moment awareness or mindfulness, the complete "owning" of each moment of your experience, good, bad, or ugly. This is the essence of full catastrophe living … it is no accident that mindfulness comes out of Buddhism, which has as its overriding concerns the relief of suffering and the dispelling of illusions'.

199 Anne Harrington and John Dunne, 'Mindfulness Meditation: Frames and Choices' *American Psychologist* <http://nrs.harvard.edu/urn-3:HUL.InstRepos:10718406> (accessed 18 November 2019), 9.

and the heart of Buddhist meditation without the Buddhism'.[200] This aspiration does not come from an anti-Buddhist perspective. Instead, Kabat-Zinn believed meditation needed to be decoupled from the cultural, religious and ideological factors associated with the Buddhist origins of mindfulness in order to present mindfulness as a method of healing accessible to those of all faiths and none. This meant removing any religious language or concepts from mindfulness practice and presenting mindfulness as a non-religious therapeutic approach.

However, for many years, Kabat-Zinn was a practitioner of forms of Buddhist meditation, including Insight Meditation, founded by Mahāsī Sayādaw.[201] This contemporary form of meditation is typical of trends in Buddhist modernism, where rituals and prayer are removed, and meditative practices aimed at cultivating mindfulness remain as the locus. This would suggest that the development of MBSR stemmed from Kabat-Zinn's own practice of meditation within the context of Buddhist modernism. Kabat-Zinn viewed the benefits of meditation separate from their original religious scaffolding of rituals, prayers and ethical framework. He practiced modern forms of meditation which themselves originated from a decoupling of teachings and traditions from their original Buddhist foundations.

However, several concerns and tensions have emerged in respect of MBSR and mindfulness as promoted by Kabat-Zinn. These critiques can be categorised as first, mindfulness as a radical decontextualisation of a Buddhist practice which has been uprooted from the wisdom and ethical tradition of Buddha's teachings that frame meditation; and second, an

200 Jon Kabat-Zinn, 'Mindfulness and the Cessation of Suffering: An Exclusive New Interview with Mindfulness Pioneer Jon Kabat-Zinn', Interview by Danny Fisher, *Lion's Roar* 7(October) (2010). <http://www.lionsroar.com/mindfulness-and-the-cessation-of-suffering-an-exclusive-new-interview-with-mindfulness-pioneer-jon-kabat-zinn/>. Accessed on 18 November 2019.

201 Yoon Suk Hwang and Patrick Kearney, *A Mindfulness Intervention for Children with Autism Spectrum Disorder: Mindfulness in Behavioural Health* (Cham: Springer International Publishing, 2015), 12. 'Jon Kabat-Zinn was a practitioner of Korean Seon Buddhism and Theravāda mindfulness meditation as taught at the Insight Meditation Society (IMS) in Barre Massachusetts, who also practised and taught yoga. During a meditation retreat in 1979 he was inspired to share what he had learnt of these practices to people who would ordinarily never enter a yoga or meditation centre'.

epistemological incoherence over whether mindfulness is a secular activity or a recontextualised form of Buddha's teaching.

First, the secularisation of mindfulness has been criticised for assuming that there is an inherent, axiomatic moral and ethical framework operative in the practice. Poirier argues that while a secular healthcare ethos and ethical foundation permeates MBSR in hospital settings,[202] such an ethos can be absent in other settings, such as commerce, where maximising productivity and wealth can be the overarching aim rather than cultivating wellbeing and reducing stress.[203] In a similar vein, Forbes argues Kabat-Zinn has sacrificed the Buddhist ethical framework intrinsically linked to the original practice of mindfulness. 'He (Kabat-Zinn) jettisoned ... the body of ethics and wisdom in which mindfulness is embedded. He cut off the insights about the nature of the self and the deeper causes of suffering. He secularised mindfulness and made it a service'.[204]

However, MBSR should not be dismissed as an opportunistic, cynical seizure of mindfulness. Kabat-Zinn has developed a resource that has demonstrably positive outcomes in areas of physical and mental health. By removing religious vocabulary, he has made accessible a source of healing to many who would never have approached mindfulness as a resource for wellness. While it certainly is a form of appropriation, this in no way denies its observable benefit to people. Moreover, in the Catholic primary school context, resources that could help to reduce anxiety and improve wellbeing in students would be valuable and life-giving in ensuring their full and holistic development, as will be discussed in a later chapter.

Buddhist scholar Bhikku Bodhi argues that ethics (*sīla*) represents one of the three higher trainings along with meditation (*samādhi*) and wisdom

202 Marc R. Poirier, 'Mischief in the Marketplace for Mindfulness', in Robert Meikyo Rosenbaum and Barry Magid, eds, *What's Wrong with Mindfulness (And What Isn't): Zen Perspectives* (Somerville, MA: Wisdom Publications, 2016), 17. 'A core ethical expectation of healing, or at least doing no harm, pervades the health care professions, keeping the interests of institutions, mindfulness instructors, and patients more aligned'.

203 Ibid.

204 David Forbes, *Mindfulness and Its Discontents: Education, Self and Social Transformation* (Nova Scotia: Fernwood Publishing, 2019), 15–16.

(*paññā*), which are part of the Fourth Noble Truth of Buddhist teachings.[205] However, it has been argued that MBIs including MBSR neglect ethics that are integral to Buddha dharma or teaching.[206] Schmidt notes that programs such as MBSR '... do not make any metaphysical or religious assumptions' and are '... not committed to substantive ethical standards about what is good, bad, right or wrong'.[207] As MBSR is a clinical health program, there should be no reason that it would hold such metaphysical assumptions.

While MBSR shares Buddhism's commitment to the reduction of stress and suffering, there is no immediate reason why MBSR as a secular health resource should axiomatically retain the ethical standards of the Buddhist tradition. Regarding the place of ethics in MBSR, Kabat-Zinn proposes that loving kindness generated in oneself during mindfulness can be shared and spread to those around us.[208] Further, Kabat-Zinn argues that it is '... the personal responsibility of each person engaging in this work to attend with care and intentionality to how we are actually living our lives, both personally and professionally, in terms of ethical behaviour'.[209]

However, this notion of mindfulness promoting a self-evident ethic standard of interconnected benevolence is problematic. While a person could attempt to share loving kindness with others, there is no underlying

205 Bhikku Bodhi, 'The Noble Eightfold Path: The Way to the End of Suffering' (2013). <http://www.accesstoinsight.org/lib/authors/bodhi/waytoend.html>. Accessed on 19 November 2019.

206 See Steven Stanley, '*Sīla* and *Sati*: An Exploration of Ethics and Mindfulness in Pāli Buddhism and their Implications for Secular Mindfulness-Based Applications', in Edo Shonin, William Van Gordon, and Nirbay N. Singh, eds, *Buddhist Foundations of Mindfulness* (Berlin: Springer, 2015), 89–113, and Lynette Monteiro, Frank Musten and Jane F. Compson, 'Traditional and Contemporary Mindfulness: Finding the Middle Path in the Tangle of Concerns', *Mindfulness 6*(1) (2014), 1–13.

207 Andreas T. Schmidt, 'The Ethics and Politics of Mindfulness-Based Interventions' *Journal of Medical Ethics 0* (2016), 1–5.

208 Jon Kabat-Zinn, *Wherever You Go, There You Are: Mindfulness Meditation for Everyday Life* (London: Piatkus, 1994), 166. 'You can direct loving kindness towards anybody, toward people you know and people you don't ... You can also practice directing loving kindness towards those groups who suffer, or whose lives are caught up in war or violence or hatred ...'

209 Jon Kabat-Zinn, 'Some Reflections on the Origins of MBSR, Skilful Means and the Trouble with Maps', *Contemporary Buddhism, 12*(1) (2011), 194.

ethical framework encouraging them to do so. Nor is there any clarity on what such kindness would look like in different situations. Moreover, the appropriation of mindfulness techniques based on MBSR by military forces challenges the loving kindness promoted by MBSR. Rather than a vehicle for benevolence and interconnectedness, military uses of mindfulness focus on making the soldier more effective in their purpose.[210] Mindfulness that is reduced to context-free 'bare attention' is at risk of being utilised for ends which are at odds with Buddhist teachings on morality and ethics (*sīla*). This equates to a radical deracination of mindfulness from its original Buddhist context of right mindfulness.

The bare attention mindfulness of MBSR removes any link to Buddhist precepts which are centred on the cessation of suffering. However, it is problematic to justify the Buddhist roots of mindfulness when the techniques are instrumentalised to make soldiers more efficient. While there are many schools and vehicles of Buddhism, it is difficult to harmonise the loving kindness promoted by Kabat-Zinn's MBSR with mindfulness techniques as a utilitarian means of increased efficiency and performance on the battlefield. As there is no distinction in MBSR between right mindfulness and wrong mindfulness, Purser argues that Buddhist mindfulness cannot be understood in isolation from the ethical development offered by the dharma of the Eightfold Path:

> The cultivation of 'right mindfulness' is only one part of the Buddha's Eightfold Path, along with 'right' understanding, intention, speech, action, livelihood, effort and concentration ... However, the other dimensions that support 'right mindfulness' – which leads to wisdom by cultivating wholesome mental states- are left out of MBSR, suggesting its teachers have misconstrued Buddhist ethics.[211]

210 Sebastjan Vörös, 'Mindfulness De- or Recontextualized? Traditional Buddhist and Contemporary Perspectives', *Taiwan Journal of East Asian Studies 13*(1) (2016), 7. 'Here, the threat of misuse and misappropriation seems to be the most pertinent, as is vividly portrayed by the ... "mindful sniper". A mindful sniper is a person who has acquired great proficiency in cultivating "bare attention" but uses this capacity for purposes that are in obvious disagreement with Buddhist ethical standards, e.g., to improve their military skills'.

211 Ronald E. Purser, *McMindfulness: How Mindfulness Became the New Capitalist Spirituality* (London: Repeater, 2019), 79.

This raises the important issue here of right mindfulness in the Buddhist tradition against the non-evaluative 'bare attention' of mindfulness approaches such as MBSR. The goal of stress reduction is laudable in Kabat-Zinn's program, as there is growing evidence of physical and mental health benefits of mindfulness practice. There is no obligation on MBSR to retain any of the ritualistic or ethical aspects of the Buddhist wisdom tradition. However, right mindfulness in Buddhism presupposes a world-view where the practitioner is committed to reducing the suffering of all and challenging structural and societal sources of injustice. The parameters for MBSR are narrower and do not necessarily translate to loving kindness being shared through Kabat-Zinn's mindfulness programme. This can potentially run the risk of MBSR being distorted into a shallow self-help tool with no regard for one's relation and commitment to reducing suffering for others, draining mindfulness of its potentially life-giving potential. In this regard, Reynolds offers a useful medical analogy for the possible dangers in filtering out the wisdom teachings and religious aspects of Buddhist teaching:

> Mindfulness Based Stress Reduction (MBSR) isolated a particular practice of Buddhism in the same way that conventional medicine takes on 'active ingredient' from herbs. It is still herbal medicine but is now packaged to treat a particular symptom- stress. The other 'bits' of traditional religion are left behind as modern medicine discards the rest of the herb. These other bits play an important role, however, in limiting a side effect of modern mindfulness practice- the fact that it could leave us as selfish as ever.[212]

Several commentators have also commented on the multiple meanings that can be attributed to mindfulness given its often open and somewhat opaque definitions, ranging from mindfulness as placeholder for Buddhist

212 Stefan G. Reynolds, *Living with the Mind of Christ: Mindfulness in Christian Spirituality* (London: Darton, Longman & Todd, 2016), 39.

dharma to a universal human capacity.[213] The reason for such ambiguity is an effort at broadening the accessibility of mindfulness and its benefits to a wider audience. Kabat-Zinn hoped that MBSR could promote the Buddha dharma as a secular, universally accessible therapeutic approach, thereby creating opportunities for non-Buddhists to engage in mindfulness to alleviate suffering. The challenge such a laudable recontextualisation presents is attempting to communicate the essence of reducing suffering or *dukkha* to a secular audience.

Suffering is a central teaching of Buddhism and is explored in The Four Noble Truths. The cessation of suffering is the ultimate goal of Buddhist dharma; the liberation from the cycle of birth and rebirth and the suffering that permeates it. Kabat-Zinn argues that secularised mindfulness can lead to liberation from suffering in the immanent sense and does not require practitioners to use the terminology of dharma. In seeking to promote mindfulness as a non-religious means of reducing suffering, any transcendental or religious concepts such as reincarnation, Nirvana and karma are removed. 'The entire *raison d'être* of the dharma is to elucidate the nature of suffering and its root causes, as well as provide a practical path to liberation from suffering. All this is to be undertaken, of course, without ever mentioning the word 'dharma''.[214]

Mindfulness in this sense is promoting teachings on suffering based on the Four Noble Truths (The truth of suffering, the truth of the origin of suffering, the truth of the cessation of suffering and the truth of the path to

213 This includes Bhikku Bodhi arguing that mindfulness '... has become so vague and elastic that it serves as a cipher into which we can read anything we want.' Bhikku Bodhi, 'What Does Mindfulness Really Mean? A Canonical Perspective', *Contemporary Buddhism, 12*(1)(2011), 22. Candy G. Brown argues that Kabat-Zinn's succinct definition of mindfulness as 'paying attention in a particular way: on purpose, in the present moment, and non-judgmentally' is deliberately open, this definition being '...capacious enough to carry 'multiple meanings' both seeming to denote a universal human capacity and also functioning as 'place-holder for the entire dharma', and an 'umbrella term''. Candy G. Brown, 'Can "Secular" Mindfulness Be Separated from Religion', in Ronald E. Purser, David Forbes and Adam Burke, eds, *Handbook of Mindfulness: Culture, Context and Social Engagement* (Basel: Springer Publishing, 2016), 77.

214 Jon Kabat-Zinn, 'Some Reflections on the Origins of MBSR, Skilful Means and the Trouble with Maps', *Contemporary Buddhism, 12*(1) (2011), 188.

the cessation of suffering) in a universally accessible manner to people of all creeds and backgrounds. However, Kabat-Zinn is guilty on several occasions of loose and ambiguous rhetoric that equates MBSR with Buddhism more generally, which brings its secular label into question.

Kabat-Zinn makes claims about mindfulness and MBSR that stretch far beyond the scientific perspective that MBSR is accepted within psychological and healthcare circles. He speaks of '... direct experience of the numinous, the sacred, the Tao, God, the divine, Nature, silence, in all aspects of life'.[215] Further, there are remarks on how the technical contents of MBSR are '... merely launching platforms or particular kinds of scaffolding to invite cultivation and sustaining of attention in particular ways that lead to "ultimate understanding" which "transcends even conventional subject object duality."'[216] While always maintaining the secularity of mindfulness practice, the content of such rhetoric is laden with a vague orientation towards some higher metaphysical or transcendent realm of being. The challenge in espousing non-scientific rhetoric about mindfulness in a secular context is that there is a blurring of the lines between what is perceived as sacred and secular. In response to Kabat-Zinn's claims that mindfulness is both secular and the essence of Buddha's teaching, Thupten Jingpa, long-standing principal translator for the Dalai Lama, argues:

> I have no problem at all with taking something, like the technique of mindfulness, out of the Buddhist context and bringing it to the larger world, so long as we don't make the next claim and say that somehow we have captured the essence of the Buddhist teachings. You can't have it both ways. You cannot say that this is Buddhism and at the same time say that this is secular.[217]

215 Jon Kabat-Zinn, '*Catalyzing Movement Towards a More Contemplative/Sacred-Appreciating/Non-Dualistic Society*,' The Contemplative Mind in Society Meeting of the Working Group, Sponsored by the Nathan Cummings Foundation & Fetzer Institute (29 September–2 October) (1994). <http://www.contemplativemind.org/admin/wp-content/uploads/2012/09/kabat-zinn.pdf>. Accessed on 20 November 2019.

216 Jon Kabat-Zinn, 'Mindfulness-Based Interventions in Context: Past, Present and Future', *Clinical Psychology: Science and Practice, 10*(2) (2003), 147–8.

217 Edo Shonin and William Van Gordon, 'Thupten Jingpa on Compassion and Mindfulness', *Mindfulness 7* (2016), 281.

Moreover, Brown argues that while MBSR is portrayed as a secular practice, it is '... an MBI infused at every level- concept, structure, teacher training, and graduate resources- with carefully camouflaged Buddhist content'.[218] In particular, certified MBSR teachers are obliged to attend lengthy retreats in Buddhist centres, including those that focus on Theravada meditation, where they reflect on the wisdom teachings, including the Four Noble Truths.[219] This raises questions as to whether MBSR is to be interpreted by teachers and students as Buddhist meditation in itself, albeit without any of the ritual, prayers or liturgy associated with Buddhism, or secular meditation which has been inspired by Buddhist precepts.

The mindfulness of MBSR is a facet of Buddhist modernism, where meditation has become detached from its traditional Buddhist framework and presented as a therapeutic healthcare approach. In the process of recontextualising Buddhist meditation, important elements of the dharma are negated in favour of universal accessibility. By disregarding '... unnecessary historical and cultural baggage,'[220] MBSR retains the 'essential' content of the '... universal dharma that is co-extensive, if not identical, with the teachings of the Buddha, the Buddhadharma'.[221] This is seen when Kabat-Zinn equates mindfulness with right mindfulness in an interview, which confuses matters as right mindfulness is an explicit Buddhist teaching located within an integrated ethical and wisdom framework:

> When we use the word mindfulness in MBSR, we mean right mindfulness. I use mindfulness as kind of an umbrella term. Woven into mindfulness is an orientation towards nonharming and seeing deeply into the nature of things, which in some way implies, or at least invites one to see the interconnectedness between the seer and the

218 Candy G. Brown, 'Can "Secular" Mindfulness Be Separated from Religion?', in Ronald E. Purser, David Forbes and Adam Burke, eds, *Handbook of Mindfulness: Culture, Context and Social Engagement* (Basel: Springer Publishing, 2016), 90.

219 Ibid, 80–4.

220 Jon Kabat-Zinn, 'Some Reflections on the Origins of MBSR, Skilful Means and the Trouble with Maps', *Contemporary Buddhism, 12*(1) (2011), 290.

221 J. Mark G. Williams and Jon Kabat-Zinn, eds, *Mindfulness: Diverse Perspectives on its Meaning, Origins and Applications* (Abingdon: Routledge, 2013), 14.

> seen, the object and the subject. It is a nondual perspective from the very beginning, resting on an ethical foundation.[222]

By claiming mindfulness has an ethical foundation in an ambiguous way, Kabat-Zinn is blurring the lines between the secular and the religious in Buddhist meditation. In doing so, people who would never have practiced meditation can do so and see benefits in their lives. This may be the case in Catholic primary schools where mindfulness is presented as a secular psychological activity. Moreover, the interconnectedness between seer and seen that Kabat-Zinn speaks of echoes the essential attitude for a sacramental awareness, a key aspect of a Catholic worldview. In this sense, the outlook Kabat-Zinn proposes may find compatibility with the sacramentality of Catholic education.[223] This will be explored in a later chapter.

However, while such an ethical approach may indeed be beneficial and potentially find an ally in a Catholic vision of education, questions remain over whether MBSR brings about the transformative effects in other and in society which are cultivated in Buddhist meditation. While MBSR may reduce stress, it does not necessarily follow that the practitioner is compelled to challenge suffering on others or in wider society. It is an experiential approach which may have significant personal benefits, but Kabat-Zinn's claims of a self-evident ethical foundation are ambiguous at best. This is a self-centred practice which is not a limitation in and of itself. Rather, the thesis of the positive transformation of society through privatised mindfulness is testing the limits of credibility.

Nicholas Lash's criticism of the contemporary interest in spirituality is similar in this regard, noting that '… it tends to soothe rather than subvert

222 Alan Senauke and Barbera Gates, 'The Thousand Year View: An Interview with Jon Kabat-Zinn', *Inquiring Mind 30* (2) Spring (2014).

223 See Thomas Carroll, 'Mindfulness as *praeparatio evangelica* in the Irish Catholic School', *Irish Theological Quarterly 88*(4) (2023), 323–39 and Thomas Carroll, 'Mindfulness in Catholic Primary Schools: An Irish Perspective', *Religions 14*(11) (2023), 1348.

our well-heeled complacency'.[224] In this sense, Lash is echoing Tomáš Halík's suspicion of contemporary spiritual movements in the previous chapter. While the growth of the 'spiritual but not religious' demographic is an observable phenomenon in a post-Christian, post-secular age, there is a danger that some forms of spirituality favour self-satisfaction over collective or societal wellbeing.

The secularisation of mindfulness in MBSR was a response by a practitioner of Buddhist meditation who saw how such techniques could relieve suffering for patients in chronic pain in a healthcare setting. By removing explicitly religious or metaphysical language and concepts that might deter patients, Kabat-Zinn laudably hoped that stress and pain might be reduced. However, in utilising techniques associated with Buddha dharma, MBSR is open to critique for decoupling the ethical and wisdom framework that undergirded Buddhist meditation. Without this framework or scaffolding, mindfulness practice can be open to abuse and misappropriation.

In terms of Catholic education, Mindfulness 1 represents Buddhist meditative practices which have been translated into secular psychological techniques with demonstrable mental and physical wellbeing benefits. In this regard, Mindfulness 1 has potential benefits to the educational endeavour of Catholic schools.

Mindfulness 2

Mindfulness has rapidly grown from a clinical tool for medical professionals to a readily available resource for consumers in wider society. While some people suffering with conditions like depression and anxiety utilise mindfulness-based interventions, many people coping with stress are also using

224 Nicholas Lash, *The Beginning and End of Religion* (Cambridge: Cambridge University Press, 1996), 174. 'My mistrust of contemporary interest in 'spirituality' arises from the suspicion that quite a lot of material set out in book stores under this description sells because it does not stretch the mind or challenge our behaviour. It tends to soothe rather than subvert our well-heeled complacency'.

mindfulness resources outside of the clinical setting. Like Mindfulness 1, this second strand of mindfulness is primarily focused on immanent goals such as improving physical and mental health outcomes for practitioners.

Mindfulness in this sense is commodified into mindfulness applications, books and products. Apps typically utilise mindfulness techniques such as body scan exercises and mindful breathing.[225] Popular mindfulness app Headspace had, according to Forbes, over 11 million downloads and a valuation of over $250 million in 2017,[226] before a $3 billion merger with online mental health platform Ginger.[227] Such numbers indicate that there is a significant demand for mindfulness-based resources to reduce stress and suffering in contemporary society. The positive impacts of mental health apps on young people have also been highlighted in the literature.[228] Apps that reduce suffering for people are a potentially life-giving resource, as anything that improves quality of life and reduces suffering is to be welcomed. Likewise, for Catholic schools, resources that can lower student anxiety and enable them to flourish should be seen as boon.

However, it is important to note that while there are some highly effective apps in reducing stress through mindfulness approaches, of 700 mindfulness-based applications researched, only 4% were identified as providing mindfulness training and education in an independent systematic review.[229]

225 Madhaven Mani, David J. Kavanagh, Leanne Hides and Stoyan R. Stoyanov, 'Review and Evaluation of Mindfulness-Based iPhone Apps', *JMIR mHealth and uHealth*, *3*(3) (2015), e82.

226 Kathleen Chaykowski, 'Meet Headspace: The App That Made Meditation a $250 Million Business'. *Forbes*, 8 January 2017. <https://www.forbes.com/sites/kathleen-chaykowski/2017/01/08/meet-headspace-the-app-that-made-meditation-a-250-million-business/#21efbc911f1b>. Accessed on 22 March 2020.

227 Daniel Hong, 'Ginger And Headspace Merge: Looks To Build Mental Resilience In All Employees By Giving Them More Choice'. *Forbes*, 7 September 2021. <https://www.forbes.com/sites/forrester/2021/09/07/ginger-and-headspace-merge-looks-to-build-mental-resilience-in-all-employees-by-giving-them-more-choice/?sh=22f2fc25146c>. Accessed on 3 March 2024.

228 See Tania Lecomte, Stéphane Potvin, Marc Corbière, Stéphane Guay, Crystal Samson, Briana Cloutier, Audrey Francoeur, Antoine Pennou and Yasser Khazaal, Mobile Apps for Mental Health Issues: Meta-Review of Meta-Analyses, *JMIR Mhealth Uhealth 8*(5) (2020), e17458.

229 Ibid.

Such a paucity of effective mindfulness apps in the smartphone marketplace raises serious questions as to whether many apps prioritise profit over reducing consumer stress. Such questionable motives in the promotion of products for consumers that cost money but offer no discernible relief from stress could be termed 'McMindfulness'. This term was conceived by Buddhist psychotherapist Miles Neale in 2010 to address what he sees as the problem of appropriating '… cherry-picked teachings from ancient, mostly threatened, wisdom cultures and mass-marketed them as consumerist goods'.[230] McMindfulness has been accused of being the antithesis of its original Buddhist outlook on the illusion of the self.[231]

Through instrumentalisation and commodification, McMindfulness represents a socio-economic force that turns mindfulness into a product to be purchased and consumed for personal benefits such as problem-solving, better health and improvements in various aspects of life. As a utilitarian commodity, it is packaged as a universal elixir to practically any situation in life that needs improvement. 'Take this workshop, buy that book or magazine. Sit still for a weekend and be happier. If this one does not make you feel better in short order, move on and buy that one'.[232] The pursuit of resources or techniques that reduce personal suffering is an important means to sustain mental and physical wellbeing for people, and as has been highlighted, mindfulness is a potentially beneficial resource in this regard. However, by streamlining and marketing mindfulness as a practical utility, mindfulness

230 <https://innertruth.org/podcast/how-to-avoid-mcmindfulness-find-your-truth-with-dr-miles-neale/>. Accessed on 5 August 2024).

231 'McMindfulness occurs when mindfulness is used, either with intention or unwittingly, for self-serving and ego-enchanting purposes that run counter to both Buddhist and Abrahamic prophetic teachings to let go of ego-attachment and enact skilful, universal compassion. Instead of letting go of the ego, McMindfulness aims to enhance it and promotes self-aggrandizement; its therapeutic function is to comfort, numb, adjust, and advance the self within a neoliberal, corporatized, individualistic society based on private gain'. David Forbes, 'Critical Integral Contemplative Education', in Ronald E. Purser, David Forbes, and Adam Burke, eds, *Handbook of Mindfulness: Culture, Context and Social Engagement* (Basel: Springer Publishing, 2016), 357.

232 Barry Magid and Marc R. Poirier, 'The Three Shaky Pillars of Western Buddhism'. In Robert Meikyo Rosenbaum and Barry Magid, eds, *What's Wrong with Mindfulness (And What Isn't): Zen Perspectives* (Somerville, MA: Wisdom Publications, 2016), 42.

runs the risk of becoming a label that creates opportunities for maximising profit rather than improving personal wellbeing.

Moreover, while the use of technology and apps may bring mindfulness to a wider audience, removing the need for social interaction means that mindfulness risks being increasingly privatised and individualised. Without need for human engagement, Mindfulness 2 can become a self-aggrandising commodity alien if not contradictory to its traditional Buddhist ethical and wisdom framework. Such a turn to radical individualism in the West was observed by the late Rabbi Jonathan Sacks as one of the defining challenges of our time.[233]

Mindfulness 2 is open to critique on two central arguments. First, Mindfulness 2 represents a fundamental deracination from its traditional liberative and ethical purposes in the Buddha dharma. Second, Mindfulness 2 maintains the social structures and factors that generate stress in a neoliberal capitalist society. Included in this critique is an examination of mindfulness applications in educational settings and whether they promote critical enquiry into causes of societal suffering or maintain a neoliberal status quo.

Like Mindfulness 1, McMindfulness has been criticised for decoupling Buddhist mindfulness techniques from their historical, ethical and wisdom context. Proponents of Mindfulness 1 in a clinical setting can claim some ethical grounding through the Hippocratic Oath and competency standards for teachers. Poirier argues that Mindfulness 1:

> … is protected from the worst effects of commodification, to some extent, by a pre-existing professional ethos in the healthcare fields; they have also developed a certification process for their instructors. There is no similar secular ethical constraint that pervades the worlds of business and law.[234]

233 Jonathan Sacks, *Morality: Restoring the Common Good in Divided Times* (London: Hodder & Stoughton, 2020), 324. 'In the liberal democracies of the West, there has been too much 'I' and too little 'We'. There has been too much individualism and too little of the moral bonds that lie at the heart of friendship, family and community'.

234 Marc R. Poirier, 'Mischief in the Marketplace for Mindfulness', in Robert Meikyo Rosenbaum and Barry Magid, eds, *What's Wrong with Mindfulness (And What Isn't): Zen Perspectives* (Somerville, MA: Wisdom Publications, 2016), 17.

In this sense, the therapies and clinical applications of Mindfulness 1 aim to heal, or at least not to harm. While Kabat-Zinn can make somewhat ambiguous statements on the ethical foundations of MBSR, it is at least safeguarded from abuse by professional and healthcare standards. The same cannot be presumed of Mindfulness 2.

The renunciation of the early Buddhist monastics and the dharma of transforming one's perception of the world differ from the potentially self-centred approach of Mindfulness 2. The individualism of McMindfulness allows for the shedding of ethical and social concerns as the focus is on the practitioner feeling satisfied. This represents a major shift in the idea of the self in Buddhist modernism and risks a fundamental pillar of the mindfulness meditation: the question of non-self. The doctrine of *anātman* (no self) relates to the dharma that there is no such thing as a fixed, permanent soul. Rather, because all things are without inherent self-existence, '… all beings are constituted by their interactions with other beings and have no independent, enduring nature in and of themselves'.[235] The Vietnamese Zen master Thich Nhat Hanh calls this teaching 'interbeing'; an interconnected web of elements that only exist through interrelation with others. 'What we call self is made only of non-self-elements'.[236] As there is no fixed, permanent self, all things are interdependent with each other. As nothing can exist in isolation, interbeing means that:

> … the growing into maturity of a human is experienced as an ever widening sense of self, from identification with the individual bodymind, to self as family, self as circle of friends, as nation, as race, as human race, as all living things, and perhaps finally to self as all that is.[237]

235 David L. McMahan, *The Making of Modern Buddhism* (Oxford: Oxford University Press, 2008), 150.

236 Thich Nhat Hanh, 'The Sun in My Heart', in Stephanie Kaza and Kenneth Kraft, eds, *Dharma Rain: Sources of Buddhist Environmentalism* (Boston: Shambala, 2000), 87. For further reading on 'interbeing', see Thich Nhat Hanh and Peter Levitt, eds, *The Heart of Understanding: Commentaries on the Prajñaparamita Heart Sutra* (Berkley: Parallax Press, 1988), 3–4.

237 Joan Halifax, 'The Third Body: Buddhism, Shamanism and Deep Ecology', in Alan Hunt Badiner, ed, *Dharma Gaia: A Harvest of Essays in Buddhism and Ecology* (Berkley: Parallax Press, 1990), 23.

Despite the fundamental differences between Buddhist and Christian outlooks on the nature of the soul, both traditions present an ethical and social framework that speaks of fostering a right relationship with others. The human person is inherently social, and it is in community that relationships are fostered and our interconnectedness with each other is affirmed. In this regard, both Christian and Buddhist teachings affirm our interdependence upon each other, albeit in very different ways.

Rather than mindfulness aiding freedom from the illusion of the self in Buddhism, Mindfulness 2 risks representing an illusory self-centred outlook. As there is no ethical framework operative within McMindfulness, meditative techniques can be commodified as a profit-driven, value-neutral product that is a panacea for private and personal stress, as opposed to challenging wider sources of suffering in society. Again, while resources for personal wellbeing are important, Mindfulness 2 risks reducing human flourishing to privatised, self-serving goals rather than many of the humanising attributes spoken of by Jon Kabat-Zinn:

> Generosity, trustworthiness, kindness, empathy, compassion, gratitude, joy in the good fortune of others, inclusiveness, acceptance and equanimity are qualities of mind and heart that further the possibilities of well-being and clarity within oneself, to say nothing of the beneficial effects they have in the world.[238]

In seeking to distance himself from the worst excesses of McMindfulness 2, Kabat-Zinn warns that mindfulness '... can never be a quick fix' and that it is problematic not to acknowledge '... the ethical foundations of the meditative practices and traditions from which mindfulness has emerged'.[239] However, the processes of secularisation, commodification and individualisation have influenced Mindfulness 2 such that it has emerged as a distinct phenomenon in contemporary culture. In Western societies characterised by consumerism, the practice of mindfulness has been appropriated and privatised into

238 Jon Kabat-Zinn, *Coming to Our Senses: Healing Ourselves and the World Through Mindfulness* (NY: Hachete, 2006), 103.

239 Jon Kabat Zinn, 'Mindfulness has Huge Health Benefits—But McMindfulness is no Panacea', *The Guardian* (20 October 2015) <https://www.theguardian.com/commentisfree/2015/oct/20/mindfulness-mental-health-potential-benefits-uk>. Accessed on 28 November 2019.

a consumer product. In this sense, mental health apps, books and resources have emerged which offer mindfulness resources and tools that can have benefits to the health and wellbeing of users. Like Mindfulness 1, resources that are clinically proven to reduce suffering and stress for people are to be welcomed.

However, Mindfulness 2 can also be misappropriated into a resource solely for performance and productivity with little regard for the cessation of suffering. Loy illustrates the dangers of Mindfulness 2 being misappropriated when it enters the corporate world. Loy writes a public letter to Goldman Sachs and Exxon Mobil board member and mindfulness advocate William George, whom the UK Financial Times has interviewed:

> William George, a current Goldman Sachs board member … started meditating in 1974 and never stopped. 'The main business case for meditation is that if you're fully present on the job, you will be more effective as a leader, you will make better decisions and you will work better with other people,' he tells me (the author, David Gelles). 'I tend to live a very busy life. This keeps me focused on what's important'.[240]

Loy asks George how he compartmentalises his meditation practice from the ethical precepts, communal nature and social responsibility of Buddhism. As a member of one of the largest banks in the US, George has been in leadership of a company involved with causing untold financial misery during the financial crisis in 2008. Moreover, as a board member at Exxon Mobil, George is part of a company that has lobbied against climate change policy and has contributed massively to environmental pollution.

> … I would like to learn how, in light of your meditation practice, you understand the relationship between one's own personal transformation and the kind of economic and social transformation that appears to be necessary today.[241]

240 David Gelles, 'The Mind Business', *UK Financial Times* (25–26 August 2012). <https://www.ft.com/content/d9cb7940-ebea-11e1-985a-00144feab49a>. Accessed on 28 November 2019.

241 David Loy, 'The Challenge of Mindful Engagement', in Ronald E. Purser, David Forbes and Adam Burke, eds, *Handbook of Mindfulness: Culture, Context and Social Engagement* (Basel: Springer Publishing, 2016), 25.

This highlights the incongruity between practicing meditation and one's own outlook and actions in life. While mindfulness can improve personal performance and lower stress, there is a disconnect between being mindful of yourself and being mindful of how your interactions in the world can cause and reinforce suffering and stress. In this regard, there is no ethical framework to call for personal or social transformation. Instead, Mindfulness 2 for George seems to be a performance enhancer.

While it must be stressed that there are positive aspects of Mindfulness 2, such as apps and websites that provide resources for wellness and improved wellbeing, McMindfulness represents a commodification of the practice that places performance and efficiency at its heart. The individualism of McMindfulness is a distortion of the clinical-based Mindfulness 1 in that it seeks to reduce programs or practices promoting positive mental and physical health to a self-help tool lacking any of the healthcare ethics underpinning programs such as MBSR. This '... serves to strengthen people's conceptions of themselves as self-contained and autonomous agents, rather than relational and interdependent- and an individualised practice requires no communal ties, moral commitments, or substantive lifestyle changes'.[242]

Aspects of Mindfulness 2 have also been critiqued as placating stress on an individual level and not confronting structural sources of suffering and stress such as economic and social inequality.[243] Critics of this development include Marxist philosophers such as Slavoj Žižek, who goes so far as to call mindfulness the '... hegemonic ideology of global capitalism'.[244] In this sense, mindfulness is understood as a privatised treatment for stress while simultaneously buffering the individual from the underlying sources of that stress. In this sense, the value of stress reduction is negated as unjust and oppressive aspects of society are left unchallenged. While Mindfulness 2 can provide many benefits to people's health and wellbeing, there is merit in this critique.

242 Ronald E. Purser, *McMindfulness: How Mindfulness Became the New Capitalist Spirituality* (London: Repeater, 2019), 101.

243 Jeremy R. Carrette and Richard King, *Selling Spirituality: The Silent Takeover of Religion* (New York: Routledge, 2005), 22.

244 Slavoj Žižek, 'From Western Marxism to Western Buddhism', *Cabinet 2* (2001).

These problematic aspects of Mindfulness 2 are observed in the large-scale incorporation of mindfulness programs in business and commercial activities. Mindfulness meditation has been appropriated by international corporations such as Google and Apple. Chaskalson highlights some benefits of mindfulness in the workplace, including stress reduction, increased communication and concentration skills, and overall better work satisfaction.[245] While improving employee wellbeing may be an objective for these companies, there is a danger that employee wellbeing becomes a means to optimum profit, rather than an end in itself. Moreover, while workplace stress is undoubtedly a contemporary problem, corporations risk abusing mindfulness as 'bare attention' to propagate economic growth and profit, no matter what the social and environmental cost. Rather than examining the inherent causes of employee stress within the company, mindfulness can be used to soothe rather than subvert the sources of such strain and pressure in the workplace. Mindfulness courses operative within corporate bodies do not necessarily offer space to question ethical or social concerns that practitioners may feel are contributing to their stress levels.

> Ordinary working people are employed in these industries. These are not fundamentally immoral people. But when they are taught meditative techniques like mindfulness, is there any attention given to the object of their labours? Are they asked to consider the actual things their corporation makes and sells- and whether it has a positive or negative social value?[246]

Further, many of these multinationals do not conduct themselves with what Buddha dharma or Kabat-Zinn would call right mindfulness. While Mindfulness 2 is a practice stemming from Buddhist meditation, it is understood as a secular activity. However, there are still tensions operative within the utilisation of techniques to provide personal stress-relief while not addressing morally dubious company actions such as tax avoidance.

245 Michael Chaskalson, *The Mindful Workplace* (Oxford: Wiley-Blackwell, 2011), 164–5.

246 Alan Hozan Senauke, 'One Body, Whole Life: Mindfulness and Zen', in Robert Meikyo Rosenbaum and Barry Magid, eds, *What's Wrong with Mindfulness (And What Isn't): Zen Perspectives* (Somerville, MA: Wisdom Publications, 2016), 76.

By sidestepping tax payment, companies are indirectly contributing to greater inequality in society, especially for those poorest and in need.[247]

Contrary to the spirit of the mindfulness revolution claimed by Boyce, corporations show no inclination towards right mindfulness in the face of profit opportunities. While not necessarily a Buddhist practice anymore, these aspects of Mindfulness 2 directly contradict Buddhist teachings on right mindfulness in that it closes enquiry into the structural causes of suffering or *dhukka*. In this sense, mindfulness becomes a complete misappropriation of its original practice and tradition. Thus, these unsavoury aspects of Mindfulness 2 act as a buffer for practitioners from the structural or systematic roots of suffering in society.

These parts of Mindfulness 2 represent an evolution in capitalist spirituality that helps to reinforce the status quo of neoliberalism. McChesney states: 'Neoliberalism is the defining political economic paradigm of our time- it refers to the policies and processes whereby a relative handful of private interests are permitted to control as much as possible of social life in order to maximise their personal profit'.[248] Further, Forbes argues that 'This ideology promotes a privatised, individualistic, market-based worldview and structure. Its ideology posits that stress, lack of attention, and reactivity are problems that lie within the individual, not society, societal institutions, or social relations'.[249]

This neoliberal paradigm accommodates Mindfulness 2 as it helps to solidify conditions of docility towards the deeper causes of suffering in society. Problems are internalised and stress is seen as an individual issue rather than an external obstacle. Forbes accuses Jon Kabat-Zinn of being complicit in this mutation of mindfulness practice, by claiming our '... entire

247 Ibid, 185. 'Full payment of taxes shows corporate ethics, social responsibility, empathy and compassion for poor members of society. The application of mindfulness in corporations has failed to address widespread public concerns about the massive sums involved in tax avoidance. There is a long list of elite and powerful businesses who pay little or no tax. They include Amazon, Apple ... Google, Goldman Sachs, JP Morgan Chase ... and numerous others'.

248 Robert W. McChesney, 'Introduction', in Noam Chomsky, ed., *Profit Over People: Neoliberalism and Global Order* (New York: Seven Stories Press, 1999), 8.

249 David Forbes, *Mindfulness and Its Discontents: Education, Self and Social Transformation* (Nova Scotia: Fernwood Publishing, 2019), 27.

society is suffering from attention deficit disorder- big time'.[250] This position risks pathologising stress into a personal problem and denying mindfulness the opportunity to provide insights into the sources of stress and challenge inequalities that emerge in neoliberal, market-based economies.

> Kabat-Zinn's individualistic analysis and solution, that mindfulness is the way to overcome virtually every societal deficit, reflects the broader cultural value of personal self-regulation or self-management as the answer to any problem ... This is designed not to change the capitalist system that contributes to stress and attention deficit, but as a way to adjust and accommodate to it.[251]

This neoliberalism paradigm has implications for how mindfulness is operative within schools. In relation to educational settings, mindfulness has been utilised as a means of improving teacher and student wellbeing.[252] These are positives, as any school that helps to form emotionally healthy young people is to be commended. Purser acknowledges that while mindfulness in schools may lower depression and anxiety as well as improve concentration, the techniques can still be misappropriated into McMindfulness. This risks reducing mindfulness practice to an instrument which reinforces an education system that is result-driven, in which students are not actively enabled to critically engage with the possible causes of their stress.

Catholic schools are among those challenged by an educational model that measures success in terms of academic performance rather than character formation or human development. This educational emergency as Pope

250 Jon Kabat-Zinn, *Coming to Our Senses: Healing Ourselves and the World Through Mindfulness* (New York: Hachete, 2006), 143.

251 David Forbes, *Mindfulness and Its Discontents: Education, Self and Social Transformation* (Nova Scotia: Fernwood Publishing, 2019), 141.

252 Willem Kuyken, Katherine Weare, Obioha C. Ukoumunne, Rachael Vicary, Nicola Motton, Richard Burnett, Chris Cullen, Sarah E. Hennelly and Felicia Huppert, 'Effectiveness of the Mindfulness in Schools Programme: Non-randomised Controlled Feasibility Study', *British Journal of Psychiatry, August, 203* (2013), 126–31.

Benedict XVI terms it has been highlighted by several commentators,[253] and mirrors the concerns of educationalist John Dewey that these processes of information dissemination have removed the educative nature of schools.[254] Mindfulness at its best can be a humanising activity in education, as Kabat-Zinn has outlined, proposing a kinder, less judgemental outlook on life. However, at its worst, McMindfulness can be a dehumanising activity, reducing human flourishing to results and academic merits, buffering the suffering student from challenging structural causes of suffering.

This raises the question of bringing mindfulness and education together, where students can enjoy better wellbeing while also being encouraged to challenge injustice and be engaged in civic and political discussion. However, such a shift would require an educational model that is not motivated by economic and market interests and instead by contemplative models. The case for contemplative education has been made by several philosophers of education, who recognise the profound educational potential of cultivating a mindful disposition, enabling students to become critical and constructive

253 See Eamonn Conway, 'Vatican II on Christian Education: A Guide Through Today's 'Educational Emergency?', in Niall Coll, ed., *Ireland and Vatican II: Essays Theological, Pastoral and Educational* (Dublin: Columba Press, 2015), 258–64; Stephen McKinney and John Sullivan, *Education in Catholic Perspective* (Ashgate, 2013) Loc.5052 and Alastair McIntyre, 'The End of Education: The Fragmentation of the American University', *Commonweal,* 133(18) (2006), 10–14.

254 See John Dewey, 'My Pedagogic Creed', *School Journal* 54(3) (January 1897), 77–80. 'I believe that much of present education fails because it neglects this fundamental principle of the school as a form of community life. It conceives the school as a place where certain information is to be given, where certain lessons are to be learned, or where certain habits are to be formed. The value of these is conceived as lying largely in the remote future; the child must do these things for the sake of something else he is to do; they are mere preparation. As a result they do not become a part of the life experience of the child and so are not truly educative'. <http://dewey.pragmatism.org/creed.htm>. Accessed on 27 December 2021.

citizens in society.[255] This turn to a contemplative education would support the view that, because education is a human process, students should be encouraged to reflect on what gives them meaning in their lives, and what constitutes authentic human flourishing for them.

> There is no such thing as a neutral educational process. Education either functions as an instrument that is used to facilitate the integration of the younger generation into the logic of the present system and bring conformity to it, or it becomes the 'practice of freedom', the means by which men and women deal critically and creatively with reality and discover how to participate in the transformation of their world.[256]

The worst excesses of Mindfulness 2 mean that it can be appropriated into an effective tool for neoliberal educational interests to create more productive, compliant human capital. In this regard, stress can be pathologised and privatised, buffering students from challenging sources of suffering. However, a contemplative approach to education would enable mindfulness to equip students with a critical, constructive disposition in addressing societal inequality. In this regard, mindfulness as contemplative education represents an important opportunity for dialogue with Catholic education.

Mindfulness 2 has developed from interactions between Mindfulness 1 and a Western culture heavily influenced by consumerism and individualism. The commodification of mindfulness practices has benefited millions of people who use these resources to manage their own mental health and improve their wellbeing. However, less beneficial aspects of Mindfulness 2, such as McMindfulness, have also emerged.

Rather than see the world as interconnected and interdependent on each other, McMindfulness privatises and individualises mindfulness applications into a panacea for all of life's problems. The widespread

255 See Philip Wexler and Yotam Hotam, eds, *New Social Foundations for Education: Education in Post-Secular Society* (NY: Peter Lang, 2015), Oren Ergas, *Reconstructing 'Education' Through Mindful Attention: Positioning the Mind at the Center of Curriculum and Pedagogy* (London: Palgrave, 2017), Aislinn O Donnell, 'Contemplative Pedagogy and Mindfulness: Developing Creative Attention in an Age of Distraction', *Journal of Philosophy of Education 49*(2) (2015), 187–202.

256 Richard Shaull, 'Introduction', in Paulo Freire, ed., *Pedagogy of the Oppressed* (New York: Continuum, 1970).

adoption of mindfulness applications in corporate life can lead to practices that promote productivity but are devoid of any greater social ethos of compassion or fairness.

Within the education sector, mindfulness can help students process their emotions and enjoy better wellbeing. However, a neoliberal paradigm risks Mindfulness 2 becoming a means of privatising student stress while improving student performance. This can lead to a reductive conception of human flourishing in education systems, where student success is disproportionately judged by academic metrics rather than their holistic development. A contemplative approach to education offers one counter to this, while also representing a site for dialogue between Catholic education and mindfulness practices.

Mindfulness 3

Mindfulness 3 represents the development of mindfulness as a secular spirituality in the contemporary Western context. As was earlier highlighted by Buddhist scholar Rupert Gethin, Mindfulness 3:

> … eschews the traditional framework of karma and rebirth, where the goal of nirvana is understood as liberation from the round of rebirth, and replaces these with a more therapeutic framework where nirvana is understood as a kind of equilibrium and state of well-being achieved by mindfulness meditation'. Such practitioners will still claim the title of being 'Buddhist' and hold that 'mindfulness', is as they see it, the essence of Buddhism.[257]

Like Mindfulness 1 and 2, Mindfulness 3 sheds any explicit religious concepts or metaphysical assumptions of Buddhism in order to be accessible to those in the Western context. However, unlike Mindfulness 1 and 2, Mindfulness 3 can be explicitly understood as a post-secular spirituality. According to Gooch, secular spirituality '… can be understood not only as a spirituality

257 Peter Tyler, *Christian Mindfulness: Theology and Practice* (London, SCM Press, 2018), 15.

divorced from its traditionally 'religious' context, but also as a response to the particular spiritual needs and challenges of the times'.[258]

However, as was outlined in the previous chapter, the contemporary Western context can be seen as post-Christian and post-secular rather than just secular. Evidence for this includes the growing recognition of the failure of the secularisation thesis and the fact that a growing demographic self-identifies as spiritual but not religious. Mindfulness thus developed as a spirituality separated from the religious or metaphysical connotations of its traditional framework. It has become a spiritual alternative for many people searching for deeper meaning and purpose in the age of fragmented, questioned and detraditionalised grand narratives. In this sense, it can be seen as a post-secular spirituality.

Mindfulness 3 is then a novel development in the story of Buddhist modernism, in that while mindfulness has become secularised and psychologised (Mindfulness 1), as well as commodified and privatised (Mindfulness 2), a distinctive strand has become for some a spirituality that speaks to their hunger for deeper meaning in life. This can mean practising mindfulness with absolutely no connection to the ethics or teachings of Buddhist wisdom traditions, instead seeing mindfulness practice as integral to human flourishing and wellbeing outside of an explicitly religious framework. In this sense, Mindfulness 3 can be a spiritual practice that originated in Buddhism but is operative outside such a category.

However, it can also include those who practice mindfulness and retain some Buddhist teachings, such as the Noble Eightfold Path, albeit through a secular lens and free of explicitly religious concepts and tenets.[259] Perhaps the best-known example of this is 'secular Buddhist' teacher and writer Stephen Batchelor who despite declaring his secularity, admits '… my secular Buddhism still has a religious quality to it, because it is the conscious expression of my "ultimate concern"—as the theologian Paul Tillich once

258 Alex Gooch, 'Mindfulness as a Secular Spirituality', in Manu Bazzano, ed., *After Mindfulness: New Perspectives on Psychology and Meditation* (London: Palgrave McMillan, 2014), 101.

259 Caroline Starkey, 'British Buddhism, Secular Mindfulness and the Politics of Sustainability', *Religion* 2023.

defined "faith"'.[260] In this sense, Mindfulness 3 has a disparate audience who share a belief that mindfulness corresponds to a vision of authentic human flourishing and provides deeper meaning in their lives. This connecting of mindfulness with the inner life of spirituality, of questions of ultimate meaning and purpose, includes those who share absolutely no affiliation to Buddhism and those who adhere to Buddhism as a secular philosophy that says nothing of a transcendent realm or religious concepts.

Mindfulness 3 is thus situated in a spiritual grey area, encompassing both transcendent spiritual beliefs and a secular spirituality that seeks depth in the mystery of everyday life. In his recent book, McMahan distinguishes elements of this form of mindfulness meditation from practices promoted as scientifically verified or framed within a naturalist context:

> … many practitioners use meditation to assure themselves that there is 'more than this', more than the desacralized world portrayed by science … It is a 'more' that affirms this-worldliness but at the same time attempts to break open secularism and show that this world exceeds what it seems to be on first glance … it occupies a field of tension between, on one hand, comfort in the dominant discourse of secularity- the naturalistic worldview taught in public schools and taken for granted in mainstream newspapers … and, on the other hand, the destabilization of that very discourse, and the bending of it toward the possibility of a kind of secular re-enchantment of the world.[261]

Mindfulness 3 serves as an example of what social anthropologist Oliver Roy terms '*formatage*' (formatting). Borrowing from computer language, Roy uses '*formatage*' to analyse how religious and spiritual traditions are gradually 'reformatted' to harmonise with the prevailing norms of the Western cultures within which they are now operative.[262] In the case of Mindfulness 3, the processes of Buddhist modernism mean that Buddhism has gradually lost much of its explicitly religious concepts and terminology to reformat to the West. However, mindfulness has reformatted to the contemporary

260 Stephen Batchelor, 'A Secular Buddhist' (2012) 3. A Secular Buddhist (gaiahouse.co.uk). Accessed on 18 December 2019.

261 David L. McMahan, *Rethinking Meditation: Buddhist Meditative Practice in Ancient and Modern Worlds* (Oxford: Oxford University Press, 2023), 21.

262 See Olivier Roy, *Secularism Confronts Islam* (New York: Columbia University Press, 2007).

post-secular conditions of belief and experience, to the extent that for some it has become a spiritual practice in and of itself. For others, like Batchelor, mindfulness is an important part of a secular Buddhism concerned with a particular vision of human flourishing.

Mindfulness 3 can be critiqued from two perspectives. First, Mindfulness 3 is not grounded in any ethical framework. This is a response to the cohort who see mindfulness as a spiritual outlook with no connection to its traditional Buddhist framework. The second critique is in response to secular Buddhists such as Stephen Batchelor's use of mindfulness, arguing that Mindfulness 3 is a problematic interpretation of Buddhist teachings.

First, for contemporary spiritual seekers, mindfulness represents a spiritual approach free of the doctrines, rules and expectations of traditional religious narratives. As was highlighted in the last chapter, this is borne out by the growing numbers that identify as spiritual but not religious, as well as the contemporary popularity of meditation and mindfulness. Sheldrake asks how practices such as mindfulness, completely removed from its traditional Buddhist framework, represents a coherent ethical and moral outlook.

> A 'spiritual tradition' implies a developed theory rather than simply a spiritual practice. This raises an interesting question of authenticity when contemporary spiritual seekers sometimes borrow practices from different traditions ... or uses a practice on its own ... and ignore its background belief system or spiritual theory.[263]

Mindfulness 3 is, in this regard a practice rather than a spiritual tradition. While the potentially life-giving benefits of mindfulness have been highlighted in this chapter, questions remain over how this mindfulness practice can be an ethically grounded spiritual outlook. Like Mindfulness 1 and 2, Mindfulness 3 is fundamentally deracinated from its traditional Buddhist ethical and wisdom tradition. However, while Mindfulness 1 can claim a healthcare ethos of care, Mindfulness 3 does not have such a foundation.

Moreover, despite the occasional opaqueness of Jon Kabat-Zinn's position on Mindfulness 1 as being secular or spiritual, he at least warns that it is problematic not to acknowledge '... the ethical foundations of the meditative

263 Philip Sheldrake, *Spirituality: A Very Short Introduction* (Oxford: Oxford University Press, 2012), 32.

practices and traditions from which mindfulness has emerged'.[264] Without acknowledgement of the Buddhist ethical and moral teachings on mindfulness, Mindfulness 3, like Mindfulness 2, risks cultivating perceptions that our autonomy and wellbeing are unaffected by the context we live in or the external factors that influence how we live.

Mindfulness 2 can be used effectively to improve physical and mental health or as a problem-solving technique. Despite these benefits, the dangers of a self-aggrandising, instrumentalist mindfulness practice have been highlighted already. However, Mindfulness 3 has different goals in that it is used as a spiritual practice to deal with spiritual problems or questions of meaning. In this regard, the lack of an ethical framework to support this practice in our relationships with others is especially felt.

> If I come to mindfulness with a practical problem such as addiction to nicotine, then all well and good, a 'problem-solving mindfulness' approach may very well help me to achieve my goal. But if I come with a more 'spiritual' problem ... an uncertainty regarding what I should do and how I should live- then 'problem-solving' mindfulness is not going to be equipped to help me.[265]

Non-evaluative 'bare attention' mindfulness can be a potentially life-giving practice that reduces stress and suffering for many. In observing thoughts in a neutral manner, the practitioner sees the impermanence of thoughts as they rise and fall. However, in questions of spirituality and meaning in life, such a neutral outlook is impossible as human perception and experience are not objective or value-free. In this regard, mindfulness in isolation cannot provide an ethic to live by, as there is no moral teaching or wisdom scaffolding to support questions of how we should live our lives in relation to others in the world. Like Mindfulness 2, this lack of an ethical foundation places Mindfulness 3 at risk of becoming the antithesis of traditional

264 Jon Kabat Zinn, 'Mindfulness has Huge Health Benefits- But McMindfulness is no Panacea', *The Guardian*, 20 October 2015. <https://www.theguardian.com/commentisfree/2015/oct/20/mindfulness-mental-health-potential-benefits-uk>. Accessed on 28 November 2019.

265 Alex Gooch, 'Mindfulness as a Secular Spirituality', in Manu Bazzano, ed., *After Mindfulness: New Perspectives on Psychology and Meditation* (London: Palgrave McMillan, 2014), 106.

mindfulness; a tool for egotistical self-aggrandisation with no regard for caring for anyone except the self.

What is being critiqued here is not mindfulness practice in itself but the idea that in isolation, mindfulness represents an ethically secure spiritual tradition. As Sheldrake differentiates, a spiritual tradition implies a developed theory whereas Mindfulness 3 remains a practice without such an evolved philosophy. Gooch argues that this form of mindfulness is not equipped to support spiritual questions, as a neutral outlook on questions of the inner life is deeply problematic.

> Mindfulness will not obviate our need to have a reliably grounded sense of identity and nor will it provide solid ground on which to base our identities. It will not relieve us of our yearning to feel that we know what the world is in order to interact meaningfully with it- and nor will it restore our crumbling capacity to what the world is … we require beliefs in order to orient ourselves towards the world and interact with it in a meaningful way.[266]

Despite these challenges, a non-evaluative mindfulness practice such as Mindfulness 3 may have potential benefits on pupil wellbeing and development in Catholic schools, enabling each child to reach their full potential. One opportunity for this is the aforementioned proposed contemplative turn in education, where students are invited to examine their inner thoughts, feelings and sources of meaning through mindfulness practice. This turn to a contemplative education would support the view that because education is a human process, students should be encouraged to reflect on what gives them meaning in their lives, and what constitutes authentic human flourishing for them. Moreover, such an approach, while being non-judgemental, could never be described as neutral, as feelings and questions of ultimate meaning are, by their nature, not neutral.

In this way, Mindfulness 3 as a post-secular spiritual practice presents an opportunity to address spiritual concerns and questions for students in Catholic schools, cultivating a contemplative disposition. This would be supported by the ethical traditions and teachings of the Church, thereby ameliorating the challenge of Mindfulness 3's lack of an ethical foundation.

266 Ibid.

Second, as was highlighted earlier, Buddhism is a dynamic and plural wisdom tradition, encompassing several schools of thought that have developed in different contexts, each with distinct readings of the Buddha's teachings. Moreover, the processes of Buddhist modernism have led to the wisdom tradition being detraditionalised, secularised and individualised as it interacts with the contemporary Western context. Mindfulness 3 as an offshoot of this development is then challenged in claiming adherence to Buddhism while re-interpreting and removing fundamental teachings.

Secular Buddhists such as Stephen Batchelor often justify their shedding of overtly religious aspects of their practice by referring to early Buddhist texts such as the *Kālāma Sutta*, where the Buddha warns followers to be 'lanterns unto themselves'; that they would not accept oral tradition, claims to religious authority or teachings out of hand. Rather, followers were encouraged to test Buddha's teaching and let their own experiences be their guiding principles. However, Buddhist scholar Bhikku Bodhi argues that this is a selective and misleading representation of the Buddha dharma to suit the needs of Buddhists who want to pick and choose what they believe in.

> ... on the basis of a single passage, quoted out of context, the Buddha has been made out to be a pragmatic empiricist who dismisses all doctrine and faith, and whose Dhamma is simply a freethinker's kit to truth which invites each one to accept and reject whatever he likes.[267]

Bodhi's critique challenges the narrative that secular Buddhism retains the most important teachings of the Buddha while dispelling unnecessary religious and cultural baggage. This is partly due to the complex history and development of Buddhism and its various schools of thought, making it difficult to imagine 'what Buddha really taught'.[268] Moreover, Scharf has argued that in the Buddhist wisdom tradition, mindfulness meditation is a monastic practice aimed at cultivating specific religious or mystical experiences in the

267 Bhikku Bodhi, 'A Look at the Kalama Sutta' (1998) <https://www.accesstoinsight.org/lib/authors/bodhi/bps-essay_09.html>. Accessed on 31 December 2019.

268 Walpolo Rāhula, *What the Buddha Taught* (NY: Grove Press, 1974). Batchelor acknowledges that this is one of the major issues for the modern 'secular Buddhism' movement.

minds of practitioners.[269] These experiences open the practitioner to the illusion of the self but also serve to help the practitioner along the cycle of rebirth before reaching a soteriological conclusion in nirvana. It is difficult to reconcile the secular Buddhism of Mindfulness 3 with these traditionally fundamental aspects of Buddhist teaching in this respect.

However, Batchelor is keen to stress that secular Buddhism and by extension Mindfulness 3 is a contemplative outlook rather than a science of the mind. While neuroscience and psychological assessments can highlight the benefits of mindfulness meditation, they cannot encapsulate the subjective contemplative experience of meditation.

> Meditation is not only a solution to a particular set of problems, but a way of penetrating into the mystery that there is anything at all rather than nothing. When a problem is solved, it disappears, but when a mystery is penetrated, it only becomes more mysterious ... By stripping all overt elements of religious behaviour and belief from the dharma, Secular Buddhism ... could also end up rejecting any sense of sublimity, mystery, awe, or wonder from the practice.[270]

In this sense, Batchelor is pointing to the importance of the spiritual dimension of Mindfulness 3. Despite the processes of secularisation and detraditionalisation, Mindfulness 3 is concerned with the mystery of life, seeking to discern meaning and authenticity through meditative practices in an increasingly postmodern context. This outlook is supported by an interpretation of the ethical framework found in Buddhist teachings, albeit shorn of any religious language or content. The development of a post-secular spirituality that envisions a humanising, contemplative outlook for people is praiseworthy, but it remains to be seen, given the radical recontextualisation of

269 Robert Scharf, 'Buddhist Modernism and the Rhetoric of Meditative Experience', *Numen*, 42(3) (1995), 228–83.

270 Stephen Batchelor, 'The Everyday Sublime', in Manu Bazzano, ed., *After Mindfulness: New Perspectives on Psychology and Meditation* (London: Palgrave McMillan, 2014), 47.

Buddhist teaching, how long approaches such as those offered by Batchelor can retain the title of 'Buddhist'.[271]

For Catholic education, the promotion of Mindfulness 3 offers both opportunities and challenges. First, the promotion of mindfulness as a contemplative practice can enable students to examine their inner feelings, thoughts and sources of meaning. This probing of the inner life can open students to deeper questions of meaning and purpose in life, thus entailing a more humanising and holistic education. In this regard, mindfulness framed as a secular practice separate from Buddhist teaching represents an opportunity for Catholic schools.

However, the interpretation of Mindfulness 3 as secular Buddhism is problematic for Catholic schools. Given the particularity of the Buddhist wisdom tradition, despite the processes of secularisation, detraditionalisation and individualisation, the promotion of Mindfulness 3 in Catholic schools is open to criticism of 'Stealth Buddhism'. This is the claim that mindfulness can act as a Trojan horse in settings such as schools, suggesting that despite the secular framing of Mindfulness 3, Buddhist dharma such as the illusion of the self will be transmitted to practitioners.[272] This implicit presence of Buddhist doctrine would be incompatible with the educational vision of the Catholic school.

Mindfulness 1 and 2 at their best can help reduce suffering for students by developing the insight of the impermanence of thoughts. However, for Catholic education, Mindfulness 3 can go too far by promoting the view that the self is illusory. But Mindfulness 3 as a post-secular contemplative practice and understood as an innate human capacity, also provides opportunities for students in Catholic schools to probe their inner thoughts and experiences in order to explore questions of meaning, values and identity.

271 Batchelor admits that the Buddhist title may eventually be removed from this developing phenomenon. 'Buddhists need to rise to the challenge of articulating a philosophically coherent and ethically integrated vision of life that is no longer tied to the religious dogmas and institutions of Asian Buddhism … they might encourage the dawning of a culture of awakening, which may or may not call itself 'Buddhist.' Ibid, 48.

272 Candy G. Brown, 'Can "Secular" Mindfulness Be Separated from Religion?', in Ronald E. Purser, David Forbes and Adam Burke, eds., *Handbook of Mindfulness: Culture, Context and Social Engagement* (Basel: Springer Publishing, 2016), 84–5.

This would also necessitate a clear distinction between the spiritual outlook of secular Buddhism and the Christian understanding of the human person. This means that a robust Catholic educational vision must be articulated in order to help students engage with contemplative practices such as mindfulness in Catholic schools.

Mindfulness 3 represents a novel development in the processes of Buddhist modernism in the contemporary Western context. It speaks to the contemporary popularity of meditation, to the growing 'spiritual but not religious' demographic and the designation of the contemporary West as post-secular and post-Christian. Mindfulness 3 is thus a response to contemporary hunger for spiritual meaning that is no longer axiomatically found in traditional religious institutions.

For those who engaged in mindfulness as a spiritual outlook, a practitioners risk falling into the same trap as those of Mindfulness 2 via the removal of an explicit ethical framework. For secular Buddhists such as Stephen Batchelor, Mindfulness 3 is supported by interpreting Buddhist teaching in a way that removes any religious or transcendental content. While this may be problematic for Buddhists who see tenets such as nirvana and karma as metaphysical concepts, it may be that secular Buddhism and by extension Mindfulness 3 are further developments in the processes of Buddhist modernism.

Aside from physical and mental wellbeing benefits, Mindfulness 3 can be a contemplative practice for students in Catholic schools, which could foster a spiritual orientation towards questions of ultimate meaning and purpose in life. This application of Mindfulness 3 can only be operative if approached as an innate human capacity rather than through stealth Buddhism, the implicit teaching of Buddhism framed through a secular lens. If Mindfulness 3 is understood as the former and not the latter, then Mindfulness 3 offers educational potential to Catholic schools as a post-secular spirituality.

CHAPTER 3

The Place of Mindfulness in Irish Education

This chapter will outline and examine how mindfulness is currently operative within Irish Catholic primary schools. In order to do this, it will first provide an overview of current research on the relationship between mindfulness and education. Following this, the role of mindfulness in the Irish education system will be explored with specific regard to the concept of wellbeing in the new Junior Cycle programme at post-primary level. It will also include the current relationship between mindfulness and the incoming SPHE curriculum at the primary level as well as the role mindfulness is set to play in the recalibration of wellbeing at the heart of the new Irish primary curriculum.

It will then detail the types of mindfulness courses and initiatives available to Irish primary school communities, including the *Paws b* programme, which offers a form of mindfulness curriculum to primary school children aged 7–11 and the *Weaving Wellbeing* programme for primary schools, which include mindfulness components. This mapping of how mindfulness interacts with Irish education will better equip us to evaluate the compatibility of mindfulness with ethos in Irish Catholic primary schools.

Mindfulness and education

Mindfulness has enjoyed exponential growth in popularity in educational discourse in recent years.[273] In the first major study of its kind, educationalists Ergas and Hadar's systematic review of mindfulness in education literature

273 Kimberley A. Schonert-Reichl, and Robert W. Roeser, eds, *Handbook of Mindfulness in Education: Integrating Theory and Research into Practice* (New York: Springer, 2016);

observes 447 peer reviewed papers published in this area between 2002 and 2017.[274] As was seen in the previous chapter, there is a growing body of research demonstrating the positive effects mindfulness has on physical and mental wellbeing. This is also the case regarding the benefits of mindfulness in educational settings. These mindfulness-attributed benefits range from higher self-esteem and enhanced social skills to improved academic performance.[275]

Moreover, several educationalists have written about the transformative potential of contemplative practices in education.[276] Roth defines contemplative practices as '... the many ways human beings have found, across cultures and across time, to concentrate, broaden and deepen conscious awareness'.[277] In this sense, mindfulness as a contemplative practice offers a profound educational potential by deepening students' awareness of their

---

Charlotte Zenner, Solveig Herrnleben-Kurz, and Harald Walach, 'Mindfulness-Based Interventions in Schools – A Systematic Review and Meta-Analysis', *Frontiers in Psychology 5* (2014), 603–16; Katherine Weare, 'Developing Mindfulness with Children and Young People: A Review of the Evidence and Policy Context', *Journal of Children's Services, 8*(2) (2013), 141–53; Isobel Killoran, 'Mindfulness in Education: Using and Teaching Mindfulness in Schools', *Childhood Education, 93* (2) (2017), 99.

274 Oren Ergas and Linor L. Hadar, 'Mindfulness in and as Education: A Map of a Developing Academic Discourse from 2002 to 2017', *Review of Education* (2019), 1.

275 Richard Amundsen, Leigh M. Riby, Colin Hamilton, Melanie Hope and Deborah McGann, 'Mindfulness in Primary School Children as a Route to Enhanced Life Satisfaction, Positive Outlook and Effective Emotion Regulation', *BMC Psychology 8* (2020), 71; Kimberley A. Schonert-Reichl and Molly Stewart Lawlor, 'The Effects of a Mindfulness-Based Education Program on Pre-and Early Adolescents' Well-being and Social and Emotional Competence', *Mindfulness, 1*(3) (2010), 137–51; Laura S. Bakosh, Renee M. Snow, Jutta M. Tobias, Janice L. Houlihan and Celestina Barbosa-Leiker, 'Maximizing Mindful Learning: Mindful Awareness Intervention Improves Elementary School Students', Quarterly Grades', *Mindfulness, 7*(1) (2016), 59–67.

276 See Oren Ergas, *Reconstructing 'Education' Through Mindful Attention: Positioning the Mind at the Center of Curriculum and Pedagogy* (London: Palgrave MacMillan, 2017); Aislinn O'Donnell, 'Contemplative Pedagogy and Mindfulness: Developing Creative Attention in an Age of Distraction', *Journal of Philosophy of Education 49*(2) (2015), 187–202; Philip Wexler and Yotam Hotam, *New Social Foundations for Education: Education in 'Post-Secular' Society* (NY: Peter Lang, 2015).

277 Harold D. Roth, 'Against Cognitive Imperialism: A Call for a Non-Ethnographic Approach to Cognitive Science and Religious Studies', *Religion East and West 8* (2008), 19.

thoughts and feelings. Ergas calls these inner emotions, experiences and thoughts the 'inner curriculum'. Such contemplative practices can enable students to make and discover meaning in the world around them. This proposed turn to contemplative education would be complementary to the vision of Catholic education, which promotes the harmonious and holistic development of the person, valuing academic excellence as well as the spiritual dimension of life.

While the benefits of school-based mindfulness practices are common, several concerns have been raised, albeit far fewer in number than studies on the positive effects of mindfulness.[278] As was detailed in the previous chapter, Purser warns of educational mindfulness programmes that reinforce societal sources of stress and suffering rather than challenge them.[279] Forbes argues that some forms of mindfulness have become a tool to bolster a neoliberal educational agenda focused on performance, productivity and efficiency.[280]

Moreover, the simplification of mindfulness to non-evaluative 'bare-attention' is referenced by Hyland. The reduction of mindfulness to an individualised, passive activity poses a danger that the individual may never move beyond their own experience of the present to reduce suffering in the

278 Hyland provides a useful overview of the development of these critiques. See Terry Hyland, 'The Limits of Mindfulness: Emerging Issues for Education', *British Journal of Educational Studies* 64(1) (2016), 97–117.

279 Ronald Purser, *McMindfulness: How Mindfulness Became the New Capitalist Spirituality* (London: Repeater, 2019), 183–4. 'The therapeutic approach is conservative, directing attention away from the outside world. Mindfulness could be an empowering and emancipatory practice, exploring ways to change social conditions and priorities. Instead, it maintains the status quo. Students are taught to meditate away their anger and accept their frustrations (non-judgementally of course). This might help them focus on work, but unless they also learn about the causes of stress in social, economic and institutional structures, links between education and democracy are severed'.

280 David Forbes, *Mindfulness and Its Discontents: Education, Self and Social Transformation* (Nova Scotia: Fernwood Publishing, 2019), 147. 'Within schools' neoliberal competitive culture, stress becomes decontextualized and interpreted as the personal failure of an individual to become successful; one must compete against others on an otherwise meaningless high-stakes test, adapt to the demands of productivity, and be a team player'.

world around them and in others.[281] This echoes the critiques of Mindfulness 1 and 2 in the previous chapter which argue that some manifestations of mindfulness privatise stress rather than challenge societal sources of stress.

Finally, there is an important note made by Ergas and Hadar on the current quality of discourse in this area. They argue: 'The nascency of the field is expressed in a surprising and potentially unhealthy paucity of critical papers in this field. The number of critical papers found seems small and possibly suggests an immature and over-optimistic phase of this discourse'.[282] This finding raises questions over the rapid growth in popularity of mindfulness-based interventions in schools. While there are growing numbers of studies outlining wellbeing benefits of mindfulness, it could be argued that the zeal in sharing the good news of mindfulness has overtaken the evidence supporting it. While mindfulness may indeed offer many positive and welcome outcomes to students' wellbeing, it is clear that critiques of mindfulness in education remain sparse. This signifies the timeliness of this exploration of the compatibility of mindfulness and Catholic ethos in Irish primary schools.

The growth of mindfulness in schools is located within the wider discourse of wellbeing and schools. Andrews et al. define wellbeing as:

> ... healthy and successful individual functioning (involving physiological, psychological and behavioural levels of organisation), positive social relationships (with family members, peers, adult caregivers, and community and societal institutions, for instance, school and faith and civic organisations), and a social ecology that provides safety (e.g., freedom from interpersonal violence, war and crime), human and civil rights, social justice and participation in civil society.[283]

281 Terry Hyland, 'The Limits of Mindfulness: Emerging Issues for Education', *British Journal of Educational Studies, 64*(1) (2016), 104. 'Enhancing awareness and fostering stillness in the present moment are not ends in themselves but need to be seen as providing the necessary conditions for engaging with the broader enterprise of cultivating the moral and spiritual virtues which can assist us in dealing with the challenges of everyday life'.

282 Oren Ergas, and Linor L. Hadar, 'Mindfulness in and as Education: A Map of a Developing Academic Discourse from 2002 to 2017', *Review of Education* (2019), 35.

283 Arlene B. Andrews, Asher Ben-Arieh, Maya Carlson, William Damon, Carol Dweck, Felton Earls, Cynthia Garcia-Coll, Robert Gold, Neal Halfon, Roger Hart, Richard M. Lerner, Bruce McEwen, Michael Meaney, Dan Offord, Donald Patrick, Magda Peck, Barbera Trickett, Thomas Weisner and Barry Zuckerman (Ecology Working Group), *Ecology of Child Well-Being: Advancing the Science and the Science-Practice Link* (Georgia: Centre for Child Well-Being, 2002), 103.

The breadth of this statement highlights the challenges associated with succinctly defining wellbeing in education, given the variety of contexts and disciplines in which the term is applied.[284] In academic research, wellbeing is often connected to the positive psychology movement,[285] and researchers '... might characterise wellbeing as "positive and sustainable characteristics which enable individuals and organisations to thrive and flourish."'[286] This reading of wellbeing has grown in recent decades and wellbeing promotion has become increasingly influential across several spheres, including education. Moreover, wellbeing itself can be understood as being composed of multiple dimensions, including physical, emotional, occupational, intellectual and spiritual wellbeing.[287] While Gillett-Swan and Sargeant acknowledge that while '... wellbeing is a highly popularised and aspirational concept in philosophical, psychological, medical and health literature ... there has not been a clearly defined and workable definition of wellbeing that incorporates its multifaceted, multidimensional and progressive elements'.[288]

Mindfulness is immediately compatible with this conception of wellbeing linked with positive psychology. As demonstrated in the last chapter, the benefits of mindfulness practice can include improved physical and mental wellbeing. Jon Kabat-Zinn's work at secularising and simplifying

284 Margaret Nohilly and Fionnuala Tynan, 'The Evolution of Wellbeing in Educational Policy in Ireland', *International Journal of Wellbeing 12*(1) (2022), 44.

285 According to the American Psychological Association Dictionary, '... positive psychology is a field of psychological theory and research that focuses on the psychological states (e.g., contentment, joy), individual traits or character strengths (e.g., intimacy, integrity, altruism, wisdom), and social institutions that enhance subjective well-being and make life most worth living.' <https://dictionary.apa.org/positive-psychology>. Accessed on 6 October 2020.

286 Gill Ereaut and Rebecca Whiting, What do We Mean by 'Wellbeing'?: And Why Might it Matter? (Department for Children, Schools and Families) (Research report) (2008), 4.

287 The Wellbeing Online Home Page for Washington State University presents the Wellbeing Wheel, highlighting the eight dimensions of wellbeing. <https://wellbeingonline.wsu.edu/#:~:text=Wellbeing%20Online%20is%20dedicated%20to,holistic%20approach%20to%20healthy%20living>. Accessed on 4 August 2020.

288 Jenna Gillet-Swan and Jonathan Sargeant, 'Wellbeing as a Process of Accrual: Beyond Subjectivity and Beyond the Moment', *Social Indicators Research 121*(1) (2015), 146.

forms of Buddhist meditation has created a clinical treatment for stress reduction among other ailments. The application of MBSR (Mindfulness-Based Stress Reduction) into cognitive behavioural therapies such as MBCT (Mindfulness-Based Cognitive Therapy)[289] has further enabled mindfulness to be framed as a psychological means to improved wellbeing rather than Buddhist meditation.[290]

In light of this contemporary interest in wellbeing promotion across several sectors of society, it can be argued that mindfulness has entered the education system through the gateway of wellbeing. When understood as the positive and sustainable characteristics enabling students to flourish, wellbeing represents an invaluable resource for schools to help pupils reach their potential. In this regard, the positive outcomes offered by mindfulness are fully compatible with the narrative of wellbeing promotion, which is to be observed in the Irish education system.

While this work focuses on mindfulness in the Catholic primary school sector, it is important to outline the post-primary school context due to policy and curricular developments regarding wellbeing. These developments may serve as a precursor to wellbeing promotion in the upcoming New Primary Curriculum, which has doubled the allocated time for Physical Education and Social, Personal and Health Education, recalibrated as a single Wellbeing subject.[291] The place of wellbeing in the New Primary Curriculum will be explored in greater detail later in the chapter. It is also important to note how secondary schools with a Catholic ethos have reacted to these developments, given the scope and aims of this work.

289 <http://www.mbct.com/>. Accessed on 4 August 2020.

290 See Stefan G. Reynolds, Mindfulness, 'Yoga and Schools: An Opportunity or a Problem?', *The Furrow* (December 2019), 678. Reynolds's description of mindfulness in schools is useful here: '... most Mindfulness teaching today has taken off its Buddhist robes. It is used ... more generally as a practice for stress relief: in schools to cultivate attention and calmness'.

291 National Council for Curriculum and Assessment, *Primary Curriculum Framework for Primary and Special Schools* (Dublin: NCCA, 2023), 38–9.

Mindfulness and Irish post-primary schools

There has been a significant focus at the policy level on wellbeing promotion in the Irish education system in recent years.[292] Despite children in Ireland ranking fifth in the most recent studies on flourishing and wellbeing,[293] there remain significant concerns on youth mental health and wellbeing. The *My World 2 Survey*, Ireland's largest and most comprehensive study of youth mental health and wellbeing, found increases in anxiety and depression as well as decreases in self-esteem and resilience among young people aged 12–25.[294] Moreover, research on the effects of the COVID-19 pandemic on child mental health highlights a legacy of increased anxiety, emotional distress and depressive symptoms in young

292 Former Department of Education and Skills Minister Joe McHugh's opening statement in the DES *Wellbeing Policy Statement and Framework for Practice* articulates this: 'The promotion of wellbeing is central to the Department's mission to enable children and young people to achieve their full potential and contribute to Ireland's social, cultural and economic development'. Department of Education and Skills, *Wellbeing Policy Statement and Framework for Practice 2018–2023* (Revised 2019) (Dublin: Rialtas na hÉireann, 2019) 1. See also Margaret Nohilly and Fionnuala Tynan, 'The Evolution of Wellbeing in Educational Policy in Ireland', *International Journal of Wellbeing 12*(1) (2022), 42–53.

293 Helen Clark, Awa Marie Coll-Seck, Anshu Banerjee, Stefan Peterson, Sarah L Dalglish, Shanthi Ameratunga, Dina Balabanova, Maharaj Kishan Bhan, Zulfiqar A Bhutta, John Borrazzo, Mariam Claeson, Tanya Doherty, Fadi El-Jardali, Asha S George, Angela Gichaga, Lu Gram, David B Hipgrave, Aku Kwamie, Qingyue Meng, Raúl Mercer, Sunita Narain, Jesca Nsungwa-Sabiiti, Adesola O Olumide, David Osrin, Timothy Powell-Jackson, Kumanan Rasanathan, Imran Rasul, Papaarangi Reid, Jennifer Requejo, Sarah S Rohde, Nigel Rollins, Magali Romedenne, Harshpal Singh Sachdev, Rana Saleh, Yusra R Shawar, Jeremy Shiffman, Jonathon Simon, Peter D Sly, Karin Stenberg, Mark Tomlinson, Rajani R Ved and Anthony Costello, 'A Future for the World's Children? A WHO–UNICEF–Lancet Commission', *The Lancet Commissions 395(10224)* (2020), 605–58. <https://www.thelancet.com/action/showPdf?pii=S0140-6736%2819%2932540-1>. Accessed on 4 August 2020.

294 Barbera Dooley, Clíodhna O' Connor, Amanda Fitzgerald and Aileen O' Reilly, *My World Survey 2: The National Study of Youth Mental Health in Ireland* (Dublin: UCD and Jigsaw, 2019).

children.[295] Wellbeing promotion is set to remain a significant theme in Irish schools, especially given the many challenges brought about by the pandemic.

Within the secondary school sector, wellbeing has emerged as a significant area of learning as part of Junior Cycle reforms.[296] According to the National Council for Curriculum and Assessment (NCCA), '… student wellbeing is present when students realise their abilities, take care of their physical wellbeing, can cope with the normal stresses of life and have a sense of purpose and belonging to a wider community'.[297] Since 2020, post-primary schools have been obliged to offer 400 timetabled hours on wellbeing. The subjects deemed fundamental to learning about wellbeing are Physical Education (PE), Civic, Social and Political Education (CSPE) and Social, Personal and Health Education (SPHE).[298] The latter subject provides a basis for mindfulness practice in schools as a means of maintaining and enhancing student wellbeing, albeit without mindfulness explicitly appearing in the SPHE curricular guidelines. The *Junior Cycle Short Course on SPHE*[299] is composed of five strands, the fourth being 'My Mental Health'. This includes learning outcomes '4.2 appreciate the importance of talking things over, including recognising the links between thoughts,

295 See Jeffrey Kluger, 'The Coronavirus Seems to Spare Most Kids from Illness, but Its Effect on Their Mental Health Is Deepening', *TIME Magazine* (23 July 2020) and Katriona O' Sullivan, Serena Clark, Amy McGrane, Nicole Rock, Lydia Burke, Neasa Boyle, Natasha Joksimovic and Kevin Marshall, 'A Qualitative Study of Child and Adolescent Mental Health during the COVID-19 Pandemic in Ireland', *International Journal of Environmental Research and Public Health, 18*(3) (2021), 1062. <https://time.com/5870478/children-mental-health-coronavirus/>. Accessed on 4 August 2020).

296 National Council for Curriculum and Assessment, *The Framework for Junior Cycle* (Dublin: NCCA, 2015).

297 National Council for Curriculum and Assessment (NCCA), *Guidelines for Wellbeing in Junior Cycle* (Dublin: NCCA, 2017) 17.

298 Ibid, 59.

299 National Council for Curriculum and Assessment (NCCA), *Specification for Junior Cycle: Social, Personal and Health Education* (Dublin: NCCA, 2016).

feelings and behaviour' and '4.3 practise some relaxation techniques'.[300] These outcomes mirror the underlying processes of mindfulness in that the students are enabled to notice and attend to thoughts as they arise, as well as calming exercises to ground themselves in the present moment, incorporating body scans and regulation of the breath.

It is noteworthy that Religious Education is not included in the grouping, despite much evidence that states belonging to and practising a religious tradition enhances one's wellbeing in many different ways.[301] Moreover, Meehan has convincingly argued that within the Irish post-primary context, pedagogically sound religious education can in fact be a legitimate source of wellbeing for students, further signifying the positive correlation between religion and wellbeing.[302]

The wellbeing paradigm of the new Junior Cycle is solidifying the place of mindfulness in Irish post-primary education. The curricular and policy reforms of the new programme enable significant numbers of children to practice mindfulness on a regular basis as a means of wellbeing promotion. But as Forbes and Purser warned in the previous chapter, mindfulness risks being instrumentalised to buffer a neoliberal agenda focused on efficiency

300 Ibid, 14. The language of relaxation techniques and recognising thoughts can reasonably be linked to mindfulness practice, which focuses on awareness of thoughts and feelings. As explored in the previous chapter, mindfulness can be a relaxation technique insofar as it reduces stress and anxiety.

301 See Emily A. Greenfield and Nadine F. Marks, 'Religious Social Identity as an Explanatory Factor for Associations Between More Frequent Formal Religious Participation and Psychological Well-Being', *The International Journal for the Psychology of Religion, 17*(3) (2007), 245–59, Patty Van Cappellen, Maria Toth-Gauthier, Vassilis Saroglou and Barbara L. Fredrikson, 'Religion and Well-Being: The Mediating Role of Positive Emotions', *Journal of Happiness Studies 17* (2016), 485–505, Tyler J. VanderWeele, 'Religious Communities and Human Flourishing', Current Directions. *Psychological Science 26*(5) (October 2017), 476–81 and Ying Chen and Tyler J. VanderWeele, 'Associations of Religious Upbringing with Subsequent Health and Well-Being From Adolescence to Young Adulthood: An Outcome-Wide Analysis,' *American Journal of Epidemiology, 187*(11) (2018), 2355–64.

302 See Amalee Meehan, 'Wellbeing in the Irish Junior Cycle: The Potential of Religious Education,' *Irish Educational Studies 38*(4) (2019), 501–18 and Amalee Meehan, 'Religion as a Source of Well-Being: Implications for Second-Level School Programs in Ireland and Beyond,' *Religious Education 115*(5) (2020), 507–21.

and productivity. In this sense, mindfulness is in danger of misappropriation for the production of improved student academic output despite of pressurised academic conditions, rather than confronting those sources of pressure and stress. Such a misappropriation would represent a reductive view of human flourishing, emptying mindfulness practice in schools of their humanising benefits, privatising rather than challenging sources of stress for students in schools.

The significant growth of mindfulness and education literature remains at an early but optimistic stage, with studies suggesting that mindfulness practice offers several benefits to pupil wellbeing and development. At a time when young people face significant challenges to mental health and wellbeing, contemplative education may offer a means to deepening student awareness. However, questions remain whether mindfulness practice will be reduced to a commodity for privatising stress and serving a neoliberal agenda of productivity and efficiency.

In the Irish context, the advent of wellbeing in the new Junior Cycle programme is significant as it provides a vehicle for mindfulness to become embedded at a curricular and policy level in Irish post-primary education. Such a focus on wellbeing in Irish education is to be welcomed as resources such as mindfulness that are demonstrated to support students' physical and mental wellbeing align with the school's commitment to pupils flourishing. However, this should not be to the detriment of Religious Education which can also be a contributor to student wellbeing.

Having examined the emergence of mindfulness in Irish post-primary schools, attention now focuses on developments in the Irish primary school context.

Mindfulness and Irish primary schools

As in post-primary education, mindfulness is an emerging phenomenon in Irish primary schools. The rationale for mindfulness practice in the classroom stems from a growing body of research indicating a host of benefits to students, including improved self-esteem, decreased anxiety, better attentiveness and enhanced academic performance.[303] This fits into the wider trends of school-based interventions to improve student wellbeing. However, questions remain over the effectiveness of school-based wellbeing interventions. This was highlighted by Durlak et al.'s meta-analysis of school-based interventions, finding '… there is a wide gap between research and practice in school-based prevention and promotion just as there is with many clinical interventions for children and adolescents'.[304] This observation is echoed in Gunawardena et al.'s recent systematic review of wellbeing interventions in Australian schools, which found that 80% of the strategies and programs examined did not report a statistically significant effect on students' wellbeing outcomes.[305]

Moreover, as was stated earlier mindfulness in schools fits into the broader discourse of wellbeing in schools. The critique of how mindfulness is operative and emerging within the Irish Catholic primary school context can be categorised into two interrelated themes. First, as has been seen at post-primary level, curricular reforms at primary level place greater emphasis on wellbeing which provides a vehicle for mindfulness practice in the classroom. Second, wellbeing programs such as *Weaving Wellbeing* and mindfulness curricula such as *Paws b* have become increasingly popular in the primary education setting as schools seek to improve pupil wellbeing. These themes together highlight how the emergence of wellbeing promotion

303 See Marc Suhrcke and Carmen de Paz Nieves, 'The Impact of Health and Health Behaviours on Educational Outcomes in High Income Countries: A Review of the Evidence', World Health Organisation (2011), Chris Bonell, Neil Humphrey, Adam Fletcher, Laurence Moore, Rob Anderson and Rona Campbell, 'Why Schools Should Promote Students' Health and Wellbeing (Editorial)', *The British Medical Journal* (13 May 2014).

304 See Joseph A. Durlak, Roger P. Weissberg, Allison B. Dymnicki, Rebecca D. Taylor and Kriston B. Schellinger, 'The Impact of Enhancing Students' Social and Emotional Learning: A Meta-Analysis of School-Based Universal Interventions', *Child Development, January/February 82*(1) (2011), 420.

305 Harshi Gunawardena, Alexander Voukelatos, Sham Nair, Shane Cross and Ian B. Hickie. 'Efficacy and Effectiveness of Universal School-Based Wellbeing Interventions in Australia: A Systematic Review', *International Journal Environmental Research and Public Health 20*(15) (2023), 6508.

has enabled Catholic primary schools, which make up the vast majority of primary schools in Ireland,[306] seedbeds for mindfulness practice.

Mindfulness, wellbeing and the new primary curriculum

Like its post-primary counterpart, wellbeing has emerged as a central theme in policy literature for Irish primary schools.[307] Moreover, during the COVID-19 pandemic, the Department of Education and Skills highlighted the centrality of wellbeing promotion in the reopening of schools.[308] The guidance included mindfulness as an option for reducing anxieties felt by children during the reopening.[309]

In recent years, mindfulness has grown increasingly popular in Irish primary schools.[310] The rationale for this popularity is based on the numerous studies highlighting the positive effects mindfulness has on student wellbeing,

306 As per the Department of Education and Skill's latest statistics, over 88% of all primary schools in the Irish state are under Catholic patronage. See Department of Education and Skills, Statistical Bulletin-August 2024 (Dublin: Dublin: Rialtas na hÉireann, 2024). <https://www.gov.ie/en/collection/annual-statistical-reports/>. Accessed on 31 August 2024.

307 See Department of Education and Skills, *Wellbeing Policy Statement and Framework for Practice 2018–2023* (Revised 2019) (Dublin: Rialtas na hÉireann, 2019), National Educational Psychological Service, *Wellbeing in Primary Schools: Guidelines for Mental Health Promotion* (Dublin: Rialtas na hÉireann, 2019).

308 'Promoting the wellbeing of our school communities is a fundamental element of the department's overall plan to ensure a successful return to school as we continue to manage the impact of the COVID-19 pandemic'. Department of Education and Skills, *Supporting the Wellbeing of School Communities as Schools Reopen: Guidance for Schools* (Dublin: Rialtas na hÉireann, 2020).

309 Ibid. 'Many will benefit from relaxation techniques and calming activities, such as mindfulness, drawing, physical activity, music and relaxation/breathing exercises'.

310 Michelle McBride, 'Breathing Bells and Mind Jars: Mindfulness Comes to School', *Irish Times*, 17 January 2017. <https://www.irishtimes.com/news/education/breathing-bells-and-mind-jars-mindfulness-comes-to-school-1.2933176>. Accessed on 12 August 2020.

development and performance, which were highlighted in the previous chapter. In this sense, it is completely understandable why schools have employed mindfulness due to the many benefits attributed to it, especially improved wellbeing. At a time where children's mental health is increasingly challenged by external factors including smartphone overuse,[311] cyberbullying[312] and the ongoing consequences of the pandemic,[313] resources that can improve child wellbeing are to be welcomed. Thus, wellbeing as a key goal of the Social, Personal and Health Education (SPHE) subject has acted as the vehicle for mindfulness practice in Irish primary schools.

This is primarily done so by making connections between mindfulness and wellbeing promotion in the SPHE subject, as well as through what is called the 'hidden curriculum'. This '… refers to the unspoken or implicit values, behaviours, procedures, and norms that exist in the educational setting'.[314] This is akin to the ethos of a school. For a Catholic school, the full and harmonious development of the child is synonymous with the child enjoying positive wellbeing as they reach their full potential. In this sense, mindfulness does not contradict the characteristic spirit of a Catholic school, as it too seeks to help children flourish. It can be understood as a

311 Samantha Sohn, Philippa Rees, Bethany Wildridge, Nicola J. Kalk and Ben Carter, 'Prevalence of Problematic Smartphone Usage and Associated Mental Health Outcomes amongst Children and Young People: a Systematic Review, Meta-analysis and GRADE of the Evidence', *BMC Psychiatry 19*(Article Number 356) (2019).

312 Jo Inchley, Dorothy Currie, Sanja Budisavljevic, Torbjørn Torsheim, Atle Jåstad, Alina Cosma, Colette Kelly, Ársæll Már Arnarsson and Oddrun Samdal, eds, *Spotlight on Adolescent Health and Well-being: Findings from the 2017/2018 Health Behaviour in School-aged Children (HBSC) Survey in Europe and Canada. International Report. Vol. 2. Key data (Copenhagen*, World Health Organisation Regional Office for Europe, 2020).

313 Katriona O' Sullivan, Serena Clark, Amy McGrane, Nicole Rock, Lydia Burke, Neasa Boyle, Natasha Joksimovic and Kevin Marshall, 'A Qualitative Study of Child and Adolescent Mental Health during the COVID-19 Pandemic in Ireland', *International Journal of Environmental Research and Public Health, 18*(3) (2021), 1062 and Margaret Curtin, Maria O' Shea and Claire Hayes, 'The Impact and Lived Experience of Covid-19 Restrictions for Vulnerable Children and Families in a Low-Income Irish Community', *Child Care in Practice 29*(4) (2023), 470–86.

314 Merfat Ayesh Alsubaie, 'Hidden Curriculum as One of Current Issue of Curriculum', *Journal of Education and Practice 6*(33) (2015), 1.

secular psychological resource for wellbeing promotion in a setting inspired by Gospel values and vivified by the person of Jesus Christ.

Wellbeing is set to become a more visible and significant curricular area in primary schools, as seen in the new *Curriculum Framework for Primary and Special Schools*[315], which replaces the 1999 Primary School Curriculum. This is observed in the placing of wellbeing as both a curricular subject and a key competency. First, the proposed curriculum changes include the merging of PE and SPHE into a single Wellbeing subject with a time allocation of 3 hour per week. This contrasts with the hour and a half per week for PE and SPHE in the previous curriculum. Second, wellbeing has been enshrined one of seven key competencies of the new curriculum, which as its overarching vision: '… aims to provide a strong foundation for every child to thrive and flourish, supporting them in realising their full potential as individuals and as members of communities and society during childhood and into the future'.[316] This identification of wellbeing as a key competency as well as a specific subject highlights a conception of education as a process of human development, enabling children to achieve success as individuals and grow to be citizens that contribute to the good of society. However, it is important that this new curricular focus on wellbeing does not become subject to a neoliberal educational agenda, seeing wellbeing as key to productive and efficient workers, rather than happy and flourishing human beings.

Such an explicit commitment to the wellbeing promotion of each child irrespective of background, ability or creed is a welcome and vital proposition for a curriculum. For children to reach their potential, positive wellbeing is an essential aspect of their development. As highlighted earlier, mindfulness practice has been shown to assist students in fostering physical and mental wellbeing, which in turn can help children thrive and reach their potential. In this sense, mindfulness as a technique to improve wellbeing is congruent with the vision of the new Primary Curriculum in its commitment to wellbeing promotion.

In the new Primary Curriculum, attributes under the aforementioned wellbeing competency include 'Being self-aware and resilient,' and 'Acting

315 National Council for Curriculum and Assessment, *Primary Curriculum Framework for Primary and Special Schools* (Dublin: NCCA, 2023), 38–9.

316 Ibid, 5.

responsibly and showing care towards self and others,' and 'Being spiritual and having a sense of purpose and meaning'.[317] While mindfulness is certainly applicable to the former two attributes, it is unclear whether it can or should be applicable to the latter in this context. Mindfulness traces its origins to forms of Buddhist meditation, but in the Western context, it has been reframed, secularised and simplified in order to make the practice more universally accessible. Mindfulness in schools is almost universally understood as a secular psychological activity, deracinated from its Buddhist origins. While Chapter 2 highlights MBSR founder Jon Kabat-Zinn's sometimes vague and problematic language on the secularity of mindfulness, programmes such as MBSR are promoted as secular and not in conflict with any religious tradition.

The National Council for Curriculum and Assessment (NCCA) states that the wellbeing competency '... also recognises the spiritual dimension of living, which enables children to experience a sense of awe and wonder and know that life has a meaning'.[318] It is unclear whether mindfulness as a psychological resource fits into this spiritual framework. This is not to dismiss the life-giving benefits that mindfulness practice can provide to people's wellbeing. Moreover, this is not to dismiss the idea that mindfulness can be a spiritual activity that cultivates a person's awareness of the sacred in life. Rather, it is important to notice the incoherence of framing forms of mindfulness such as Mindfulness 1 as secular and psychological while also implying spiritual benefits.

However, Mindfulness 3 as a post-secular spiritual resource can assist in locating mindfulness as a psychological activity which also operates as a contemplative practice for students. This approach would challenge any presupposed spiritual/secular binary in mindfulness, instead providing a resource that contributes to students' wellbeing while also nurturing a contemplative outlook. In the Catholic school, this would translate as cultivating

317 Ibid, 13.
318 Ibid, 9.

a sacramental imagination[319] in students, where there is an encouragement to see the world as engraced, God's presence mediated across every possible facet of our experiences. In this sense, students became aware of the deeper sources and questions of meaning and authenticity in life, which echoes Michael Paul Gallagher's argument that being present in moments of silence allows the person to become consciously aware of mystery, a sense of otherness that transcends their everyday experience and social imaginary. This approach offers opportunities for dialogue between forms of mindfulness practices and the sacramentality of Catholic education, which will be explored in the next two chapters.

At a time of significant concerns over child wellbeing, mindfulness is emerging as a beneficial resource to help lower anxiety and improve attention albeit in need of further robust study. Thus, mindfulness in schools fits into the broader discourse of wellbeing in schools. With this in mind, and similar to post-primary level, curricular reforms seek to embed wellbeing as a foundational theme in primary schools. As mindfulness has been demonstrated to offer a raft of wellbeing benefits, schools utilise mindfulness as an aid to child wellbeing. In this sense, this explicit focus on wellbeing is a welcome development as holistic wellbeing must be at the heart of the educational endeavour.

It remains unclear whether mindfulness as a secular psychological activity is meant to have benefits to a student's spiritual wellbeing in the New Primary Curriculum. Mindfulness 3 represents a means to addressing this question as it presents mindfulness as a post-secular spirituality. For the Catholic school, resources that are shown to help students enjoy a holistic educational approach and improve wellbeing are welcome. Moreover, Mindfulness 3 presents an opportunity to nurture a sacramental imagination in students, which will be explored in the next two chapters.

319 According to theologian Thomas Groome, the principle of sacramentality '... reflects the central Catholic conviction that God mediates Godself to us and we encounter God's presence and grace coming to meet us through the ordinary of life'. ... See Thomas Groome, 'What Makes a School Catholic?' In Terence McLaughlin, Joseph O' Keefe and Bernadette O' Keeffe, eds, *The Contemporary Catholic School: Context, Identity and Diversity* (Oxfordshire: RoutledgeFarmer, 1996), 112.

Mindfulness and wellbeing programs in Irish primary schools

In recent years, several initiatives and programmes have emerged focusing on wellbeing enhancement and mindfulness practice in Irish primary education. These programmes include the Paws b course and the Weaving Wellbeing program. These two initiatives have been chosen for investigation as the Paws b course is an explicitly mindfulness-based course consisting of real-time lessons, pedagogy sessions and a wide selection of resources. Paws b is relevant here as it is the first mindfulness programme designed for use in primary schools in Ireland and the United Kingdom. The second program, Weaving Wellbeing is underpinned by the principles of positive psychology and is the first Irish-designed mental health programme of its kind, aimed at enhancing pupil wellbeing. Among the components of Weaving Wellbeing are resilience skills, including mindfulness practices. These are contemporary programs relevant to current discourse on mindfulness in Irish primary schools. As such, both programs will be examined to map out how they are operative within the Irish primary school context.

Paws b

The Paws b mindfulness programme was developed for children aged 7–11 by the UK national non-governmental organisation Mindfulness in Schools Practice (MiSP) in 2013, with the aim of improving mental health and wellbeing.[320] Following reported positive outcomes of the .b programme for

320 'Our aim is to improve the lives of a generation of children and young people by making a genuine, positive difference to their mental health and wellbeing'. <https://mindfulnessinschools.org/about/>. Accessed on 29 August 2020.

teens,[321] MiSP differentiated the content and materials to enable younger children to engage in the mindfulness practices within the .b curriculum. MiSP state that Paws b 'Promotes wellbeing and resilience, offers knowledge and skills applicable to the child's life, can be individually tailored to suit each child, and extends the thinking skills learning which is promoted in the national curriculum such as neuroscience and metacognition'.[322]

The course content of Paws b is six 1-hour lessons delivered weekly, or alternatively split into twelve 30-min lessons.[323] The first lesson introduces the subject of the brain and a discussion of our ability to make decisions. This is followed by a breath counting mindfulness exercise. The second lesson introduces the 'searchlight' of attention, an introduction to the philosophy of mindfulness and includes two mindfulness breathing exercises. The third lesson is made up of a grounding mindfulness exercise and a conversation on 'wobbly feelings'. The fourth lesson contains a 'count and add two' mindfulness breathing exercise and a conversation on how to avoid reacting badly to situations. The fifth lesson includes a discussion of worries and how such worries can be supported by the previously learnt mindfulness practices. Finally, the sixth lesson concludes with a review of learning from the course and practising all of the previously learnt mindfulness exercises.[324]

321 Felicia A. Huppert and Daniel M. Johnson, 'A Controlled Trial of Mindfulness Training in Schools: The Importance of Practice for an Impact on Well-being', *The Journal of Positive Psychology* 5(4) (2010), 264–74; Willem Kuyken, Katherine Weare, Obioha C. Ukoumunne, Rachael Vicary, Nicola Motton, Richard Burnett, Chris Cullen, Sarah Hennelly and Felicia Huppert, 'Effectiveness of the Mindfulness in Schools Programme: Non-Randomised Controlled Feasibility Study', *British Journal of Psychiatry* 203(2) (2013), 126–31.

322 <https://mindfulnessinschools.org/teach-paws-b/>. Accessed on 29 August 2020.

323 <https://mindfulnessinschools.org/teach-paws-b/paws-b-curriculum/>. Accessed on 29 August 2020.

324 George Thomas, 'Evaluating the Impact of the Paws b Mindfulness Programme on Mainstream Primary School Aged Pupils' Suppressing and Sustaining Attention Skills, and their Academic Proxy Measures', (University of Manchester PhD Thesis) (2015), 78. Alternatively, Paws b can be offered via a twelve-lesson curriculum, which is outlined by Wimmer and Dorjee. 'Lesson one provides basic information about the human brain 10 and how mindfulness training can change the brain. Lesson two shows how we

The content of these mindfulness lessons is underpinned by learning about neuroscience with children learning about different areas of the brain such as the frontal cortex and the hippocampus. Also, children learn how our thoughts are connected to our bodies, emotions and actions. Attention is introduced through the analogy of a puppy, which can be trained through an attitude of kindness, gentleness and patience. Children are encouraged to be mindfully aware of their thoughts and to nurture dispositions of kindness and openness to experiences, as well as the importance of keeping the mind and body safe when making decisions.

The tone of these lessons is influenced by positive psychology, especially seen in the final two lessons which focus on growing and savouring happiness. This includes cultivating ways that we can best care for ourselves and others, as well as developing specific ways to savour happiness. These final two lessons in particular focus on conversations about wellbeing and how best to flourish into a happy, kind and grateful person.

Any program that cultivates a content, benevolent and thriving child deserves praise as child mental health and wellbeing continue to be challenged by factors such as cyber-bullying, smartphone overuse, as well as the impact of COVID-19. Lessons that promote kindness and self-care are also praiseworthy in this regard, in that they present an implicit ethic that kindness is not only generated but can be shared with others. The mindfulness practices introduced are intended to improve children's wellbeing and

---

can concentrate and make helpful choices using mindfulness. In lesson three, children experience how they can broaden and narrow their attentional focus with a mindful attitude. Lesson four is about the application of mindfulness in everyday situations. In lesson five pupils learn about the nature of dynamic changes in our mental and bodily states. Lesson six teaches how mindful attention can help us stabilize our mind and body. Lesson seven explores how we tend to cope in challenging situations. In lesson eight children learn how mindfulness can help them nurture their well-being. Lesson nine is about the power of thoughts and the habits of our minds. Lesson 10 teaches how the mind is connected to emotions, behaviour, and bodily reactions, and how this connection can be modulated with the help of mindfulness. In lesson eleven pupils learn how to mindfully take care of themselves and others. Lesson 12 is about how to cherish moments of joy and happiness'. Lena Franziska Wimmer and Dusana Dorjee, 'Towards Determinants and Effects of Long-Term Mindfulness Training in Pre-adolescence: A Cross-Sectional Study Using Event-Related Potentials', *Journal of Cognitive Education and Psychology 19* (2020), 10.

resilience through nurturing an awareness of the present moment and of their thoughts and feelings. In this way, Paws b may offer potential benefits to primary school children, not least Catholic schools, in terms of emotional wellbeing.

It is also stressed several times on the Paws b website that the participants in the course may not teach fellow educators the Paws b programme. Moreover, for acceptance into the course, there are five specific pre-requisites to meet.

The first is that applicants must have completed an 8-week mindfulness course. There is a prescribed list of suitable courses, including MBSR (Kabat-Zinn's Mindfulness-Based Stress Reduction) and MBCT (Mindfulness-Based Cognitive-Therapy). The rationale for this criterion is that 'This training forms an essential foundation and experiential understanding of a range of mindfulness practices that are necessary for teaching Paws b, and it is assumed that you have engaged in these practices extensively before attending a Teach Paws b course'.[325] This criterion assumes that applicants understand mindfulness practices within the secular psychological framework of Mindfulness 1.

The second and third pre-requisites outline the necessity of applicants having a rigorous and extensive personal mindfulness practice, encompassing 5 out of 7 day a week for 2–3 months. The rationale for this is that the greater the personal practice, the greater the teacher's capacity to model mindfulness in the classroom.[326] The fourth requirement is full attendance at the 3-day Paws b course. The fifth and final requirement is a commitment to personal practice as well as teaching mindfulness to the highest professional standards.

Research on the effects of Paws b in the classroom remains at an embryonic stage. Moreover, while the current research suggests improvements in

325 <https://mindfulnessinschools.org/prerequisites/paws-b/>. Accessed on 31 August 2020.

326 Ibid. This period of 2–3 months embedding helps to stabilise and deepen your practice, which leads to a level of familiarity with the subtle workings of your mind. This in turn strengthens your capacity to model mindfulness in holding the experience of others and to respond skilfully if difficult situations arise for young people in the classroom.

child wellbeing, there are several limitations evident in the literature that at least temper some of the research findings.[327]

To date, there have been several small, controlled studies on the effects of Paws b, two of which NHS Scotland deemed to be inconsistent in a 2017 review of health and wellbeing interventions in schools.[328] This review was limited to research from Ireland and the United Kingdom to ensure findings were as relevant to Scottish schools as possible. One study[329] found that teacher-rated outcomes, including self-reflection and self-awareness improved significantly for children who had completed the Paws b programme compared to those who had received usual school provision. However, parents did not report the same positive improvements and found no positive changes in their children's emotional wellbeing.[330] This finding was in contrast to a study that found Paws b had decreased negative affect and improved meta-cognition in pupils.[331] While findings that offer potential benefits for child wellbeing are welcome, this study itself had several limitations, including

327 Chilcott's review of Paws b literature found significant limitations across each of the studies, meaning caution is necessary when interpreting purported benefits of the practice. These limitations included many reports using self-reporting measures and all reports hamstrung by insufficient long-term follow-up measures. See Lloyd Chilcott, 'Academic Critique of Paws b, a Mindfulness Based Intervention for Children', University of Southampton Blog, (2021). <https://blog.soton.ac.uk/edpsych/files/2021/07/PAWS-B-Jan-2021-Lloyd-Chilcott.pdf>. Accessed on 18 March 2024.

328 Janet White, *Rapid Evidence Review: Reducing the Attainment Gap – The Role of Health and Wellbeing Interventions in Schools* (Edinburgh: NHS Health Scotland, 2017), 9.

329 George Thomas and Cathy Atkinson, 'Measuring the Effectiveness of a Mindfulness-Based Intervention for Children's Attentional Functioning', *Educational & Child Psychology 33*(1) (2016), 51–64.

330 Janet White, *Rapid Evidence Review: Reducing the Attainment Gap – The Role of Health and Wellbeing Interventions in Schools* (Edinburgh: NHS Health Scotland, 2017), 9.

331 Charlotte E. Vickery and Dusanna Dorjee, 'Mindfulness Training in Primary Schools Decreases Negative Affect and Increases Meta-Cognition in Children', *Front Psychology* 6 (2016), 2025.

a small sample size, no control group and no randomisation[332] and did not explicitly find improvements in child wellbeing.[333]

More recent studies on the effects have found that the Paws b programme was sufficient to improve pupils' attention skills[334] as well as superior response inhibition and emotion regulation to peers who did not practice mindfulness.[335] These findings are welcome as they suggest that Paws b offers several benefits to child wellbeing and enable greater attention skills. However, several limitations are also found in these studies including small sample size.[336] Crompton et al.'s

332 Ibid. This study did not allow for randomisation of groups and further research is needed using a more stringent design. In addition, this study did not utilise an alternative active control (in addition to treatment as usual control) which somewhat reduces the validity of conclusions concerning benefits of the mindfulness program on emotional well-being and effect sizes being attributable to mindfulness alone, or other non-specific intervention factors such as novelty. A further limitation of this study was the use of non-blind teacher and parental ratings which limited the reliability of findings for meta-cognition. However, the parallel use of both raters aimed to increase the internal validity of informant-based measures and enabled us to exercise caution in the interpretation of significant improvements for meta-cognition regarding discrepancies between teacher and parental ratings at follow-up. Although this study used a follow-up design, it was limited to 3 months.

333 Ibid. 'We did not find significant longitudinal changes in measures of mindfulness, PA, emotional awareness and expressive reluctance, and positive well-being'.

334 George Thomas, '*Evaluating the Impact of the Paws b Mindfulness Programme on Mainstream Primary School Aged Pupils' Suppressing and Sustaining Attention Skills, and Their Academic Proxy Measures*', PhD Thesis, University of Manchester, 2015, 283.

335 Lena Franziska Wimmer and Dusana Dorjee, 'Towards Determinants and Effects of Long-Term Mindfulness Training in Pre-adolescence: A Cross-Sectional Study Using Event-Related Potentials', *Journal of Cognitive Education and Psychology 19*(1) (2020), 22.

336 Nevertheless, several limitations restrict the interpretation of the results. Firstly, the sample size, even though appropriate for an ERP study, was relatively low for self-report comparisons, which limits statistical power. Hence, the study was not able to detect small effects. Secondly, differences between MG (Main Group) and CG (Control Group) cannot be interpreted as causal effects of mindfulness training due to the cross-sectional design/self-selection of groups. Systematic group differences other than degree of mindfulness experience could be confounding factors. For instance, both groups were based in two schools that used different media of instruction MG received school lessons in English, whereas CG were taught in Welsh. Since all children were fluent in English, this means that most CG were proficient bilinguals. Bilingualism, in turn, has been found to be associated with improved EF ... Hence, working with these controls may have prevented us from detecting mindfulness-based benefits on EF'. Ibid, 22.

study found that the programme could increase some aspects of prosociality, as judged by peers and teachers, but had no effect on self-assessed empathy. Again, several important limitations were identified, reinforcing the need for caution in analysing the results.[337]

This is not to deny the potentially life-giving benefits of mindfulness for children in the classroom. Rather, in order to ensure that child wellbeing is cultivated and enhanced in the classroom, research must be robust in order to justify the claims of wellbeing improvement through classroom-based mindfulness interventions. While some findings may find positive outcomes for child wellbeing, it is imperative that these findings can be replicated on a larger scale, utilising necessary research methods to ensure the feasibility of the results. In this way, mindfulness can become an evidence-based method of helping children to flourish, which would be a boon for all schools, not least Catholic schools.

The only available Irish study on Paws b was conducted with 48 children aged 10–11 in a large urban Dublin primary school.[338] While many children enjoyed the mindfulness practice, the researchers found that 'The children's accounts suggest that mindfulness offers symptomatic relief, and that mindfulness is becoming entangled with a neoliberal agenda—creating better learners and test takers who are more in control of their emotions'.[339] While this was a small-scale study, the children's accounts echo Forbes and Purser's arguments that mindfulness may provide relief without addressing the sources of their stress. There is a danger that an educational system that focuses on productivity and efficiency could utilise mindfulness as a performance enhancer rather than a means of cultivating children's wellbeing.

337 Katie Crompton, Daphne Kaklamanou, Allesandra Fasulo and Eszter Somogyi, 'The Effects of a School-Based Mindfulness Programme (Paws b) on Empathy and Prosocial Behaviour: A Randomised Controlled Trial', *Mindfulness 15*(3) (2024).

338 Catriona O'Toole and Fiona O'Connor, 'A Reprieve but not a Fix for Childhood Stresses: A Participatory Study of Schoolbased Mindfulness in an Irish Primary School' (ECER 2017 Conference) <https://www.maynoothuniversity.ie/sites/default/files/assets/document/ECER%202017%20Conference%20-%20Presentation%20by%20Dr.%20Catriona%20O%27Toole_0.pdf>. Accessed on 1 September 2020.

339 Ibid. (Slide 16.)

The available research suggests that while Paws b may have benefits to child wellbeing, current data is not rigorous enough to state this definitively. The research thus far has been hampered by different limitations such as small sample sizes, no control groups or lack of randomisation. These issues mean that established critical research on the benefits of Paws b remains scarce, reflecting Ergas and Hadar's earlier observation on mindfulness and education literature.[340] This should not serve as a dismissal of Paws b as a potential mindfulness resource for cultivating child wellbeing. Resources that enhance the child's capacity to flourish are a welcome and increasingly important currency in Irish education. However, caution is required over the benefits of the programme thus far, until more rigorous, large-scale research and stringent research methods are applied. O'Toole and O'Connor's conclusions are apt in this regard.

> We should be cautious about uncritical acceptance of mindfulness programmes in school settings … Caution about overselling mindfulness and overstating the potential of individual students to transcend their difficult circumstances.[341]

In this sense, while Paws b may offer positive outcomes for child wellbeing, it is imperative that the enthusiasm for mindfulness practice in the classroom does not overtake what current research can establish on the Paws b course. Moreover, it is equally imperative that research on the programme is critical, rigorous and subject to the highest academic standards.

While there are some emerging studies that promote the positive emotional wellbeing of pupils, there is need for larger studies using a range of research methods to ensure the integrity of findings. Resources that are

340 'The nascency of the field is expressed in a surprising and potentially unhealthy paucity of critical papers in this field. The amount of critical papers found seems small and possibly suggests an immature and over-optimistic phase of this discourse.' Oren Ergas and Linor L. Hadar, 'Mindfulness in and as Education: A Map of a Developing Academic Discourse from 2002 to 2017', *Review of Education* (2019), 35.

341 Catriona O'Toole and Fiona O'Connor, 'A Reprieve but not a Fix for Childhood Stresses: A Participatory Study of School based Mindfulness in an Irish Primary School' (ECER 2017 Conference) <https://www.maynoothuniversity.ie/sites/default/files/assets/document/ECER%202017%20Conference%20-%20Presentation%20by%20Dr.%20Catriona%20O%27Toole_0.pdf> (accessed on 1 September 2020) (Slide 19).

evidenced to decrease anxiety and cultivate a child's ability to flourish is welcome. Mindfulness could then be a life-giving practice that reduces suffering and stress. More comprehensive research on Paws b would ensure that enthusiasm for mindfulness does not oversell what are the established evidence on Paws b benefits.

Paws b offers a resource to Catholic schools insofar as it enables students to greater attentiveness to the present moment. However, in order to live out the Catholic ethos of a school, mindfulness cannot be just a self-centred or self-focused activity.[342] Noel Keatings's Christian Meditation project offers such an Other-centred approach to meditation.[343] However, as was highlighted in both this and the previous chapter, there remains a danger of mindfulness in schools being misappropriated to buffer a neoliberal educational agenda, privatising and individualising stress.

In order to interrogate the compatibility of mindfulness and Catholic ethos, a robust Catholic educational vision must then be presented in the next chapter. This will outline the operative anthropology and epistemology in the Catholic school, mapping out areas for evaluating the relationship between Catholic ethos and mindfulness.

Paws b seeks to use mindfulness to develop resilience and positive mental and emotional wellbeing in children. Similar to Mindfulness 1, the curriculum content has a psychological framing, with children learning

342 This is not a criticism of mindfulness. Rather, it is a descriptive term, as in secular mindfulness the intention of the practitioner is primarily the wellbeing of the practitioner. This distinction is expressed in the Irish Catholic Bishops' Conference's reflection on mindfulness, which explores how meditation in a Christian sense is rooted in a loving relationship with Christ. In this sense, the aim of Christian meditation is to become aware of the Spirit of God at work in our hearts. See Council for Catechetics, Irish Catholic Bishops' Conference, *A Reflection on Mindfulness: Rediscovering the Christian Tradition of Meditation and Contemplation* (Dublin: Veritas, 2018).

343 For Keating, the intention of meditation is of fundamental importance. In Christian Meditation, the intention is Other-centred in that it is rooted in deepening a relationship with God, 'In the Christian tradition, this Other is named as Christ. The Christian tradition teaches that one of the deep fruits of Christian contemplative practice is that it leads to a more authentic, more compassionate, Christ-centred way of being in the world'. See Noel Keating, *Meditation with Children: A Resource for Teachers and Parents* (Dublin: Veritas, 2017), 40.

about techniques, neuroscience and how our thoughts are connected to our bodies, emotions and actions. Children are encouraged to be attuned to their thoughts and to nurture dispositions of kindness and gratitude to help them flourish and find meaning in their lives. While there may be some early developments on how Paws b positively impacts pupil wellbeing, many of these studies have often been hampered by research limitations. In this sense, courses like Paws b cannot be revered as a breakthrough in supporting child wellbeing just yet.

The attentiveness to the present moment makes possible for the pupil a deeper awareness and appreciation of God's presence in their lives. However, for mindfulness to make an authentic contribution to Catholic ethos, it is necessary that these practices translate into meaningful actions as followers of Christ, through striving for social justice and displaying a preferential option for the poor and marginalised. For a Catholic school, Christian mindfulness must be self-forgetting and ultimately mindful of the other. In this regard, a detailed overview of a Catholic educational vision is needed to help us answer the question at the heart of this work.

Weaving Wellbeing

Founded by primary teacher Fiona Forman and life coach Mick Rock, Weaving Wellbeing is a mental health and wellbeing programme underpinned by positive psychology, which includes mindfulness techniques in its curriculum content. According to its website, it is '… the first Irish designed positive mental health programme of its kind which aims to enhance wellbeing in children aged from 8 to 12 years'.[344] Since its launch, Weaving Wellbeing has grown beyond its original Irish primary education market into Australian schools also.[345,346]

344 <https://weavingwellbeing.com/>. Accessed on 7 September 2020.
345 <https://www.hbe.com.au/hb5343.html>. Accessed on 7 September 2020.
346 <https://weavingwellbeing.com/current-news/>. Accessed on 7 September 2020.

The programme is completed over 10 weeks, with 10 lessons per class level from 2nd Class to 6th Class, and each lesson is completed over one week. As the content of these lessons is on wellbeing promotion, Weaving Wellbeing aligns with the stated aims of the SPHE subject as well as wellbeing policy statements by the Department of Education and Skills highlighted earlier. However, in order to examine Weaving Wellbeing, it is first necessary to outline the concept of positive psychology, which Forman makes clear has had a profound impact on the programme.[347]

Positive psychology has been described as '… the scientific study of optimal functioning. It seeks to identify the strengths and skills that enable individuals and communities to thrive'.[348] Widely associated with the work of American psychologist Martin Seligman, this approach seeks to complement traditional forms of psychology which primarily focus on disease and healing deficits in human functioning. Seligman argues that unlike these approaches which deal almost exclusively with repairing pathological damage, the aim of positive psychology is to go beyond this, '… to catalyse a change in the focus of psychology from preoccupation with the worst things in life to also building positive qualities'.[349] Positive psychology is thus concerned with developing a scientific lens on how people flourish and live happy, fulfilling lives. In this sense, positive psychology can be described as the science of optimising wellbeing.

The positive qualities associated with improving wellbeing and flourishing are categorised by Seligman and psychologist Christopher Peterson

347 'To enhance children's well-being by teaching them evidence-based skills and strategies from positive psychology, to help them to become resilient and flourishing members of society'. Fiona Forman, *'An Introduction to positive psychology and The Weaving Well-Being Programme',* CPD Presentation for Scoil an Spioraid Naoimh, Layton (2018). <http://ssnlaytown.ie/wp-content/uploads/2018/08/Laytown-Weaving-Well-Being-002.pdf> (Slide 44) (accessed on 7 September 2020).

348 Joseph Ciarrochi, Paul W. B. Atkins, Louise L. Hayes, Baljinder K. Sahdra and Philip Parker, 'Contextual Positive Psychology: Policy Recommendations for Implementing Positive Psychology into Schools,' *Frontiers in Psychology*, 10 October 2016.

349 Martin E. P. Seligman and Mihaly Csikszentmihalyi, 'Positive Psychology: An Introduction', *American Psychologist* 55(1) (2000) 5.

into twenty-six Character Strengths and six core Virtues (CSV).[350] This categorisation of virtues resembles to an extent Aristotelian virtue ethics and their appropriation by St Thomas Aquinas in the sense that the overarching theme is on living 'the good life', or a virtuous life. Scientific studies to understand and promote human flourishing are welcome as endeavours that propose ways to help people leave meaningfully and virtuously are needed at a time when mental health concerns are increasingly prevalent in society. Moreover, the virtues listed in the framework are proposed as transcultural and universal in order to be accessible to as many people as possible. However, this universalising and decontextualising of human virtues risks undermining contextual factors that influence the capacity to flourish such as culture, family and social class. This concern was raised in the previous chapter by Forbes and Purser regarding the radical decontextualisation of mindfulness in MBSR from its traditional Buddhist framework to widen its accessibility.[351] The content of a radically decontextualised mindfulness risks privatising and individualising stress rather than challenging societal and contextual sources of suffering. This same 'content over context' critique could also be applicable to universalising virtues while potentially

350 Martin E. P. Seligman and Christopher Peterson, *Character Strengths and Virtues: A Handbook and Classification* (Oxford, Oxford University Press, 2004). The virtues and character strengths are listed as:

1. *Wisdom and Knowledge*: creativity, curiosity, open-mindedness, love of learning, perspective, innovation
2. *Courage*: bravery, persistence, integrity, vitality, zest
3. *Humanity*: love, kindness, social intelligence
4. *Justice*: citizenship, fairness, leadership
5. *Temperance*: forgiveness and mercy, humility, prudence, self-control
6. *Transcendence*: appreciation of beauty and excellence, gratitude, hope, humour, spirituality <http://www.ldysinger.com/@books1/Peterson_Character_Strengths/character-strengths-and-virtues.pdf>. Accessed on 8 September 2020.

351 'The cultivation of "right mindfulness" is only one part of the Buddha's Eightfold Path, along with "right" understanding, intention, speech, action, livelihood, effort and concentration ... However, the other dimensions that support 'right mindfulness'— which leads to wisdom by cultivating wholesome mental states- are left out of MBSR, suggesting its teachers have misconstrued Buddhist ethics. See Ronald E. Purser, *McMindfulness: How Mindfulness Became the New Capitalist Spirituality* (London: Repeater, 2019), 79.

undermining contextual contingencies that influence an individual's flourishing. This can have implications for Catholic schools which have a distinctive underlying anthropology and conception of human flourishing explicitly taught in religious education.

Seligman's pioneering work in positive psychology has heavily influenced the development of Weaving Wellbeing, with co-author Fiona Forman citing Seligman's proposed PERMA[352] model of wellbeing as the guiding framework of the programme.[353]

The programme is divided into class levels each with an overarching theme which is then subdivided into several themes for exploration as outlined in the framework map[354] in Figure 1. Mindfulness is explicitly located at the 4th Class level associated with the Resilience theme.

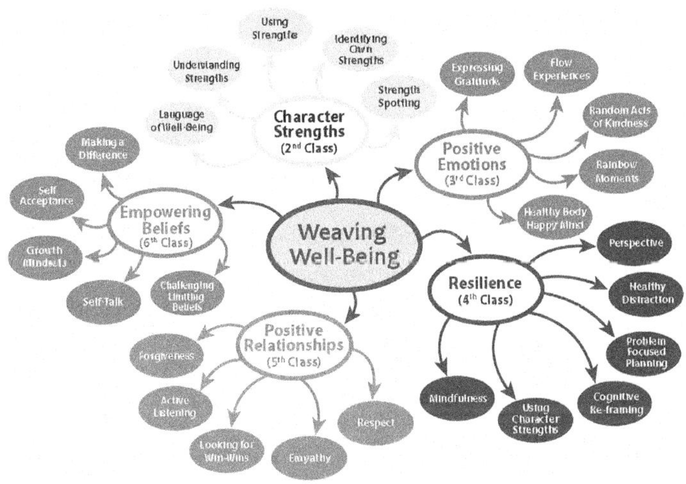

Figure 1: Weaving wellbeing mind map.

352 Positive Emotion, Engagement, Relationships, Meaning, Accomplishment. See Martin E. P. Seligman, *Flourish: A Visionary New Understanding of Wellbeing and Happiness* (NY: Free Press, 2011).

353 Fiona Forman, '*Summary of Findings of the Pilot Stage of the Weaving Wellbeing Programme*' (NUIG Health Promotion Conference 2019). <http://www.nuigalway.ie/media/healthpromotionresearchcentre/conference2019/Fiona-Forman.pdf> (Slide 6). Accessed on 8 September 2020.

354 <https://weavingwellbeing.com/wp-content/uploads/2015/07/Mndmap-Weaving-Well-Being-Dec-2016-Low-Res.jpg>. Accessed on 8 September 2020.

The Weaving Wellbeing lessons are designed for implementation within the guidelines and objectives of both the current SPHE and the upcoming Wellbeing curricular subject. The multi-year structure entails development and progression of these themes and sub-themes (including mindfulness) using age-appropriate pedagogies, resources and practices.[355] Arguably the greatest strength of this programme is providing children with a vocabulary to understand, recognise and talk about wellbeing. Examples of this include working definitions of resilience as:

> … being able to bounce back from all of the normal set-backs, disappointments and failures which are part of everyday life. We can strengthen our resilience by learning about certain skills which we can think of as our very own Tools of Resilience.[356]

This also includes introducing the concept of wellbeing as:

> … feeling good and strong in our minds and bodies, having energy, getting along with and helping others, knowing our strengths and feeling proud because we are doing our best. It means we can cope with the little problems and disappointments of life. It means enjoying life, being grateful for what we have and accepting ourselves just as we are![357]

This development of child-friendly language and activities on wellbeing is a welcome and humanising resource for many classrooms, providing concrete teaching materials to help children acknowledge how and why to improve their wellbeing.

The Weaving Wellbeing structure essentially seeks to enable children to weave positivity into their daily lives in thoughts, feelings and outlook. This is achieved through the reinforcement and revision of seven key psychological concepts across the Weaving Wellbeing multi-year program: Growth Mindset, Language of Wellbeing, Self-Efficacy, Character Strengths,

355 Free samples of the workbooks used across the different classes are available on the Weaving Wellbeing website. <https://weavingwellbeing.com/sample-books/>. Accessed on 14 September 2020.

356 <https://www.actnow.ie/wp-content/uploads/2018/04/Tools-of-Resilience-Pupil-Book-Sample-Copy.pdf 2>.

357 <https://www.actnow.ie/wp-content/uploads/2018/04/Character-Strengths-Pupil-Book-Sample-Copy.pdf 1>.

Cognitive Reframing, Emotional Competence, Social Competence and Making a Difference. Figure 2 details this process.[358]

Reinforcement and Progression of Core Concepts through the Weaving Well-Being Programme

Weaving Well-Being

Growth Mindset	Language of Well-Being	Self-Efficacy	Character Strengths	Cognitive Reframing	Emotional Competence	Social Competence	Making a Difference
2nd Class: All Lessons	2nd Class: Lessons 1 & 2	2nd Class: Lesson 2	2nd Class: Lessons 3 - 10		2nd Class: Lessons 4, 5 & 10	2nd Class: Lessons 5, 6 & 10	2nd Class: Lesson 10
3rd Class: All Lessons	3rd Class: Lesson 1	3rd Class: Lesson 3	3rd Class: Lesson 4		3rd Class: Lessons 2 - 10	3rd Class: Lessons 4 & 6	3rd Class: Lesson 6
4th Class: All Lessons	4th Class: Lesson 1	4th Class: Lessons 2 - 10	4th Class: Lesson 6	4th Class: Lesson 5	4th Class: Lessons 7 - 10	4th Class: Lesson 10	4th Class: Lesson 1
5th Class: All Lessons	5th Class: Lesson 1	5th Class: Lesson 10	5th Class: Lesson 6	5th Class: Lesson 8	5th Class: Lesson 3	5th Class: Lessons 2 - 10	5th Class: Lesson 9
6th Class: All Lessons	6th Class: Lesson 1	6th Class: Lessons 1-10	6th Class: Lesson 5	6th Class: Lessons 1, 2 & 4	6th Class: Lesson 7	6th Class: Lesson 7	6th Class: Lesson 8

Reference (Weissberg, R. P., Goren, P., Domitrovich, C., & Dusenbury, L. (2013). CASEL guide: Effective social and emotional learning programs: Preschool and elementary school edition. Chicago, IL: CASEL)

Figure 2: Weaving wellbeing concept reinforcement and progression table.

In Weaving Wellbeing, mindfulness practices are seen as tools to help build resilience in students, enabling them to deal with adversity while protecting their wellbeing. In this way, mindfulness practice can be embedded as a method of cultivating resilience and improving wellbeing. Like Paws b, mindfulness practice is strongly linked to teaching children about neuroscience and how mindfulness affects certain parts of the brain. In this sense, both approaches are psychologically based understandings of mindfulness as a tool for awareness and regulation of thought processes. However, unlike Paws b, mindfulness in Weaving Wellbeing is one of several activities for building resilience and improving pupil wellbeing.

Unlike Paws b, there are no pre-requisites for the implementation of Weaving Wellbeing, such as completion of a mindfulness course, personal mindfulness practice or compulsory training. EPV approved and non-EPV

358 <https://weavingwellbeing.com/wp-content/uploads/2015/07/WWB-Reinforcement-Progression-tableV4-for-WEB.jpg>. Accessed on 14 September 2020.

approved courses[359] in Weaving Wellbeing are available for teachers via face-to-face courses at regional teacher education centres or online courses. However, unlike the pre-requisites of Paws b, completion of these courses is not obligatory for teachers implementing Weaving Wellbeing.

A major advantage of courses in Weaving Wellbeing is their proposed applicability to the School Self-Evaluation (SSE) process.[360] SSE is promoted as a collaborative, reflective process of internal school review, enabling teachers to systematically review their teaching and learning in order to help schools improve student learning outcomes. The implementation of Weaving Wellbeing on a whole-school basis offers several possible advantages to SSE, including the development of school policies on wellbeing, strategies to improve wellbeing across the school community and exploring resources to improve teacher wellbeing.

In this sense, the broader goal of Weaving Wellbeing is to develop schools rather than individual classes in weaving facets of positive psychology into the educational endeavour, improving teaching, learning and wellbeing. This turn to nurturing a child's awareness and understanding of wellbeing is to be welcomed as in light of growing concerns over child mental health and anxiety, schools must be equipped to help each child thrive and reach their full potential. This should be seen as complementary rather than

359 According to the Department of Education and Skills, 'Under rule 58 of the Rules for National Schools, teachers are entitled to Extra Personal Vacation (EPV) on foot of attending approved summer courses'. <https://www.education.ie/en/Education-Staff/Services/Breaks-Leave/Extra-Personal-Vacation-Days/>. Accessed on 14 September 2020. Typically, these courses are offered during July and August and completion of one EPV course entitles a teacher to three additional days of paid leave, often called 'course days'.

360 <https://www.education.ie/en/Schools-Colleges/Services/Quality-Assurance/SSE-Primary-and-Post-Primary/School-Self-Evaluation.html#:~:text=School%20self%2Devaluation%20(SSE),to%20improve%20outcomes%20for%20learners>. Accessed on 14 September 2020. For further reading, see Department of Education and Skills, *Circular 0040/20: Arrangements for Inspection and School Self-Evaluation for the 2020/2021 School Year* (2020). <https://www.education.ie/en/Circulars-and-Forms/Active-Circulars/cl0040_2020.pdf> and Department of Education and Skills, *Looking at our Schools 2016: A Quality Framework for Primary Schools* (Dublin: Rialtais na hÉireann, 2016).

contradictory to the work of the Catholic school in nurturing each child to reach their full potential. In this sense, schools should critically reflect on the values promoted in Weaving Wellbeing and the underlying values and virtues that contribute to the distinctiveness of the school's characteristic spirit to ascertain their compatibility.

However, further research is required to discern the relationship between positive psychology programs and religious education in Catholic schools. While programs like Weaving Wellbeing may, given sufficient research, support pupil wellbeing, it is a secular resource that can complement but not replace the commitment to support the holistic development of pupils in the Catholic school, which includes nurturing the spiritual development of pupils in light of the Good News. As such, this is an area of research that merits further consideration elsewhere.

Research on the Weaving Wellbeing programme is at an early stage. According to programme co-founder Fiona Forman, there are several research projects underway at colleges and universities, including Mary Immaculate College, Trinity College Dublin, NUI Galway and University College Dublin.[361] While much of this research is currently publicly unavailable, it highlights a growing interest in the programme and its impact in schools.[362] The programme has grown in popularity over recent years, with over two hundred Irish primary schools estimated to have used Weaving Wellbeing in 2017.[363] The popularity of teacher education courses in Weaving Wellbeing, along with the increased focus on wellbeing at the curricular and policy

361 Fiona Forman, *'Summary of Findings of the Pilot Stage of the Weaving Wellbeing Programme'* (NUIG Health Promotion Conference 2019) (Slide 22) <http://www.nuigalway.ie/media/healthpromotionresearchcentre/conference2019/Fiona-Forman.pdf>. Accessed on 15 September 2020.

362 Caitríona Mulcahy, *Does the Weaving Well-Being Programme (WW) Affect the Academic Achievement and Engagement of Irish Primary School Students?* PhD Thesis, Mary Immaculate College, 2023. <https://dspace.mic.ul.ie/handle/10395/3165>. Accessed on 20 April 2024.

363 John Manning, "'Weaving well-being' Fiona Forman and Mick Rock talk to John Manning about the ground-breaking school programme they developed to teach the power of positivity", *Fingal Independent, 29* April 2017. <https://www.independent.ie/regionals/fingalindependent/lifestyle/weaving-well-being-35649138.html>. Accessed on 15 September 2020.

level, highlights that it is likely many hundreds more primary schools have engaged with the programme. The growing emergence of wellbeing promotion in schools will likely lead to significant increases in research on Weaving Wellbeing.

Available research literature on Weaving Wellbeing is thin. Outcomes of this study included enhanced levels of efficacy, problem-solving and positivity, along with a significant reduction in anxiety, but the results were not generalisable due to a small sample size.[364] However, Forman states that current research projects include larger sample sizes, including one with one hundred and fifty students. Forman's own research includes a pilot study of over one hundred and fifty children nationwide to inform further development of the Weaving Wellbeing programme.[365] Teacher, pupil and parental feedback were very positive, suggesting that Weaving Wellbeing which includes mindfulness exercises, has many potential benefits to child wellbeing. This further strengthens the argument for further research in this area, using larger sample sizes and research methods to provide an objective evaluation on the possible benefits of the programme. For the Catholic school, it is imperative that children have access to evidence-based resources that cultivate a capacity to flourish as the holistic development of the child is central to a Catholic vision of education.

While research on Weaving Wellbeing remains at an early stage, there is a significantly larger body of literature on the effects of other Positive Psychology Interventions (PPIs), similar in scope to Weaving Wellbeing. Waters presents a systematic review of 12 PPIs in schools in international primary and post-primary school contexts.[366] Like Mindfulness-Based Interventions (MBIs) such as Paws b, these PPIs were operative within individual classrooms as opposed to on a whole-school basis. The PPIs included mindfulness meditation curricula offered at an American Catholic high

364 Fiona Forman, *'Summary of Findings of the Pilot Stage of the Weaving Wellbeing Programme'* (NUIG >Health Promotion Conference 2019) (Slide 22). <http://www.nuigalway.ie/media/healthpromotionresearchcentre/conference2019/Fiona-Forman.pdf>. Accessed on 15 September 2020.

365 Ibid, (Slide 23).

366 Lea Waters, 'A Review of School-Based Positive Psychology Interventions', *The Australian Educational and Developmental Psychologist 28*(2) (2011), 75–90.

school[367] and an English private school as part of their religious education programme.[368] These two studies included larger sample sizes than those seen in studies on Paws b (ranging from 120 to 173), included a pre-test and post-test design and used controlled groups. Results included greater emotional-regulation, calmness and self-acceptance.[369] Other PPIs, such as the Penn Resiliency Programme (which includes relaxation techniques and cognitive reframing) and the Strathhaven Positive Psychology Program, have yielded outcomes such as decreased anxiety[370] and increased positive emotions and optimism.[371] It is noteworthy that the quality of research into PPIs is generally higher than that of some MBIs and the vast majority of studies examining Paws b in the sense that there are rigorous research methods applied.[372] This includes control groups being used, generally larger sample sizes of hundreds of students, retests after several years and some studies effectively using a double-blind method for teacher evaluations of student behaviour.

367 Patricia C. Broderick and Stacie Metz, 'Learning to BREATHE: A Pilot Trial of a Mindfulness Curriculum for Adolescents. Advances', *School Mental Health Promotion, 2* (2009), 35–46.

368 Felicia A. Huppert and Daniel M. Johnson, 'A Controlled Trial of Mindfulness Training in Schools: The Importance of Practice for an Impact on Well-being', *The Journal of Positive Psychology 5*(4) (2010), 264–74.

369 Lea Waters, 'A Review of School-Based Positive Psychology Interventions', *The Australian Educational and Developmental Psychologist 28*(2) (2011), 80.

370 Steven M. Brunwasser and Jane E. Gillham, '*A Meta-Analytic Review of the Penn Resiliency Programme*', presented at the Society for Prevention Research, San Francisco, CA, May 2008; Martin E. Seligman, Randall M. Ernst, Jane E., Gillham, Karen J. Reivich and Mark Linkin, 'Positive Education: Positive Psychology and Classroom Interventions', *Oxford Review of Education, 35* (2009), 293–311.

371 Martin E. Seligman, Randall M. Ernst, Jane E, Gillham, Karen J. Reivich and Mark Linkin, 'Positive Education: Positive psychology and Classroom Interventions', *Oxford Review of Education, 35* (2009), 293–311.

372 However, the quality of PPI research has been debated. See Laura Haynes, Owain Service, Ben Goldacre and David Torgerson, *Test, Learn, Adapt: Developing Public Policy with Randomised Controlled Trials* (London: Cabinet Office, 2012) and Gerald M. Rosen and Gerald C. Davison, 'Psychology Should List Empirically Supported Principles of Change (ESPs) and not Credential Trademarked Therapies or Other Treatment Packages', *Behavior Modification 27* (2003), 300–12.

While research on Weaving Wellbeing remains at an early stage, it is likely that similar outcomes could be predicted due to the programme being based on Seligman's PERMA model, which is prominent in many PPIs currently operative in schools internationally. Moreover, Water's review found that the PPIs studied had significant positive impacts on wellbeing and academic performance. Further research on the effects of Weaving Wellbeing is required to evaluate whether these benefits are to be observed in the programme.

Weaving Wellbeing broadly fits into contemporary conceptualisations of education as having an increased emphasis on student wellbeing instead rather than solely academic performance. Moreover, several educationalists have spoken of the renewed importance of education as developing the whole student, that is, encompassing the intellectual, moral, emotional and spiritual development of the student.[373] This has also been expressed by Ergas, O'Donnell and Wexlar earlier in this chapter. In order to assess whether programmes that include mindfulness such as Weaving Wellbeing complement or contradict Catholic ethos, a robust vision of Catholic education is needed, which will be developed in the next chapter.

The influence of Seligman's work on positive psychology on Weaving Wellbeing is profound. It is worth noting that Seiligman identifies as non-religious,[374] but is interested in how religious people have been found to be

373 See Barbera L. McCombs, 'The Learner-Centered Psychological Principles: A Framework for Balancing Academic Achievement and Social-Emotional Learning Outcomes', in Joseph E. Zins, Michelle Bloodworth, Roger Weissberg and Herbert Walberg, eds, *Building Academic Success in Social and Emotional Learning* (New York: Teachers College Press, 2004), 23–9, Nel Noddings, 'A Morally Defensible Mission for Schools in the Twenty First Century', *The Phi Delta Kappan, 76* (1995), 365–8, Parker Palmer, 'Teaching with Heart and Soul: Reflections on Spirituality in Teacher Education', *Journal of Teacher Education, 54* (2003), 376–85.

374 Wendy Schuman, 'The Psychology of Real Happiness: Psychologist Martin Seligman helped change his profession's focus from what's wrong with people to what's right with them. (Interview with Martin Seligman)'. 'But part of my concern is the enormous number of people who, like myself, have no religious beliefs, and yet want to lead a meaningful life'. <https://www.beliefnet.com/wellness/health/2003/01/the-psychology-of-real-happiness.aspx>. Accessed on 1 October 2020.

more optimistic and satisfied with life.[375] In this sense, Seligman is interested in developing a humanistic framework for flourishing and living a meaningful life. While positive psychology is by its nature rigorously scientific and materialist, there remain opportunities for programmes such as Weaving Wellbeing to make a significant contribution to the Catholic school ethos.

Abecina has offered observations on the interaction between positive psychology and Christian schools[376], arguing that Christian schools should welcome the language of virtue and flourishing embedded in positive psychology, as there is a rich Christian intellectual tradition on living a virtuous life, including writings by Augustine and Thomas Aquinas.[377] Moreover, there may be opportunities for this scientifically validated language of flourishing in programmes such as Weaving Wellbeing to complement the holistic development offered in Catholic schools. For Catholic education, Christ as the human *par excellence*, is the source of living in a fuller and more authentically human way. Jesus tells his followers 'I have come that they may have life, and have it to the full'.[378] In this sense, the scientific language of flourishing can assist in articulating the operative anthropology underpinning the Catholic school, offering a distinctive vision of life.

However, Abecina contends that Christian schools should not uncritically accept as trans-cultural and universal the character strengths and virtues of positive psychology, applying the work of moral philosopher Alistair McIntyre on the particularity and historical contingency of virtues.[379]

375 Martin Seligman and Sethi Sheena, 'Optimism and Fundamentalism', *Psychological Science 4*(4) (1993), 256–9. More recent studies have found similar results. See Anne Berthold and Willibald Ruch, 'Satisfaction with Life and Character Strengths of Non-Religious and Religious People: It's Practicing One's Religion That Makes the Difference', *Frontiers in Psychology 5* (14 August 2014)

376 Alex Abecina, 'Whose Virtues? Which Character Strengths? Positive Psychology in Christian Schools' (2014) <http://www.ethos.org.au/online-resources/engage-mail/whose-virtues-which-character-strengths-positive-psychology>. Accessed on 17 September 2020.

377 See W. Jay Wood, 'Christian Theories of Virtue', in Nancy E. Snow, ed., *The Oxford Handbook of Virtue* (Oxford: Oxford Press, 2018).

378 Ibid.

379 For further reading, see Alister McIntyre, *After Virtue After a Quarter of a Century* (NY: Bloomsbury, 2011).

Therefore, Christian schools committed to integrating positive psychology into their wellbeing programs and curricula must articulate for themselves:

> Whose virtues? Which character strengths? Which positive psychology are we actually seeking to encourage? Those shaped by Christ, or of liberal modernity? … Which practices? Whose traditions are we actually commending to our students as we seek their wellbeing? Those of the Spirit of Christ or rival ones that conform to the spirit of the age?[380]

Abecina is right to point out that there is a danger in the assumption that the content of positive psychology virtues and character strengths is universally applicable in every context. Similar, albeit more polemical, critiques have been made of the mindfulness movement by Purser and Forbes in the previous chapter. By decontextualising experiential practices, there is a risk that the practitioner focuses on their experience of mindfulness or positivity while the contextual factors that influence their wellbeing are undermined. For mindfulness practice (which forms part of positive psychology programmes), this means ignoring the structural and societal sources of stress and suffering. However, Weaving Wellbeing offers a potentially life-giving resource to students, enabling them to thrive and improve their resilience. The approaches are humanising, encouraging students to see their wellbeing as important to living a meaningful life.

For Catholic schools, flourishing has a more profound, ultimate aim, concerning the person growing in relationship with God. This conception of human flourishing is taught explicitly in faith formation and while positive psychology can present a humanistic framework for flourishing, it cannot undermine the distinctiveness of Catholic school ethos. In this sense, Catholic schools can incorporate the many life-giving benefits of programs such as Weaving Wellbeing. However, they first need to be able to articulate how their Catholic ethos enables children to flourish, and how wellbeing programmes (with its mindfulness components) enhance their mission rather than replace it.

380 Alex Abecina, 'Whose Virtues? Which Character Strengths? Positive Psychology in Christian Schools' (2014). <http://www.ethos.org.au/online-resources/engage-mail/whose-virtues-which-character-strengths-positive-psychology>. Accessed on 17 September 2020.

Weaving Wellbeing is a contemporary and popular Irish positive psychology intervention (PPI) operative in Irish primary schools. Weaving Wellbeing seeks to improve resilience and positive wellbeing in children, including the use of mindfulness exercises. The programme provides schools with a resource to help children improve their wellbeing and lower their anxiety, which remains a key concern in Irish youth mental health discourse. Unlike Paws b, there is no requirement to be a mindfulness practitioner to teach the mindfulness concepts to a class.

While research on Weaving Wellbeing remains at an embryonic stage, broader studies and reviews of PPIs in schools have yielded promising results in terms of improved pupil wellbeing. Many of these studies examine larger sample sizes than Paws b and employ rigorous research methods.

The scientific validation of positive psychology should be welcomed by Catholic schools as it could complement the schools' efforts to help children flourish. However, it is important that Catholic schools also critically examine the virtues and character strengths of positive psychology interventions in order to discern what is valuable in positive psychology and corresponds with a Catholic educational vision.

CHAPTER 4

Criteria for a Vision of Catholic Education

In the last chapter, we explored how mindfulness is operative within the Irish primary education system. To evaluate the compatibility of mindfulness with the ethos of Irish Catholic primary schools, it is imperative to develop criteria to ground such an evaluation. Accordingly, this chapter will outline criteria that constitute a vision of Catholic education applicable to the Irish Catholic primary school context.

First, Catholic ethos must be defined in the context of Irish Catholic primary schools, as well as relating ethos to the educational vision of the Catholic school. Second, there is a need to differentiate between Catholic education and Catholic schooling, given the myriad of contexts in which Catholic education operates. Following this, we move on to developing the criteria for our evaluative task.

This will be done by examining three significant Church publications on Catholic education since the Second Vatican Council: *Gravissimum Educationis (1965)*, *The Catholic School (1977)* and *The Religious Dimension of Education in a Catholic School (1988)*. These documents have been chosen for investigation due to the significance attributed to them by several prominent researchers in Catholic education.[381] Additionally, more recent Church documents including *Educating to Intercultural Dialogue in Catholic Schools: Living in Harmony for a Civilisation of Love (2013)* and *Educating to Fraternal Humanism: Building a 'Civilisation of Love' 50 Years*

381 See Sean Whittle, *A Theory of Catholic Education* (London: Bloomsbury, 2015), 34–44, Stephen McKinney, 'A Rationale for Catholic Schools', in Leonardo Franchi and Stephen McKinney, eds, *A Companion to Catholic Education* (Herefordshire: Gracewing, 2011), 147–61, John Sullivan, *Catholic Education: Distinctive and Inclusive*, PhD Thesis, Institute of Education, University of London, 1998 and Mario D'Souza, *A Catholic Philosophy of Education: The Church and Two Philosophers* (Quebec: McGill-Queen's University Press, 2016).

after Populorum Progressio (2017) will examine how Catholic education is to engage with contemporary developments in society. These aforementioned documents will provide a broad summary of the aims and rationale of Catholic education, informing the creation of criteria later in the chapter.

The efforts at supporting and promoting Catholic education in Ireland will also be explored, with reference to the work of the Catholic Education Partnership and the documents *Vision 08: A Vision for Catholic Education in Ireland (2008)* and *Share the Good News: The National Directory for Catechesis (2011)*. This will contextualise the efforts being made in articulating a Catholic educational vision in Irish schools.

Following this, the framework for the distinctiveness of Catholic education proposed by Catholic theologian and educationalist Thomas Groome will be explored. The themes offered by Groome will be examined in dialogue with those of other significant contemporary writers on Catholic education, including John Sullivan, Patricia Kieran and Stephen McKinney. Reflections on Catholic education in the writings of Pope Francis will also be included.

Finally, the characteristics of a vision of Catholic education from post-Conciliar Church publications and influential writers on Catholic education will be distilled into a set of criteria suitable for judging the compatibility of mindfulness with ethos in Irish Catholic primary schools. In doing so, we are equipped to answer the research question at the heart of this work.

Catholic ethos, education and schooling

At the outset of this chapter, it is important to first explore the concept of Catholic school ethos. Derived from a Greek word (*εϑοσ*) for habit or custom, the ethos of the Catholic school can be defined as '… the pattern of belief and practice of a learning community united in the conscious pursuit of the ultimate end of human life, revealed and made possible by Jesus Christ'.[382]

382 David Albert Jones and Stephen Barrie, *Thinking Christian Ethos: The Meaning of Catholic Education* (Oxford: Catholic Truth Society, 2015), 145. Jones and Barrie also offer a general definition of ethos as '… the pattern of belief and practice of a community that embodies and expresses its fundamental dispositions and objectives'.

In this sense, ethos is the characteristic spirit of the Catholic school which animates its ideas, customs and fundamental values. Randles summarises how ethos is vivified by persons and is generated gradually through these repeated patterns of behaviour, habits and values:

> Ethos will form the framework within which people operate and at the same time the ethos is continually being re-established and sustained by the actions and attitudes and values of those people and the practices which embody those values, the beliefs and attitudes promoted by the school and the goals aspired to, valued and celebrated by the school community. Ethos is dynamic, a way of being and of acting which becomes embedded while at the same time remaining delicate and sensitive to change.[383]

Each school lives out its Catholic ethos in a unique way as each school, despite its shared Catholic tradition and mission, is unique and operates within a particular context, influenced by school leadership, governance and the faith commitment of staff and students. Stock argues that despite this diversity, Catholic schools are united in their efforts to offer a distinctive vision of human flourishing and education.

> In short, an 'ethos' is a way of living, behaving and doing things by people who, though diverse, follow common values and are united by a shared vision of life. It is often therefore used in a way that is closely linked with 'culture' and 'philosophy'.[384]

In this sense, Catholic school ethos is the lived expression of a Catholic educational vision, embodying the conduct, customs and vision of life that Catholic education aspires to offer to each pupil. It is the living out of a distinctive conception of what it means to be human and what constitutes human flourishing. Given the uniqueness of each Catholic school in the manner it lives out its characteristic spirit, exploring the educational vision of the Catholic school offers a more fruitful approach, given that all of these schools are united by a shared Christian vision of life. By evaluating the

383 Eileen Randles, 'The Ethos of the Catholic Primary School' in *Catholic Primary Schools Management Association Board of Management Handbook 2012*, 51. <https://education.dublindiocese.ie/wp-content/uploads/sites/5/2012/02/CPSMA_Handbook_2012.pdf>. Accessed on 18 April 2025.

384 Marcus Stock, *Christ at the Centre: Why the Church Provides Catholic Schools* (Oxford: Catholic Truth Society, 2012), 18. <https://www.catholiceducation.org.uk/images/Christ_at_the_Centre_1.pdf>. Accessed on 29 May 2021.

compatibility of mindfulness with a Catholic educational vision, it is then possible to judge whether mindfulness is congruent with the lived expression of this educational vision, which is the Catholic school ethos.

At the outset of this chapter, it is also necessary to first differentiate between Catholic education and schooling as these terms while related are not equivalent to each other. As McKinney argues, the contemporary concept of education includes several modes of teaching and learning, encompassing formal learning in schools among others.[385] Catholic education also includes different processes of teaching and learning, including formal learning in educational institutions as well as less formal learning in the homeplace and in a parish setting. In this sense, while education certainly occurs in the Catholic school, education and schooling are not synonymous in the Catholic tradition. In the context of this work, Catholic education refers to the formal educational activities and processes operative within the Catholic primary school in the Irish state.[386]

Moreover, it is important to stress that the criteria being established are for *a* vision of Catholic education, not *the* vision of Catholic education. As Kieran and Hession argue, 'A brief survey of contemporary literature on Catholic education is sufficient to support the viewpoint that there is no homogenous, universally endorsed vision of Catholic education'.[387] In the Irish context, Catholic primary schools play a major role in this educational endeavour. However, no two Catholic primary schools are the same, with each school interpreting and living out a Catholic vision of education in a distinctive way through their ethos. Moreover, given the gamut of contexts globally in which Catholic education is operative, proposing a monolithic, prescriptive vision of Catholic education would prove deeply problematic.

385 Stephen McKinney, 'A Rationale for Catholic Schools', in Leonardo Franchi and Stephen McKinney, eds, *A Companion to Catholic Education* (Herefordshire: Gracewing, 2011), 147.

386 Philosopher John Haldane offers a useful definition of the educational endeavour which occurs in the school. 'In the context of schooling, education is a deliberate process whereby the cognitive, affective and practical potentialities of the pupil are realized and given deliberate content'. John Haldane, 'Philosophy and Catholic Education', *The Sower 16*(3) (1995), 30–1.

387 Patricia Kieran and Anne Hession, *Children, Catholicism and Religious Education* (Dublin: Veritas, 2005), 116.

Despite this plurality of interpretations of a vision of Catholic education, Kieran and Hession argue that post-Conciliar Church documents have '... incrementally developed a largely consistent vision of the nature of Catholic education'.[388] These teachings provide a basis to outline core tenets of a vision of Catholic education. In this sense, criteria will be developed from themes consistent with post-Conciliar teachings on a vision of Catholic education which the Irish Catholic primary school should espouse and live out through their ethos. These criteria will also interact with key insights from contemporary theologians of Catholic education including Thomas Groome, Stephen McKinney and John Sullivan. In doing so, we will have developed suitable criteria which can be used to evaluate the relationship between mindfulness and ethos in Irish Catholic primary schools. We will first examine those post-Conciliar documents.

Post-Conciliar teaching on Catholic education

The transformative impact of the Second Vatican Council (1962–1965) on the development of the contemporary Catholic Church cannot be overstated.[389] Church historian Adrian Hastings argues 'There can be no question that the Vatican Council was the most important ecclesiastical event of this century ... It so greatly changed the character of by far the largest communion of Christendom'.[390] Called by Pope John XXIII, the Council set out to update and spiritually renew the Church, heal rifts with other Christian

388 Ibid.

389 See Shaun Blanchard and Stephen Bullivant, *Vatican II: A Very Short Introduction* (Oxford: Oxford University Press, 2023).

390 Adrian Hastings, *A History of English Christianity 1920–1990* (London: SCM Press, 1991), 525. For further reading on this paradigm shift in the life of the Church, see James E. McEvoy, *Leaving Christendom for Good: Church-World Dialogue in a Secular Age* (Maryland: Lexington Books/Rowman and Littlefield, 2014).

churches and promote a more positive outlook within the Church to the modern world.[391]

The whole set of sixteen Conciliar documents has come to be interpreted as an interconnected, coherent corpus, offering '... a rich tapestry illustrating what the church, in continuity with its past, seeks to be, proclaim and teach in the world'.[392] This compilation of Church teaching envisions a renewed self-understanding of Catholic identity in the contemporary world, of *ressourcement* (returning to the sources) in continuous interaction with *aggiornamento* (updating). The Conciliar document *Gravissimum Educationis* presents the Church's self-understanding of Catholic education in relationship with the modern world.[393]

Entitled in English, the 'Declaration on Christian Education', *Gravissimum Educationis* (hereafter *GE*), was promulgated on 28 October 1965 having received 2,290 votes for and only 35 against. According to Pohlschneider, the question of the public funding of faith schools was one of the key motives in the Council addressing Christian education.[394] Moreover, according to Conway and Finegan, '... the final text of *GE* reflects the fact that throughout debates over its various schemata numerous bishops had voiced criticism of a State monopoly on schools and expressed support for the public funding of faith schools.'[395]

391 Dermot Lane offers a concise synopsis of these structural shifts that emerged at the Council, including a call to dialogue with the modern world, the presence of seeds of the Word in other religions and a new appreciation of anthropology to proclaiming the Good News. See Dermot A. Lane, *Catholic Education in the Light of Vatican II and Laudato Si'* (Dublin: Veritas, 2015), 18–19.

392 Gareth Byrne, 'The National Directory of Catechesis in Ireland: An Outworking of the Council', in Niall Coll, ed., *Ireland and Vatican II: Essays Theological, Pastoral and Educational* (Dublin: Columba Press, 2015), 298.

393 All references from *Gravissimum Educationis* and all Conciliar documents thereafter have been sourced from Austin Flannery, ed., *Vatican Council II: The Basic Sixteen Documents* (Dublin: Dominican Publications, 1996), and unless otherwise stated, *Gravissimum Educationis* will be referenced as *GE* thereafter.

394 Johannes Pohlschneider, 'Declaration on Christian Education,' in Herbert Vorgrimler, ed., *Commentary on the Documents of Vatican II* (NY: Herder & Herder, 1967–1969), 1–2.

395 Eamonn Conway and Thomas Finegan, 'Public Funding and Divestment of Public Schools', *Melita Theologica 66/1* (2016), 51.

While belonging to the Vatican II corpus, Whittle notes that *GE* is a declaration and does not enjoy the same dogmatic status as other statements.[396] Moreover, *GE* has been critiqued by several commentators for weakness in content[397] as well as its lack of prominence at the Council.[398] However, an important point in the context of this work is that one of the fruits of *GE*, despite its stated weaknesses, was the development of a post-Conciliar commission, the Congregation for Catholic Education (hereafter referred to as CCE).[399] Along with the episcopal conferences, this body was tasked with articulating and applying the philosophy of Catholic education to local contexts. Several of the guidance documents published by the CCE will be examined later.

Several commentators have framed *GE* as reaffirming much of Pope Pius XI's 1929 encyclical letter *Divini Illius Magistri*, albeit without the encyclical's more defensive, conservative tenor.[400] Moreover, while *Divini Ilius Magistri* was addressed to the Catholic faithful, *GE* was outward

396 Sean Whittle, *A Theory of Catholic Education* (London: Bloomsbury, 2015), 35.

397 Future Pontiff Joseph Ratzinger described the Declaration as '... unfortunately, a rather weak document'. See Joseph Ratzinger, *Theological Highlights of Vatican II* (NJ: Paulist Press, 2009), 254.

398 Historian John O' Malley noted that '... the document never entered centre stage at the Council' in John W. O' Malley, *What Happened at Vatican II?* (MA: Harvard University Press, 2010). O' Malley makes the important point that one of the key issues was that the concept of education was understood differently across the different cultures represented at the Council. Conway makes a similar point regarding the huge variation in the relationships between church and state globally in regard to education. See Eamonn Conway, 'Vatican II on Christian Education: A Guide Through Today's 'Educational Emergency?' in Niall Coll, ed., *Ireland and Vatican II: Essays Theological, Pastoral and Educational* (Dublin: Columba Press, 2015), 253–4.

399 As of May 2022, the Congregation for Catholic Education has been merged with the Pontifical Council for Culture to form the Dicastery for Culture and Education. For the purposes of this work, the original CCE reference will be used.

400 See V. Alan McClelland, 'Wholeness Faith and the Distinctiveness of the Catholic School' in Terence McLaughlin, Joseph O' Keefe and Bernadette O' Keeffe, eds, *The Contemporary Catholic School: Context, Identity and Diversity* (Oxfordshire: RoutledgeFarmer, 1996), 155 and Sean Whittle, *A Theory of Catholic Education* (London: Bloomsbury, 2015), 30–9.

looking, addressing the Church and the world. There are also several themes in the encyclical that receive much less emphasis in *GE*, such as references to the place of Original Sin in education or the preparation for death and the afterlife. In this sense, *GE* presents a positive Church stance on education, structured in broad and optimistic general statements.

Gravissimum Educationis (1965)

GE offers a systematic overview of the Church's basic positions on education.[401] The declaration begins by locating Catholic education within the mission of the Church to spread the Good News of the life, death and resurrection of Jesus Christ to all peoples.[402] This evangelising mission entails the Church's obligation for commitment to the whole of human life, including the educational realm. *GE* defends the inalienable right to education for all people, as the true purpose of education is the formation of the human person, enabling them to flourish towards their ultimate end and to contribute to the common good.[403] This telos in Christian education is eternal life with God as proclaimed by Christ.

In declaring this universal right to education, *GE* also argues that all Christians have a right to Christian education[404] and that Catholic parents, children and communities share the right to the State's support for the

401 This can be seen in the decision made by the Council to establish the Congregation for Catholic Education as a vehicle for developing and reflecting on these basic positions on Catholic education and the distinctiveness of Catholic schools.

402 'To fulfil the mandate she has received from her divine founder of proclaiming the mystery of salvation to all men and of restoring all things in Christ, Holy Mother the Church must be concerned with the whole of man's life, even the secular part of it insofar as it has a bearing on his heavenly calling … Therefore she has a role in the progress and development of education'. *GE* Par 1.

403 Ibid, Par 1.

404 Ibid, Par 2.

provision of Catholic schools.[405] However, *GE* seeks to delineate the borders of state involvement in Catholic education, by re-affirming the primacy of parents and family as primary educators, where the children are raised in the faith and taught how to love God and their neighbour.[406]

The Church argues that principle of subsidiarity[407] should apply in the State's involvement in education to counter a monopolising of education in a country and to ensure the liberty and rights of a citizen to receive a suitable education of their choice.[408] This principle means that each member of an organisation or society recognises and respects their different roles and duties, while working collaboratively and respectfully with each other. In this sense, the Church affirms the distinctive responsibilities of all of the stakeholders in the Catholic educational endeavour.

The Church's commitment to education incorporates both religious and moral education. It is religious education, in that it is explicitly about faith formation and nurturing the person into coming to know, love and worship God, of a life '… inspired by the spirit of Christ'.[409] This means the Church supports parents in their educational and catechetical responsibility to their children. It is moral education in that it develops people of the Christian family to bear witness to their faith and work with civil society to contribute to the common good.

405 Parents should be '… free to choose according to their conscience the schools they want for their children'. Ibid, Par 6.

406 Ibid, Par 3.

407 See Andrew B. Morris, 'Selected Official Church Documents and Statements', in Andrew B. Morris, ed., *Catholic Education: Universal Principles, Locally Applied* (Newcastle: Cambridge Publishing, 2012), 23 (n1). Morris identifies the basis of this principle, stretching back to its development in the 1931 encyclical *Quadragesimo Anno*. 'It postulates that all social bodies exist for the sake of the individual, so that whatever functions individuals can discharge effectively should not be taken over by society'.

408 'But it (the state) must always keep in mind the principle of subsidiarity so that there is no kind of school monopoly, for this is opposed to the rights of the human person, to the development and spread of culture, to the peaceful association of citizens and to the pluralism that exists today in ever so many societies'. *GE* Par 6.

409 Ibid, Par 3.

While Catholic education can occur in a variety of settings, but the declaration highlights the 'special importance'[410] of the Catholic school. Like other schools, Catholic schools are committed to human formation, but the life of the Catholic school is underpinned by '… a special atmosphere animated by the Gospel spirit of freedom … to help youth grow … and to let knowledge acquired be illuminated by faith'.[411]

GE also recognises the importance of highly qualified teachers, fluent in secular and religious pedagogies. In this sense, Catholic education in the school includes religious instruction in the faith but also a comprehensive curriculum of knowledge in keeping with the holistic development of the child. In faith formation, the Catholic school partakes in the evangelising mission of the Church to '… lead pupils from the current situation to promote the good of the earthly city and also prepare them for service to the spread of the Kingdom of God … to be saving leaven in the human community'.[412] The secular knowledge and reason gained in the school which is illuminated by faith, enables the pupils to engage faith with contemporary culture and be enabled to spread the Christian message.

Paragraph 9 highlights the aforementioned ambiguity of a prescriptive vision of Catholic education by recognising that there can be a variety of forms of Catholic schools. *GE* also draws attention to Catholic schools being receptive to non-Catholics who attend the school and providing educational service to the poor.[413] The provision of Catholic education to non-Catholics does not entail faith formation but remains rooted in the Gospel spirit of freedom, recognising the religious other and seeking to contribute to the common good through dialogue and mutual respect.

Bruguès accepts the enduring legacy of *GE*, despite its rushed development and lack of prominence at the Council.[414] Central to this legacy was the establishment of the CCE, tasked with developing the foundational themes

410 Ibid, Par 5.

411 Ibid, Par 8.

412 *GE* Par 8.

413 Ibid, Par 9.

414 Jean-Louis Bruguès 'La Declaracion Gravissimum Educationis del Concilio Vaticano II', in Vicente Vide and José R. Villar, eds, *El Concilio Vaticano II: Una Perspectiva Teologica* (Madrid: Sao Paulo, 2013), 525–43.

of Christian education laid out in the declaration. Several key themes emerge from the document, which are especially relevant to our research question.

First, a vision of Catholic education has an anthropological concern in that it is committed to the holistic and harmonious formation of the human person in pursuit of their ultimate end in God. This vision recognises the universal right to education for all and the dignity of every human being as being made in the *imago Dei.* This graced nature anthropology commits Catholic education to appreciate and develop the uniqueness of each person in their totality and to be responsible partners in God's creation.

Second, the Catholic school is recognised as a site of special importance to the educational endeavour, rooted in the person of Jesus Christ. This embodying of the Gospel message is fundamental to a vision of Catholic education, as its students are called to be Christ-like in their thoughts, words and actions, living out the Gospel message and contributing to the common good. This includes special care towards the poor and marginalised. Jesus tells his followers 'I have come that they may have life, and have it to the full'.[415] In this sense, Christ as the human *par excellence* is the source of living in a fuller and more authentically human way.

Third, Catholic education is to be located within the context of the mission of the Church, proclaiming the Good News to the world, inextricably linking education and evangelisation together. The family is recognised as an important setting for evangelisation, bearing witness to a life of faith. This call to conversion in school does not entail proselytisation or indoctrination. Rather, it sets about presenting and embodying the Christian story and tradition to help students develop a mature and vibrant Christian faith.

Fourth, Catholic education envisions the autonomy of various branches of knowledge, '… that by their very constitution individual subjects be pursued according to their own principles, method, and liberty of scientific inquiry'.[416] Although the declaration is here referring explicitly to higher education, the underlying point is relevant to education in the Catholic primary school. Each subject enjoys the academic freedom to pursue knowledge that is pedagogically sound which can be illuminated by faith.

415 John 10:10.
416 *GE* Par 10.

Finally, in keeping with the spirit of *aggiornamento* that characterised Vatican II, a vision of Catholic education incorporates an engagement in dialogue between faith and culture. Catholic schools are challenged to interact creatively and critically with a society characterised by pluralism and secularisation. This involves rejecting elements of contemporary society contrary to the Gospel message, while accepting aspects that are congruent with it. This includes providing an open and welcoming education inspired by Gospel values to non-Catholics who attend schools while also respecting their religious freedom.

The themes outlined above represent the Council's attempt to codify a Catholic educational vision, but they are not comprehensively articulated in *GE*. The Council Fathers recognised both the aspirations and limitations of the document and established the CCE to reflect upon and develop the work begun in *GE*. The five themes briefly explored can be broadly categorised by John Sullivan's summation that 'Behind a Catholic philosophy of education there is an anthropology, a theology of creation and a Christology and an ecclesiology'.[417]

GE provides a starting point in discerning principles for a post-Conciliar vision of Catholic education, which can later be used as criteria for evaluating the relationship between mindfulness and ethos in Irish Catholic primary schools. We continue to discern these principles in other significant Church documents on Catholic education, now turning to *The Catholic School*.

The Catholic school (1977)

The first major publication following the establishment of the CCE, *The Catholic School* (hereafter referred to in the text as *CS*),[418] reasserts the need for the Church to be a creative and constructive dialogue partner with the

417 John Sullivan, *Catholic Education: Distinctive and Inclusive*, PhD Thesis, Institute of Education, University of London (1998), 147. <https://ethos.bl.uk/OrderDetails.do?uin=uk.bl.ethos.287956>. Accessed on 10 December 2020.

418 Congregation for Catholic Education, *The Catholic School* (1977). The document is hereafter referenced as *CS*.

world and demonstrate a Christian presence in society. This entails bearing witness to the Church and its values, particularly in light of corrosive and damaging forces in contemporary society such as relativism, materialism and a technocratic consciousness.[419]

CS reflects upon and develops the thought of *GE*, and two themes emerge here. First, there is a clear recognition of Jesus Christ as foundational to the educational enterprise in the Catholic school.[420] This means that the Catholic school is called to provide opportunities for students to encounter Christ through prayer, sacraments and scripture. This Christocentric embodiment must also be expressed in witness to the Christian life. At the heart of this endeavour is the formation of students who encounter the Gospel message, being called to create an inclusive and welcoming community based on agapic love and service to the other. It also aspires to the nurturing of a personal relationship with Jesus through prayer, cultivated both individually and communally. In this sense, the Catholic school acts as an extension of the evangelising mission of the Church, spreading the salvific message of Christ.

Kieran and Hession argue that this Christ-centred vision of education displays a distinctive anthropology. 'Inspired by the vision of Christ, who is the perfect embodiment of what it means to be human, Catholic schools have as their aim the education and development of the whole human person'.[421] This integral approach to education has implications for religious education. As Christ is the basis of the educational endeavour, encountering Christ can never be compartmentalised into occurring just in religious education lessons. Rather, Christ is the catalyst for what McKinney calls 'the Christian self-actualisation of the Catholic school'.[422] This means that the life of the school, its policy decisions, its teaching and learning have numerous

419 *CS* Par 12.

420 Ibid, 55. 'There should be constant reference to the Gospel and frequent encounter with Christ'.

421 Patricia Kieran and Anne Hession, *Children, Catholicism and Religious Education* (Dublin: Veritas, 2005), 123.

422 Stephen McKinney, 'A Rationale for Catholic Schools', in Leonardo Franchi and Stephen McKinney, eds, *A Companion to Catholic Education* (Herefordshire: Gracewing, 2011), 152.

opportunities for encounter with the person of Jesus Christ in reflection and prayer, both personal and collective.

A second theme that emerges is the declaration that the Catholic school has a dual duty to work towards 'a synthesis of faith and culture and a synthesis of faith and life'.[423] This aspiration while complex and somewhat vague,[424] refers first to a synthesis whereby knowledge is integrated through the prism of the Gospel. For Catholic education, this means each academic subject enjoys the integrity to search for the truth. This epistemological endeavour when conducted authentically, and dependent on the role of the teacher,[425] will eventually open students up to Truth itself.[426] This first synthesis has a highly educational purpose, in that it seeks to form students holistically into an orientation towards Christian life: bearing witness to the Gospel message, social justice and a rejection of dehumanising and materialist views of humanity operative in society.

The second synthesis, that of faith and life, involves the Christian formation of pupils. Catholic education is a lifelong process, and '... while this synthesis has the maturity of faith in its sight, it also provides a broader vision in distinguishing between what enhances personhood and what compromises

423 *CS Par 37*.

424 Such vagueness in elucidating the nature of the Catholic school runs the risk of generating slogan-like claims which fail to capture the distinctiveness of a vision of Catholic education.

425 Contemporary research has highlighted the significance of emerging generations of teachers in Ireland who are either non-practising Catholics or irreligious along with their hesitancy or insecurity in teaching religious education. See Sheridan, John-Paul Sheridan, 'Catholic Teacher Formation in the Republic of Ireland', in Leonardo Franchi and Richard Rymarz, eds, *Formation of Teachers for Catholic Schools: Challenges and Opportunities in a New Era* (Singapore: Springer, 2022), 55–66, Patricia Kieran and Aiveen Mullaly, 'Beyond belief? Pre-service teachers' perspectives on teaching RE in Ireland', *Journal of Religious Education 69* (2021), 423–37 and Manuela Heinz, Kevin Davison and Elaine Keane, 'I will do it but religion is a very personal thing': Teacher Education Applicants' Attitudes Towards Teaching Religion in Ireland', *European Journal of Teacher Education 41* (2018), 232–45.

426 This is based on a fundamental belief in a world that has been created by God and for God and, ultimately all knowledge will lead back to God. See Stephen McKinney, 'A Rationale for Catholic Schools', in Leonardo Franchi and Stephen McKinney, eds, *A Companion to Catholic Education* (Herefordshire: Gracewing, 2011), 152–3.

it'.[427] The Catholic school is then called to translate the Gospel into the everyday lives of its students and teachers as a community of service. This involves creative and constructive dialogue with contemporary culture, working towards an integral view of the human person. This also means students and teachers embodying the Gospel message in their lives, putting faith into action.

The religious dimension of education in a Catholic school (1988)

The Religious Dimension of Education in a Catholic School (hereafter referred to as *RDECS*)[428] presents a set of guidelines for reflection and renewal. In exploring the positive intersections of the religious and educational realms in the Catholic school, *RDECS* explores several themes relating to a vision of Catholic education similar to those examined in *GE* and *CS*.

First, the autonomy of the different academic subjects and their respective methodologies is recognised, with the understanding that the various branches of knowledge cannot '... be seen merely as subservient to faith'.[429] The Catholic school is never reduced to a site of apologetics or proselytism. While faith is nurtured through appropriate religious instruction and the passing on of the Gospel story, the transmission of knowledge cannot be undermined. To this end, *RDECS* stresses the distinction between religious instruction and religious education: religious instruction as a lifelong process of Christian maturity as part of a local church community, and

427 Mario D'Souza, *A Catholic Philosophy of Education: The Church and Two Philosophers* (Quebec: McGill-Queen's University Press, 2016), 151.

428 Congregation for Catholic Education, *The Religious Dimension of Education in a Catholic School* (1988). Likewise, the document will be referenced as *RDECS*.

429 *RDECS*, Par 53.

religious education as conveying a sense of how Christians try to live their lives according to their faith.[430]

This distinction, while open to critique[431], is important as in a post-Christian and post-secular society (as was explored in Chapter 1), more non-Catholic children attend Catholic schools than ever before. A Catholic vision of education balances the religious freedom of the child with an obligation to provide religious instruction to Catholic students as part of the evangelising mission of the Church. By stressing the academic integrity of curricular subjects, any charge of indoctrination is shown to be *anathema* to the educational enterprise of the Catholic school. This is not to compartmentalise secular knowledge from the religious ethos of the Catholic school. Rather this genuine pursuit of truth, reliant on the role of the teacher and the ethos of the school will eventually open students up to Truth itself. Moreover, religious instruction cannot be limited to the school context and there is an expectation that this lifelong formation also occurs in the home and parish settings.

Second, *RDECS* stresses the integral formation of the person, underpinned by a theological anthropology. As stated above, the imparting of knowledge remains the mandate of the Catholic school. However, the education of the whole person includes the intellectual but also the relational, spiritual and affective dimensions. For a Catholic vision of education, the person is '... created in "the image and likeness" of God; elevated by God to the dignity of a child of God; unfaithful to God in original sin, but redeemed by Christ; a temple of the Holy Spirit; a member of the Church; destined to eternal life'.[432] This theocentric view of humanity presents each person gifted with dignity and with the capacity for right relationship, working

430 'The aim of catechesis, or handing on the Gospel message, is maturity: spiritual, liturgical, sacramental and apostolic; this happens most especially in a local Church community. The aim of the school however, is knowledge. While it uses the same elements of the Gospel message, it tries to convey a sense of the nature of Christianity, and of how Christians are trying to live their lives'. Ibid, Par 69.

431 Whittle identifies two concerns with this statement as first, the content of both forms of religious teaching is sourced from the Catechism of the Catholic Church, blurring the lines between instruction and education. Second, there is an implication that school-based instruction may differ from catechesis received outside of school. See Sean Whittle, *A Theory of Catholic Education* (London: Bloomsbury, 2015), 41–2.

432 Ibid, 84.

in solidarity with each other to build an inclusive and welcoming society. This graced nature anthropology is located in the integral formation of the person that Catholic education envisions.

Finally, *RDECS* presents an outlook on the synthesis of faith and culture, stressing the need for faith to be embodied and actualised through culture.[433] Such an outlook proposes that faith and culture can interact in a constructive and creative manner, and that religious values and dispositions can be nurtured through interaction with aspects of society, such as art, history and technology. Such a synthesis is deemed especially necessary by the document given the contemporary cultural context within which the Christian narrative is operative, where a lack of conceptions of human flourishing and human relationships means many young people today are challenged by loneliness, uncertainty and a sense of meaninglessness in their lives.[434] Many of these debilitating cultural conditions set out in *RDECS* match the sense of spiritual *ennui* explored by Gallagher and Boeve earlier.[435] Thus, *RDECS* aspires to create a society centred on the dignity of the human person, translating and assimilating the Gospel values of justice and solidarity into a culture challenged by relativism and cultural pluralism.

Recent church documents on Catholic education

In the past decade, the CCE has published further guidance on the role of Catholic education can play in an increasingly complex and multi-faceted contemporary society. Catholic education has been challenged to respond to the various crises prevalent in the world today, including the climate emergency and economic inequality. Two such documents are *Educating*

433 'Faith which does not become culture is faith which is not received fully, not assimilated entirely, not lived faithfully'. Ibid, 42.

434 See Ibid, Par 10–23. These themes are explored over several paragraphs.

435 For Gallagher, there is a hunger for spiritual nourishment which is stymied by forms of cultural unbelief. For Boeve, the 'culture of the kick' embodies this desire for experience that transcends the forces of postmodernism.

to Intercultural Dialogue in Catholic Schools: Living in Harmony for a Civilisation of Love (2013) and *Educating to Fraternal Humanism: Building a 'Civilisation of Love' 50 Years after Populorum Progressio* (2017). These merit examination as they are comparatively more recent documents than the trio examined thus far, providing insight into a vision of Catholic education in relation to contemporary society. Pope Francis' 2019 *Global Compact on Education* and the CCE's 2022 instruction, *The Identity of the Catholic School for a Culture of Dialogue* are briefly outlined as well. Their inclusion is instructive to this work as they help to articulate a Catholic educational vision relevant to the contemporary Irish Catholic primary school.

Educating to intercultural dialogue in Catholic schools: living in harmony for a civilisation of love (2013)

According to Leonardo Franchi, this publication (hereafter referred to as *EIDCS*)[436] is '... a significant moment in the history of the Holy See's teaching on education in that the document proposes "intercultural dialogue" as an overarching aim of Catholic schooling'.[437] *EIDCS* offers guidelines to Catholic schools to promote intercultural and interreligious dialogue, while also stressing the important distinction between the reality of pluralism and the promotion of relativism.[438] Several themes are evident in this document, congruent with those already explored.

First, *EIDCS* highlights the Catholic school as an important setting for dialogue between faith and culture. Given the contemporary trends of secularisation and pluralisation, Catholic education is called to offer its worldview to all with an interest in human flourishing. This means that schools

436 Congregation for Catholic Education, *Educating to Intercultural Dialogue in Catholic Schools: Living in Harmony for a Civilisation of Love* (2013) is likewise referenced as *EIDCS*.

437 Leonardo Franchi, 'Catholic Education and Intercultural Dialogue', *Logos: A Journal of Catholic Thought and Culture 19*(4) (2016), 117.

438 'Being aware of the relative nature of cultures and opting for relativism are two profoundly different things' *EIDCS* Par 22.

have a clear recognition of their own Catholic identity in order to engage in an intercultural dialogue of mutual recognition. In this sense, '"Catholic schools" primary responsibility is one of witness ...'[439] to a constant personal network of relationships cultivating greater solidarity and fraternity. In doing so, Catholic education enables students to become engaged civic actors who contribute to the common good.

Second, the document stresses that this intercultural education is rooted in the person of Jesus Christ, who is the human *par excellence*. Catholic education is holistic in that it caters for every dimension of human potential. Christ as the exemplar of authentic humanity models right relationship with others, where the dignity of the other is recognised and affirmed. Catholic schools are challenged to embody Christ's life and ministry in their activities, including intercultural dialogue.[440] By placing Christ at the heart of their educational endeavour, Catholic education can help to ensure diversity is celebrated and each person is seen as unique and valued as part of an inclusive common human family.

Educating to Fraternal Humanism: building a 'Civilisation of Love' 50 years after Popolorum Progressio (2017)

Fifty years on from Pope Paul VI's encyclical on the development of all peoples, *Educating to Fraternal Humanism* (hereafter referred to as *EFH*)[441] challenges Catholics to solidarity and dialogue in challenging social inequalities. Catholic education is called to present a humanising education that is

439 Ibid, Par 57.

440 Ibid. 'The contribution that Catholicism can make to education and to intercultural dialogue is in their reference to the centrality of the human person, who has his or her constitutive element in relationships with others. Catholic schools have in Jesus Christ the basis of their anthropological and pedagogical paradigm; they must practise the "grammar of dialogue."'

441 Congregation for Catholic Education, *Educating to Fraternal Humanism: Building a 'Civilisation of Love' 50 Years after Populorum Progressio* (2017). This document is hereafter referenced as *EFH*.

centred on a holistic view of the human person while nurturing relationships that form a community. *EFH* highlights several themes consistent with those offered in the documents explored thus far.

First, *EFH* proposes an integral education that is profoundly anthropological, with the human person placed at the heart of the educational endeavour. It is a counter to corrosive anthropometric notions seen in society such as excessive materialism and individualism, instead viewing the person as being '... in a framework of relationships that make up a living community, which is interdependent and bound to a common destiny. This is fraternal humanism'.[442] This anthropological perspective means that Catholic education is called to cultivate the moral and social potential of pupils, enabling them to realise their talents and gifts as active participants of the human family. Contrary to anthropocentric tendencies in modern culture, *EFH* charges Catholic school to be a community of person-centred education, modelling right relationship and '... extending the classroom to embrace every corner of social experience in which education can generate solidarity, sharing and communion'.[443]

Second, *EFH* stresses that Catholic education must generate a culture of dialogue rooted in solidarity and openness. In a culture punctuated by pluralisation and globalisation, Catholic education must inculcate a dialogue that transcends information exchange.[444] The capacity for a shared conversation, rooted in equality and fairness must be demonstrated in Catholic education. By recognising the inherent human dignity of the other in inter-religious dialogue, students can discover and promote shared ideals and values, fulfilling a vital civic duty. This means that students are formed to possess a grammar of dialogue, the capacity to connect the ethical principles of their faith to the public square and the common good.

442 *EFH* Par 8.

443 *EFH* Par 10.

444 '... the participants ... must be free from their contingent interests and must be prepared to recognise the dignity of all parties. These attitudes are supported by the consistency with one's own specific universe of values'. Ibid, Par 12.

Global compact on education (2019) and the identity of the Catholic school in a culture of dialogue (2022)

In 2019,[445] Pope Francis proposed a *Global Compact on Education*, inviting stakeholders in society '… to dialogue on how we are shaping the future of our planet and the need to employ the talents of all, since all change requires an educational process aimed at developing a new universal solidarity and a more welcoming society'.[446] Motivated by dissatisfaction at the societal division and hatred, along with the continuing environmental emergency, Pope Francis calls for a renewed educational vision, recognising education's transformational potential for solidarity, mutual understanding and freedom.[447] This vision mirrors the hitherto recent CCE publications in the promotion of fraternal humanism and dialogue.

In 2022, the CCE published an instruction, *The Identity of the Catholic School in a Culture of Dialogue*,[448] motivated by the '… need for a clearer awareness and consistency of the Catholic identity of the Church's educational institutions all over the world'.[449] The publication is written in the key of the Global Compact on Education, sharing a concern at '… the breakdown of the "educational compact" among institutions, families and individuals. These tensions also reflect a crisis in the relationship and communication between generations, and a social fragmentation made even more evident by the primacy of indifference'.[450] In this sense, the Catholic school offers a site for a corrective to such corrosive societal trends, in which each a culture of care is instead proposed. This is an educational vision that recognises

445 Pope Francis, *Message for the Launch of the Global Compact on Education* (Rome: Vatican, 12 September 2019).

446 Pope Francis, *Vadecanum – Global Compact on Education* (Rome: Vatican, 2019), 4.

447 Luiz Fernando Klein, Philippe Richard and Quentin Wodon, 'Pope Francis' Vision for Education and the Call for a Global Compact on Education', *The Review of Faith and International Affairs 21* (2023), 13.

448 Congregation for Catholic Education, *The Identity of the Catholic School in a Culture of Dialogue* (2022).

449 Ibid, Par.1.

450 Ibid, Par 33.

the innate dignity of each human person, creed, ethnicity, community and fundamental human rights such as freedom and justice. Like previous documents, the CCE publication proposes Catholic education as a process of encounter and dialogue towards the common good.

Post-Conciliar themes for a vision of Catholic education

The purpose of this chapter section has been to identify defining principles for a vision of Catholic education located within several influential Conciliar and post-Conciliar documents on the subject. By investigating *Gravissimum Educationis (1965), The Catholic School (1977)* and *The Religious Dimension of Education in the Catholic School (1988)* along with recent influential publications *Educating to Intercultural Dialogue in Catholic Schools (2013)* and *Educating to Fraternal Humanism* (2017), several criteria emerge which appear fundamental to an authentic vision of Catholic education. These criteria will be necessary in the next chapter for answering our key question: evaluating the compatibility of mindfulness and ethos in Irish Catholic primary schools.

The criteria for a vision of Catholic education emerging from the post-Conciliar literature examined in this chapter can be broadly categorised as follows.

1. Academic integrity:
   The Catholic school, as a special site of Catholic education, fully respects the autonomy of curricular subjects. The Catholic school has a commitment to the transmission of knowledge through an integral education, nurturing an outlook of critical reflection and discernment. A Catholic vision of education encourages the genuine pursuit of truth as it can lead to the student being opened to encounter God, the source of Truth.

2. Christocentricity:
   The educational enterprise of the Catholic school is rooted in the person of Jesus Christ. Inspired by the vision of Christ as the human *par excellence*, the school is committed to education that cultivates pupils in their totality to be Christ-like. This means being inspired to build right relationships with others based on the Gospel values of agapic love and

self-forgetfulness. This Christocentric basis means that Catholic education enables students to develop a personal relationship with Christ, through liturgy, scripture, the sacraments and prayer both personal and communal.

3. Theological anthropology:
A Catholic vision of education views each pupil as being created in the likeness and image of God, born with an innate human dignity and goodness. Such a vision affirms that through God's grace, we have the capacity for love and right relationships with others, with the world around us and with God. This vision means the promotion of the holistic development of the pupil, to reach their full potential and realising their gifts and talents.

4. Faith and culture in dialogue:
A Catholic educational vision involves faith being in a critical and creative encounter with contemporary culture. The Church seeks to work with society towards the common good while rejecting aspects of culture that diminish human flourishing. A Catholic educational vision offers a counter-narrative to the debilitating effects of relativism, materialism and excessive consumerism, which can reduce education to a technocratic system rather than a holistic process of human development.

The promotion of a Catholic educational vision in Ireland

In recent years, several initiatives have been developed to support, resource and evaluate the educational vision of Catholic schools in Ireland. First, *Vision 08: A Vision for Catholic Education in Ireland (2008)* articulates the role of Catholic education in contemporary Ireland and initiated the foundation of the national Catholic educational service, the Catholic Schools Partnership, now the Catholic Education Service.[451] Second, *Share the Good*

451 Formerly the Catholic Schools Partnership (CSP), the body was reorganised and established as the Catholic Education Service in May 2020. As several publications listed were published prior to this establishment, CSP will be used in references.

News: National Directory for Catechesis in Ireland (2010) is a definitive contribution to evangelisation, catechesis and renewal in the Irish Church in the spirit of the Second Vatican Council.

Vision 08: a vision for Catholic education in Ireland

The Irish Catholic Bishops' Conference's pastoral letter *Vision 08* is set against the backdrop of debate about the role of the Church in education, and the shifting of Catholic school administration from Religious to trusts dominated by laity. It outlines a rationale for the place of Catholic education in an increasingly pluralised and multicultural society, including Catholic schools' commitment '... to reflect a distinctive vision of life and a corresponding philosophy of education ... based on the Gospel of Jesus Christ'.[452] This means the promotion of the holistic development of the child, where students are nurtured to reach their full potential as part of an inclusive and welcoming school community. The Catholic school works in partnership with home and parish in educating and forming Catholics in their faith while also welcoming students of all faiths and none.

Vision 08 re-affirms post-Conciliar teachings on Catholic education, particularly the importance of academic integrity. The document stresses the compatibility of intellectual development and scientific thinking with the mission of the Church as well as the compatibility of faith and reason.[453] However, it '... rejects those diminished and mechanistic notions of rationality which attempt to limit the concept of truth to what can be scientifically

452 Irish Catholic Bishops' Conference. *Vision 08: A Vision for Catholic Education in Ireland—Pastoral Letter* (2008), 2.

453 Ibid, 3. 'Catholic education has always placed a high value on reason, both intellectual and practical. In continuity with the earliest traditions of the Church, it regards education and the cultivation of intellectual life as precious in themselves. It sees the use of rational thought and scientific analysis as essential to the advancement of technology and human progress ... Faith and reason must be seen as vibrant partners in the human quest for understanding and ultimate fulfilment which is pursued in Catholic schools'.

established and the concept of human progress to what can be technologically achieved'.[454] In this regard, an instrumentalised rationalist view of education is rebutted on the basis that it reduces human progress or fullness to materialist or technocratic ends. Religious education is thus a vital aspect of the Catholic educational curriculum in inviting students to be inspired by the transcendent mystery of God in their lives and see themselves as being called to full and eternal life in God which is made possible through Christ's life, death and resurrection. This also means scrutinising trends in education and society that inhibit human flourishing and are counter to Gospel values.

Finally, a significant development arising from *Vision 08* is the Irish Catholic Bishops' Conference's commitment to the formation of a national Catholic educational service to support the ethos of Catholic schools in Ireland.[455] This led to the foundation of the Catholic Schools Partnership (CSP), which has since been reformulated as the Catholic Education Service (CES), which supports the advancement of Catholic education in Ireland.[456]

In 2015, the CSP launched '*Understanding and Living the Ethos in a Catholic Primary School: A Process Centred on Conversations*', an ethos self-evaluation resource for Catholic primary schools.[457] Involving all members of the school community, this document sets out a comprehensive process for Catholic schools to reflect upon and evaluate their own ethos. The five characteristics of Catholic ethos outlined by the CSP are:

454 Ibid.

455 Ibid, 10. 'It is the Bishops' intention to provide in cooperation with the Religious Trustees further support in the near future for those involved in the work of Catholic education by establishing a national Catholic Education Service for the whole of Ireland'.

456 According to their website, the Catholic Education Partnership will '... support the advancement of Catholic religion and the advancement of education in accordance with Catholic Ethos through support and promotion of Catholic faith-based education, and supporting and developing Catholic schools and other relevant environments within the Irish education system, all in accordance with the requirements and statutes for education issued from time to time by the Irish Episcopal Conference'. <https://catholiceducation.ie/about-us/>. Accessed on 9 June 2024.

457 <https://www.catholicschools.ie/understanding-and-living-the-ethos-in-a-catholic-primary-school/>. Accessed on 1 May 2021.

1. The school is founded on a Catholic understanding of education.
2. The school is a Catholic community.
3. The school is an agent of personal growth and social transformation.
4. Religious education is an integral part of the school.
5. We are called to be followers of Christ.[458]

This ethos reflection process is ongoing in Catholic schools in several dioceses in Ireland. However, since the COVID-19 pandemic, the momentum of this process has slowed, stymieing it from developing in many dioceses across the country.

The Catholic Schools Partnership has also published documents on Catholic schools in Ireland, including *Catholic Schools- Looking to the Future.*[459] This document provides a rationale for Catholic schools today, highlighting the different challenges and opportunities facing the role of these schools in any increasingly secular and pluralistic Ireland.

Share the good news: national directory for Catechesis in Ireland

Published by the Irish Catholic Bishop's Conference, *Share the Good News* '... provides the Irish Church with a framework indicating principles and guidelines for evangelisation, catechesis and religious education today'.[460]

458 Ibid, 16–20. Several targets are outlined under each characteristic to help schools explore what is distinctive about how they understand and live their Catholic ethos.

459 Catholic Schools Partnership, *Catholic Schools – Looking to the Future* (2012) <https://www.icatholic.ie/wp-content/uploads/2012/07/CSP-Future.pdf>. Accessed on 20 February 2022.

460 Irish Catholic Bishops' Conference, *Share the Good News: National Directory for Catechesis in Ireland* (Dublin: Veritas, 2014), ix.

Rooted in the spirit of Vatican II[461], the document is a resource to all involved in catechesis and evangelisation in Ireland, calling them to see their efforts as constituents of the broader faith development and mission of the Church in contemporary Irish society.

As part of this framework, *Share the Good News* offers objectives to evaluate the goals, methods and resources in the renewal of catechesis, evangelisation and religious education at all levels of the Irish Church. In terms of faith development in Catholic schools, this entails seven objectives with accompanying indicators of achievement for all members of the school community. These objectives are:

1. The members of the Catholic Church in Ireland will contribute energetically to developing a holistic understanding of education in school.
2. The Catholic school will operate according to a Mission Statement and Ethos Policy that openly reflects its Catholic spirit.
3. The Catholic school, primary or post-primary, will be characterised by respect, generosity, justice, hospitality and critical reflection.
4. The Board of Management in a Catholic school will take responsibility, on behalf of the Patron/Trustees, for developing the school, overseeing its Catholic ethos, and supporting the Principal in the daily management of the school, according to that ethos.
5. The Principal will ensure that the decisions of the Board of Management, and particularly the ethos statement set out by the Board, are lived out in the day-to-day running of the school.
6. Staff in a Catholic school will know, understand and sustain the Catholic ethos within which they are employed.
7. Religious education and faith formation will be evident in the schooling provided by a Catholic school.[462]

The partnership between home, school and parish is highlighted as being essential in nurturing and sustaining the religious education and formation

461 Gareth Byrne, 'The National Directory of Catechesis in Ireland: An Outworking of the Council', in Niall Coll, ed., *Ireland and Vatican II: Essays Theological, Pastoral and Educational* (Dublin: Columba Press, 2015), 298.

462 *Share the Good News*, 204–10.

of Catholic children.[463] As the debate over Catholic educational provision and divestment continues in Irish society, Byrne argues that '... the time and space necessary to negotiate the variety of ways in which these relationships might ... be conceived of into the future needs to be attended to with renewed energy and care'.[464] *Share the Good News* then proposes a renewal of catechesis and faith development across home, school and parish instead of an overreliance on Catholic schools as the locus of religious education and formation.

Having set out criteria for a post-Conciliar vision of Catholic education and mapped the efforts to support and evaluate Catholic education in Ireland, we now turn to influential theologian Thomas Groome's writings on a framework for Catholic education.

Thomas Groome and the distinctiveness of Catholic education

Thomas Groome offers a framework highlighting how the distinctive characteristics of Catholicism permeate a vision of Catholic education.[465] Drawing upon the work of Baptist theologian Langdon Gilkey, Groome proposes eight characteristics of Catholicism which pervade education that could be called 'Catholic'. Catholic education cannot be understood as being constituted of several segregated or compartmentalised themes specific to Catholicism. Rather, Groome's proposed model is best understood as

463 Ibid, 142.

464 Gareth Byrne, 'The National Directory of Catechesis in Ireland: An Outworking of the Council', in Niall Coll, ed., *Ireland and Vatican II: Essays Theological, Pastoral and Educational* (Dublin: Columba Press, 2015), 310.

465 Thomas Groome, 'What Makes a School Catholic?' in Terence McLaughlin, Joseph O' Keefe and Bernadette O' Keeffe, eds, *The Contemporary Catholic School: Context, Identity and Diversity* (Oxfordshire: RoutledgeFarmer, 1996), 107–23. The themes explored here are elaborated in more detail in Thomas Groome, *What Makes Us Catholic: Eight Gifts for Life* (NY: HarperCollins, 2002) and Thomas Groome, *Educating for Life: A Spiritual Vision for Every Teacher and Parent* (Allen, Texas: Thomas More, 1998).

a configuration of interconnected characteristics which are all present in Catholicism and permeate a Catholic educational vision. Sullivan's analogy is instructive here, suggesting that we '... hear these elements as notes in a symphony rather than bricks in a building'.[466] Groome's proposed themes will be explored below, with particular attention to their implications for a vision of Catholic education.

Anthropology

Catholic anthropology relates to the theocentric understanding of the human condition, recognising that our capacity for sin, while grave, is still less than our innate goodness. In this sense, Groome locates Catholic anthropology as a mediating stance of 'realistic optimism' between the polarities of Pelagian self-sufficiency and Calvinistic total depravity.[467] Despite the stain of Original Sin on human nature, we are gifted by God's unmerited grace to be made in the *imago Dei*, the likeness and image of God[468], which means to be created with the capacity for right relationship and self-forgetting love. Thus, humanity is made to lovingly relate to others, to creation and to God.

Our creation in the *imago Dei* actualises the inalienable dignity of the human person and the sacredness of human life. Humanity is of such profound dignity that God chooses to become one out of love, as revealed in the person of Jesus Christ. Groome argues that as reflections of God, Catholics must strive to promote the dignity of life for all. 'Our dignity in God's own

466 'The analogy highlights the fact that the ultimate constituents of a symphony are both the notes and their relations. In a piece of music sounds are not heard in isolation from one another; rather we 'co-hear them in the auditory atmosphere of their mutual interrelationships and reciprocal resonance'.

John Sullivan, *Catholic Education: Distinctive and Inclusive*, PhD Thesis, Institute of Education, University of London, 1998, 69. <https://ethos.bl.uk/OrderDetails.do?uin=uk.bl.ethos.287956>. Accessed on 10 December 2020.

467 Thomas Groome, 'What Makes a School Catholic?', in Terence McLaughlin, Joseph O' Keefe and Bernadette O' Keeffe, eds, *The Contemporary Catholic School: Context, Identity and Diversity* (Oxfordshire: RoutledgeFarmer, 1996), 109.

468 For further reading, see Thomas Groome, *What Makes Us Catholic: Eight Gifts for Life* (NY: HarperCollins, 2002), 55–60.

image gives us all inalienable human rights but correspondingly, our capacity to be partners and historical agents gives us the responsibility to defend and promote similar rights for all humankind'.[469] This is a call to affirm the inherent goodness of life, emphasising that no person is irredeemable as they have been made for love, freedom and right relationship with God.

In the person of Jesus Christ, God has become incarnate within human history and according to Groome is '... the definitive catalyst of God's life and love irrevocably turned towards us'.[470] Christ is the revelation of true humanity, what it means to be fully and authentically human by virtue of his historical life. Christ is also the revelation of true divinity, in that humans are of such dignity that God empties Godself out of love into our human reality and offers humanity a personal relationship that is salvific. For Groome, the grace of God in Christ transforms '... our inner selves and empowering our human efforts to do God's will ... without violating our freedom or alleviating our responsibilities'.[471]

Catholic education, like any other model of education, has a distinctive anthropology embedded within it. A Catholic vision of education views the person as a unique individual with intrinsic dignity and made in God's image and likeness. Students have inherent goodness and the capacity for love, which must be fostered in a Catholic school, along with their sense of self-worth and dignity. In the Incarnation, Jesus as the embodiment of humanity and divinity builds upon this intrinsic dignity and offers each person a vision of what it means to be truly human through his life and teachings. As Himes argues, it is the Incarnation that reveals to us that to become more Christlike in our living brings us closer to God, simultaneously cultivating us to become more fully human.

> ... whatever humanises, divinises. That is to say, whatever makes you more genuinely human, more authentically, richly, powerfully human, whatever calls into play all the

469 Thomas Groome, 'What Makes a School Catholic?', in Terence McLaughlin, Joseph O' Keefe and Bernadette O' Keeffe, eds, *The Contemporary Catholic School: Context, Identity and Diversity* (Oxfordshire: RoutledgeFarmer, 1996), 110.

470 Ibid.

471 Ibid.

> reaches of your intellect, your freedom, energy, your talents and creativity, makes you more like God.[472]

In this sense, Catholic education is both a call to holiness and a humanising endeavour. This means that Catholic anthropology calls for an education that promotes the holistic development of the child in all realms of their being, including the intellectual, moral, spiritual, relational and affective. The commitment to forming students as reflections of God thus entails a vision of Catholic education that upholds and promotes human dignity and rights, fully forming students as responsible and collaborative agents of change in society, working with others towards the common good and promoting the goodness and dignity of every person.

Finally, Catholic anthropology demands an education that promotes a conception of human flourishing that has ultimate meaning and significance. This means rejecting notions of humanity that reduce flourishing to materialist or economic ends. Pope Francis has identified the educational challenge of this reductive contemporary anthropocentrism in *Laudato Si',* where compulsive consumerism highlights the absence of human self-awareness in the twenty-first century.[473] This unfettered consumerism cannot nourish this lack of self-awareness and identity, which '… engenders a feeling of instability and uncertainty,'[474] … 'causing people to become self-centred and self-enclosed'.[475] This locking out of any sense of the transcendent in our lives can lead to a spiritual restlessness or sense of futility.

An anthropological vision of Catholic education challenges such an immanent frame by promoting life as having ultimate meaning and worth living, with each student a unique person who can make a positive and meaningful impact in the world. As a reflection of God, students are enabled to be positive and transformational agents of grace in the world. In this sense,

472 Michael J. Himes, 'Living Conversation: Higher Education in a Catholic Context', *Conversations on Jesuit Higher Education 8* (1995), 22. For further reading on Himes' reflection on the Incarnation, see Michael J. Himes, *The Mystery of Faith: An Introduction to Catholicism* (Cincinnati OH, Saint Anthony Messenger Press, 2004) 19–28.

473 Pope Francis, *Laudato Si': On Care for Our Common Home* (Dublin: Veritas, 2015), Par 203. Hereafter, this text will be referred to as *Laudato Si'*, unless otherwise stated.

474 Ibid, Par 204.

475 Ibid, Par 208.

Catholic anthropology demands an education that counters this contemporary anthropocentrism with a conception of humanity as reflections of God, marked by freedom, responsibility and relationality.

Sacramentality

For Groome, the principle of sacramentality reflects the central Catholic conviction that '... God is present to humankind and we respond to God's grace through the ordinary and every day of life in the world'.[476] This distinctive claim arises from the Christian belief that God as self-giving love is the foundation of all that exists. In order to genuinely appreciate anything that exists, Christians are called to see that it is held in existence by God's grace. God as Creator is radically different to the creature; hence, God mediates Godself into our lives in the '... bits and pieces of Every day'.[477] This sacramental awareness enables people to encounter God in any moment of life, rather than restricting God's life to liturgical activities, church life or to holy places. In this sense, any presumed boundary between secular and sacred life is dissolved as for the sacramentality principle, all of creation is engraced.

Groome argues that a sacramental consciousness nurtures a sacramental imagination, enabling the Christian to imagine what God wills for the world, seeing and discerning how to embody Christ's teachings of love, mercy and a preferential option for the poor in everyday life in thoughts, words and actions.

476 Thomas Groome, *What Makes Us Catholic: Eight Gifts for Life* (NY: HarperCollins, 2002), 68. Groome argues that the ordinary of life includes encountering God '... through our minds and bodies, through our work and efforts, in the depth of our own being and through relationships with others, through the events and experiences that come our way, through all forms of human art and creativity, through nature and the whole created order, through everything and anything of life'. Thomas Groome, 'What Makes a School Catholic?', in Terence McLaughlin, Joseph O' Keefe and Bernadette O' Keeffe, eds, *The Contemporary Catholic School: Context, Identity and Diversity* (Oxfordshire: RoutledgeFarmer, 1996), 112.

477 Patrick Kavanagh, *The Great Hunger* (London: Penguin, 2018).

> Christian sacramental consciousness has the disposition 'to see' who should be seen, especially people overlooked or made invisible by society, and to respond as agents of God's reign; it encourages a faith that does justice.[478]

A sacramental imagination goes beyond an awareness of God's grace in any given moment of our existence. However, as Hession argues, imagination here is not to be confused with fantasy.[479] A sacramental imagination thus entails that we embody the agapeic love of God in creation by living out Christ's teachings. In this sense, we are not passive receivers of God's love but active instruments of God's grace in the world.

All education examines the world through a particular viewpoint. In the case of Catholic education, this perspective is sacramental. This means that a vision of Catholic education is committed to encouraging students to become what Himes calls 'sacramental beholders'[480], seeing God's presence in all aspects of their life. Such a commitment cannot be relegated to religious education as the basis of sacramentality is that God's presence can be experienced anywhere and at any time.[481] For teachers, this means instilling in children a sense of wonder and imagination in their everyday lives. Lane emphasises the importance of imagination to Catholic education, and

478 Thomas Groome, 'What Makes a School Catholic?', in Terence McLaughlin, Joseph O' Keefe and Bernadette O' Keeffe, eds, *The Contemporary Catholic School: Context, Identity and Diversity* (Oxfordshire: RoutledgeFarmer, 1996), 113.

479 'Imagination (as opposed to fantasy) does not lead us into the unreal: on the contrary, imagination is precisely that gift which allows us to truly know the real. It is the faculty of seeing reality in depth, in a new way. Ultimately, imagination is the power we have to enter into the divine dimension of reality, the fact that it is held in being in love'. Anne Hession, 'Come and See': The Process of Catechesis', in Anne Hession and Patricia Kieran, eds, *Exploring Religious Education: Catholic Religious Education in an Intercultural Europe* (Dublin: Veritas, 2008), 201.

480 Michael J Himes, 'Living Conversion', *Conversations on Jesuit Higher Education, Fall* (1995), 21–7.

481 For Godzieba, the sacraments and sacramentality '... desire to provoke not only our participation in the saving work of Christ, but also the recognition of our deep resonance with the structure of creation, our sympathetic attunement to the overwhelming love of God who has chosen this time, this place, this materiality, in order to transform us into lovers of grace and truth'. See Anthony J. Godzieba, 'The Catholic Sacramental Imagination and the Access/Excess of Grace', *New Theology Review 21/3* (August 2008), 25.

echoing Michael Paul Gallagher's earlier sentiments, recognises the crisis of imagination observed today.[482]

A sacramental imagination is the antithesis of what Pope Francis calls the 'technocratic imagination' which is the dominant worldview currently operative in Western culture, characterised by utilitarianism and anthropocentrism.[483] Such an imagination has potentially grave implications for education as it can reduce it from the development of the human person to mere knowledge transmission for economic or materialist ends.[484] A sacramental Catholic educational vision challenges conceptions of education that sustain this technocracy, arguing that creation is imbued with God's presence, and that humans are not autocrats but stewards of creation. In this sense, sacramentality provides students with a critical and creative perspective on the world around them, enabling them to be instruments of grace by embodying self-giving love in their actions, especially towards the poor and oppressed.

This sacramentality also seeks to lessen the divide between religious education and secular subjects while also respecting the academic integrity of every subject. As Sullivan argues, through a sacramental lens, 'Every subject in the curriculum has the potential … to allow us to see some feature of the world as a way into appreciating at least part of God's nature, purpose, call

482 Dermot A. Lane, *Challenges Facing Religious Education in Contemporary Ireland* (Dublin: Veritas, 2008), 45. 'Excessive emphasis on doctrine has often led to the neglect of the Catholic imagination. Too many commentators talk about a crisis in Christian doctrine, without realising that the crisis in doctrine may be due to a severing of doctrine from the religious and theological imagination. What is needed is a recovery of the imagination that informs Catholic doctrine'.

483 See *Laudato Si'*, Par 101–36.

484 As Antony Seldon writes, 'A liberal education has too often been replaced by an indoctrination of the young in the answers they need to memorise and regurgitate for exams. It is so all-pervasive that we simply do not see any longer what has happened, and the education establishment -teachers, academics, administrators and those in the quango penumbra- does not acknowledge the impoverishment rather than the flowering of the lives of our young people. See Antony Seldon, 'Our Education System is Collapsing into a Form of Mass Indoctrination', *Independent* (23 October 2011). <https://www.independent.co.uk/voices/commentators/anthony-seldon-our-education-system-collapsing-form-mass-indoctrination-2028709.html>. Accessed on 24 December 2020.

and presence'.[485] This means that a Catholic vision of education can never be reduced to a relativistic transmission of information. Rather, a sacramental perspective means that students are encouraged to look deeper into the mystery of life, a critical aspect in providing children with a holistic education.[486]

Moreover, each subject can offer teaching opportunities to stimulate an awareness of the Holy Mystery, be that science lessons examining the complexities of the universe or the arts which engage the creativity of students.[487] In this sense, religious education is a critically important subject in a Catholic school as it helps to sublate all curricular subjects into a higher unity of opening each student to an awareness of a loving and relational God in their lives.

Community

For Groome, the Church, as community is a significant characteristic of Catholicism in: '… that we encounter God as a community of faith, that the primary mode (not the only one) of God coming to us and our going to God

485 John Sullivan, 'Philosophy of Catholic Education', in Anne Hession and Patricia Kieran, eds, *Exploring Religious Education: Catholic Religious Education in an Intercultural Europe* (Dublin: Veritas, 2008), 30.

486 'What is at stake here is the human capacity to seek the truth, even to inquire about the ultimate mystery of existence. Granted that the pupils in Second Class will not be struggling with the higher reaches of metaphysics, but if they are not taught to deal with mystery and to wonder at things that cannot be proved or experimented upon by the scientific method, and if they are not helped to listen to the tradition of faith which sees God's presence and God's love everywhere in creation, they are not being educated as whole persons'. Address by Bishop Donal Murray, 'Catholic Primary Education in Contemporary Ireland: Facing New Horizons', 2009. <https://www.catholicbishops.ie/2009/05/22/address-by-bishop-donal-murray-bishop-of-limerick-and-chair-of-the-bishops-department-of-catholic-education-and-formation-at-the-mcauley-conference-series-catholic-primary-education-in-cont/>. Accessed on 16 February 2022.

487 See Guillermo Marini and Carmelo Galioto, 'The Way of Beauty' in Catholic Schools: Keys of Understanding and Pedagogical Orientations', *International Studies in Catholic Education* (2023), 1–16.

is as "Church"'.[488] The Church as the Body of Christ is then charged with bringing about the Kingdom of God in society, creating communities based on love of God and love of neighbour, in anticipation of the full realisation of God's Reign at the end of time.[489] As Kilbride puts it:

> ... the Church has a role as bearer and herald of the Kingdom of God, understood not as a place or a state of being, but rather as a dynamic action on God's part, present and guiding the Church, the world and, indeed, the whole of Creation, towards its fulfilment.[490]

For Groome, the communality of Catholicism extends beyond communal worship. It means the Church must be a community that is transformative and liberative in society, of whose members bear witness to the Good News in their lives through effective actions to bring about peace and justice.[491]

488 Thomas Groome, 'What Makes a School Catholic?', in Terence McLaughlin, Joseph O' Keefe and Bernadette O' Keeffe, eds, *The Contemporary Catholic School: Context, Identity and Diversity* (Oxfordshire: RoutledgeFarmer, 1996), 114–5.

489 At the aforementioned 2009 address, Bishop Donal Murray articulated the relationship between community and identity in the Church. 'The sense of community-belonging with the whole of oneself is found in a civilisation or a culture or a religious commitment. When Christians gather for worship, for instance, we gather with the recognition that we are mortal, that we are sinful, that our own resources cannot save us from evil and death, that our very existence is a gift of God the Creator and that our hope is in Christ who died so that we might live the life of the new creation. This is a statement about who we are, not just in one or other aspect or sphere; it is a statement of our whole identity, our very being'. Donal Murray, 'Catholic Primary Education in Contemporary Ireland: Facing New Horizons' 2009. <https://www.catholicbishops.ie/2009/05/22/address-by-bishop-donal-murray-bishop-of-limerick-and-chair-of-the-bishops-department-of-catholic-education-and-formation-at-the-mcauley-conference-series-catholic-primary-education-in-cont/>. Accessed on 16 February 2022.

490 Thomas Kilbride, Understanding the Church Today', in Leonardo Franchi and Stephen McKinney, eds, *A Companion to Catholic Education* (Herefordshire: Gracewing, 2011), 61.

491 'For its mission to the world, the "mind of the Church" seems clearer than ever that it is to be a community of effective action and witness- a sacrament- of God's reign of peace and justice to the world, a catalyst for the "common good"'. Thomas Groome, 'What Makes a School Catholic?', in Terence McLaughlin, Joseph O' Keefe and Bernadette O' Keeffe, eds, *The Contemporary Catholic School: Context, Identity and Diversity* (Oxfordshire: RoutledgeFarmer, 1996), 115.

Catholicism retains a commitment to contribute to the common good, promote social justice and instil in society a preferential option to the poor and the outsider.[492] In this sense, this communality is the embodiment of faith in Christian communities. These communities bear witness to his mission to bring humanity into right relationship with God and with their neighbour through worshipping together and being active agents in creating a society underpinned by the vision of the Good News.[493]

This demands a Catholic school and educational vision that is both a public community and an extension of the teaching Church.[494] The distinctive ethos of each Catholic school socialises people through the inner or hidden curriculum into a community with a holistic view of the human person and rooted in the person of Jesus Christ. This means that there is a distinctive purposefulness to this public community, that the Catholic school is permeated by a spirit of love and social justice in both implicit and explicit curricula. The explicit teaching and learning in this community are implicitly grounded by a spirit of openness, relationship and partnership.

Moreover, this means that the educational vision in a Catholic school must challenge values in society antithetical to the common good such as individualism and moral relativism. Sacks argues that a critical threat to Western liberal democracy is this shift from a societal moral concern the

492 However, as Groome points out, this concept, which emphasises both person and community has often fell short of balancing the two, giving rise to clericalism or an undermining of synodality. 'It (Catholicism) can be so intent on touting the Church that it forgets the rights and responsibilities of individual members. It is unrivalled for making its clergy a favoured elite- clericalism- with complete power in all matters of sanctifying, teaching and ruling'. Thomas Groome, *What Makes Us Catholic: Eight Gifts for Life* (NY: HarperCollins, 2002), 117.

493 For further reading, see Thomas Groome, *What Makes Us Catholic: Eight Gifts for Life* (NY: HarperCollins, 2002), 105–32.

494 Thomas Groome, 'What Makes a School Catholic?' in Terence McLaughlin, Joseph O' Keefe and Bernadette O' Keeffe, eds, *The Contemporary Catholic School: Context, Identity and Diversity* (Oxfordshire: RoutledgeFarmer, 1996), 115.

welfare of others to a buffered self-interest.[495] Challenging this turn, students should be socialised to be members of communities underpinned by collective responsibility rather than personal self-interest, where individual wellbeing is understood as being fundamentally connected to the wellbeing of others. This means challenging all forms of discrimination, hatred and dehumanising trends in society.[496]

A Catholic school community is also an extension of the common life shared by those who are called out to be in right relationship with God, the Church that is the body of Christ. In this sense, the school remains a place of formation for students in the Catholic faith and into relationship with Jesus Christ. This means providing opportunities for communal prayer, engagement with the Word of God and an administrative approach that recognises the innate human dignity of each person. In doing so, as Barrie and Jones argue, Catholic education must propose a conception of the human person that is made for right relationship with each other and with God.[497]

495 See Jonathan Sacks, *Morality: Restoring the Common Good in Divided Times* (London: Hodder & Stoughton, 2020), 1. 'If we focus on the "I" and lose the "We", if we act on self-interest without a commitment to the common good, if we focus on self-esteem and lose our care for others, we will lose much else … We will lose our feelings of collective responsibility and find in its place a culture of competitive victimhood. In an age of unprecedented possibilities, people will feel vulnerable and alone'.

496 'Stated negatively, if a school does not challenge and encourage its students to oppose racism, sexism, militarism, ageism, and all other such "isms" that bedevil our society and world, its education is not Catholic'. Thomas Groome, 'What Makes a School Catholic?', in Terence McLaughlin, Joseph O' Keefe and Bernadette O' Keeffe, eds, *The Contemporary Catholic School: Context, Identity and Diversity* (Oxfordshire: RoutledgeFarmer, 1996), 116.

497 Teaching is understood as to persons by persons. Every approach to education presupposes an understanding of the human person and a Christian approach will be based on an understanding of the person as existing in communion, not only in relation to other people but in relation to God. Furthermore, it is the vertical communion in God in Christ that shapes and sustains the horizontal communion with other people'. David Albert Jones and Stephen Barrie, *Thinking Christian Ethos: The Meaning of Catholic Education* (Oxford: Catholic Truth Society, 2015), 122–3.

Tradition

Catholic education is committed to sharing with the world the Good News of salvation, which is the mission of the Church. This news is rooted in the conviction that in the Incarnation, God becomes man in the person of Jesus Christ. Groome argues that Christ as the Word made flesh '… is at the heart of Catholic education. Encounter with the person of Jesus Christ and his "good news of salvation" is mediated now through Christian Story and Vision'.[498] This reality of the Christian faith is seen in Scripture and Tradition, developed and handed down through Church teaching. This historical reality of Christian faith is reflected and carried on through the pluriform of Catholic elements that symbolise this continuing revelation of the Incarnation.[499] This narrative is in constant and ongoing dialogue with the Christian Vision, presenting a living encounter with God's revelation. This continuing journey of Tradition into divine truth is a significant theme of Vatican II, expressed clearly in the document *Dei Verbum*.[500]

The Christian Vision then represents how Catholics live out the reign of God in response to the Christian Story. This means being shaped by our continuing encounter with Jesus Christ and being effective witness to the Good News in thought, word and action. Such a commitment to Christian life is '… the ongoing coming to fulfilment of God's intentions of shalom and fullness of life for humanity, history and all creation'.[501] This Vision is the application and translation of the Christian story to our own lives, a continuing encounter with Jesus Christ who is the revelation of the salvific

498 Thomas Groome, 'What Makes a School Catholic?', in Terence McLaughlin, Joseph O' Keefe and Bernadette O' Keeffe, eds, *The Contemporary Catholic School: Context, Identity and Diversity* (Oxfordshire: RoutledgeFarmer, 1996), 117.

499 Ibid, 117–118. These elements include '… its scriptures and liturgies; its creeds, dogmas, doctrines and theologies; its sacraments and rituals, symbols, myths, gestures and religious language patterns; its spiritualities, laws and expected lifestyles …'.

500 'The tradition which comes from the apostles develops in the Church with the help of the Holy Spirit. For there is a growth in the understanding of the realities and the words which have been handed down … (A)s the centuries succeed one another, the Church constantly moves forward towards the fullness of divine truth', Vatican II, *Dei Verbum* (1965), Par 13.

501 Ibid, 118.

will of God. In this sense, Tradition represents the ongoing formation of the person in light of the Good News, made possible through the entering of God in the human condition in the Incarnation.[502]

A vision of Catholic education must commit to a sharing of the Christian Story and Vision through religious education in the Catholic school. This means that people are encouraged to see that the Christian Vision and Story gives meaning to their lives and that following Jesus' ways and teachings fulfils our innermost yearnings.

Evangelisation and religious education are not to be misinterpreted as indoctrination, where students are presented with uncritical or unreasoned propaganda for Catholicism to be treated as unquestionably true. As Whittle argues, such an approach is *anathema* to Catholic education[503] and as has been noted earlier, Church teachings have stressed the autonomy and academic freedom of curricular subjects in Catholic schools, as well as the religious freedom of each person. In the school setting, Catholic religious education, while sensitive to the diverse religious backgrounds and worldviews of students, has a mandate to provide faith formation and instruction to Catholic students. Hession argues that children are enabled:

> … to immerse themselves in Christian religious beliefs, practices and values, inviting them to live inside the Christian vision of the good life. The goal, in the schooling context, is religious understanding and promotion of belonging and commitment to the Catholic religious tradition and to the Church community.[504]

This passing on of the Christian tradition is a holistic endeavour, nurturing the formation of students in light of God's revelation in Jesus Christ. This

502 For further reading on the Catholic characteristic of tradition, see Brendan Leahy, 'Tradition', in Anne Hession and Patricia Kieran, eds, *Exploring Theology: Making Sense of the Catholic Tradition* (Dublin: Veritas, 2007), 90–8.

503 Whittle summarises the understanding of indoctrination as incompatible with authentic education. 'To be indoctrinated is normally taken to be the antithesis of being properly educated. Indoctrination involves acquiring beliefs in non-rational ways whereas education involves acquiring them through rational ways. If Catholic schools, as faith schools, involve indoctrination then this amounts to a major philosophical objection to their existence'. Sean Whittle, *A Theory of Catholic Education* (London: Bloomsbury, 2015), 18.

504 Anne Hession, *Catholic Primary Religious Education in a Pluralist Environment* (Dublin: Veritas, 2015), 148.

entails that students are given the opportunity to reflect upon the symbols, values and beliefs of the Catholic faith, and nurtured into developing a personal relationship with Christ. Catholic education requires students that are formed to be critical and creative citizens in society, translating the Good News into their lives and into the culture around them and challenging individualistic and relativist trends in contemporary culture.

While Tradition is passed on in religious education, a vision of Catholic education means that the entire curriculum must be underpinned by the evangelical character of a Catholic school. The school, working in partnership with the parents and the parish is a microcosm of the Body of Christ, the educating Church that continues in its task of evangelisation. Such a commitment means that the education provided can never be reduced to the service of the labour market, or that openness to the sacred be replaced by closed, instrumentalist reasoning. For Catholic children, the handing on of Tradition instead means that they are nurtured into a Christian narrative in which God, through the person of Jesus Christ has revealed His love and salvific will for all.

Rationality

Groome argues a distinctive characteristic of Catholicism is its commitment to scholarship and reason, that faith and reason need and augment each other.[505] Faith needs reason to avoid falling into religious fundamentalism while reason is enhanced and enriched by faith opening the mind to the mystery of God and the spiritual dimension of the human person. A Catholic commitment to rationality presupposes that knowledge, reason and judgment are neither objective nor value-free. Rather, the pursuit of

505 Thomas Groome, 'What Makes a School Catholic?', in Terence McLaughlin, Joseph O' Keefe and Bernadette O' Keeffe, eds, *The Contemporary Catholic School: Context, Identity and Diversity* (Oxfordshire: RoutledgeFarmer, 1996), 119.

knowledge is shaped by a Catholic worldview and ethic, stressing the need for reason to serve human flourishing.[506]

In this sense, a Catholic view of rationality is to be applied to contributing to the common good and bearing witness to the Christian life. The symbiosis of faith and reason is a path to critical and creative interaction with the world, putting our critical faculties at the service of others to bring about the inclusive and welcoming society that is the Kingdom of God.

Rationality in the Catholic tradition is thus a humanising enterprise, based on a multidimensional Catholic anthropology that sees the person as made for right relationship with the world and with God. This holistic view of the human person means that intellectual development can never be separated from the relational, moral or affective aspects of being human. Rather, it is but one element of an integral understanding of what it means to be human.

A vision of Catholic education is committed to the holistic development of students, which includes the nurturing of the intellect and critical faculties. This Catholic approach to reason and knowledge means that Catholic education can never be reduced to a means of training individuals for economic or market purposes, as Murray argues.[507] Catholic education is a humanising endeavour in which reason is illuminated by faith, where knowledge is underpinned by a Christian ethic and perspective. As Evans argues, this dynamic relation between faith and reason means that students are offered:

506 Ibid, 120. In this it rejects the disembodied rationality of Cartesianism, and avoids the dichotomous schema of Kant that separates theoretical from practical reasoning, and thus science from ethics. It rejects the now common assumption that reasoning is 'objective' and 'value free'. Instead, Catholicism sees reason as a gift of God that is to bring us to both understanding and moral responsibility.

507 Donal Murray, *A Special Concern – The Philosophy of Education: A Christian Perspective* (Dublin: Veritas, 1991), 6–7. 'If education were to convey the idea that the purpose of human life is to be found in examinations passed and jobs obtained it would communicate a shallow and impoverished falsehood. It is one of the prime purposes of education to communicate and to deepen an appreciation of the nature and dignity of the human person'.

> … an understanding of the richness of what it is to be human. Human beings are individual but complex. Each has a unique identity and many have a capacity for understanding, desire and an appreciation of beauty. Though knowledge may begin with simple perception it requires mental skill, ingenuity and creativity to bring it to completion in wisdom, which allows people to comprehend the totality of the world, the depths of the human heart and mind and the mystery of God.[508]

Catholic education sees rationality as one of the many dimensions of what it means to be human. The person, being made in the likeness and image of God is enabled to develop their intellect in the process of becoming more human, acquiring knowledge and making reasoned judgements and choices in freedom. This Catholic rationality is underpinned by a belief that reason is graced to us by God and to be put to use for the wellbeing of society. This means that students are not passive recipients of knowledge but active learners, critically appraising knowledge using their imagination and reason, enabling them to reach informed and responsible decisions for the common good. As D'Souza puts it, '… the intellectual mandate of the Catholic school must always be at the service of human unity, and more fundamentally, at the service of Christ and his call to pick up one's cross and follow him'.[509] Students are thus called to put their intellectual faculties at the service of others, embodying Christ's life and teaching in their actions and decisions.

A Catholic vision of education is committed to the transmission of knowledge in light of God's revelation in Jesus Christ. Thus, students are taught truths of the Catholic faith in religious education that are a handing on of the Christian narrative. This means that rationality in a Catholic perspective is counter cultural to postmodern or relativist positions that there is no ultimate truth. Rather than utilise rationality as a means to apologetics, the Catholic school enables students to critically engage with the Christian story, to think independently and apply the Gospel message to their lives though reasoned moral actions. Moreover, students are fostered into seeing knowledge as a gift that can flourish into wisdom and awareness of the presence of God in their lives.

508 David Evans, 'Faith and Reason: The Route to Wisdom', in Stephen McKinney and John Sullivan, eds, *Education in a Catholic Perspective* (Surrey: Ashgate, 2013).

509 Mario D'Souza, *A Catholic Philosophy of Education: The Church and Two Philosophers* (Quebec: McGill-Queen's University Press, 2016), 214.

Personhood

Groome argues that Catholic education is concerned with epistemology but also ontology. Catholic schools then focus on the transmission of knowledge but also provide a conception of what is to be human, what it means for a person to flourish, lead a good life and contribute to the common good of society. 'Catholic education intends to inform and form the very "being" of its students, to mould their identity and agency- who they are and how they live'.[510] This Catholic ontological commitment engages the human person in their totality, shattering conceptions of knowledge as non-perspectival or value-free.

For Groome, this Catholic commitment to personhood acknowledges the Christian and Jewish tradition of epistemology and ontology as unified in the full development of the human person, shaped by a theological anthropology. '… in the Hebrew and Christian traditions, "to know" means a wisdom that brings one's very 'being' into right relationship with God, self-others, and creation; ultimately, to know is to love …'[511] In this way, knowledge becomes a path to wisdom and to deeper relationship with God, through the holistic development of the person. A Catholic concern for personhood acknowledges the multidimensionality of each individual, and that they are made for love and for freedom. In Jesus Christ, every person is then given the opportunity to have life in abundance, to flourish and embody right relationship.

The Catholic school as a site of Catholic education must then be concerned with both epistemology and ontology. Jesus Christ is at the heart of this dyad. McKinney argues that this means that for the entire school community, '… being is with, in and for Christ. This is not necessarily an introverted understanding of being but a being that welcomes others and invites them to share, insomuch as they wish to, the richness of this theological

510 Thomas Groome, 'What Makes a School Catholic?', in Terence McLaughlin, Joseph O' Keefe and Bernadette O' Keeffe, eds, *The Contemporary Catholic School: Context, Identity and Diversity* (Oxfordshire: RoutledgeFarmer, 1996), 121.

511 Ibid.

vision of education'.[512] In this sense, being in Catholic education is a community of persons rooted in Christ, sharing in a distinctive vision of what it means to be human.

For McLaughlin, central to the rationale for a Catholic school is:

> ... a 'Christian personalism' involving a moral conception of social behaviour in a just community, a concern for social justice and the common good in an ecumenical and multicultural world and the development of personal responsibility and social engagement.[513]

This commitment to personhood means students are nurtured to reach their full potential to contribute to the wellbeing of society. This means the developments of students as reasoned, imaginative and socially conscious citizens that put their skills and talents at the service of others, to bring about a more just society. In this way, they are translating the Good News into the culture around them. This also means recognising and challenging aspects of culture that dehumanise and depersonalise others.

Finally, this ontological concern means that a vision of Catholic education cannot be compromised by instrumentalist reasoning based on competitiveness and effectiveness. A person cannot be reduced to a vessel for upskilling at the service of a market economy. Personhood means recognition of reason but also creativity, relationality, imagination, social justice and personal responsibility. A Catholic educational vision challenges schools to cultivate in pupils all of these dimensions to their fullest potential as integral formation of the human person.

Justice

Groome argues that social justice is a key tenet of Catholicism. This entails a responsible and proactive approach to practical charity and the

512 Stephen McKinney, 'A Rationale for Catholic Schools', in Leonardo Franchi and Stephen McKinney, eds, *A Companion to Catholic Education* (Herefordshire: Gracewing, 2011), 151.

513 Terence McLaughlin, 'The Distinctiveness of Catholic Education', in Terence McLaughlin, Joseph O' Keefe and Bernadette O' Keeffe, eds, *The Contemporary Catholic School: Context, Identity and Diversity* (Oxfordshire: RoutledgeFarmer, 1996), 142.

pursuit of justice, putting the Gospel teachings into action.[514] The 1971 World Synod of Bishops express the centrality of justice to the Church's mission, arguing:

> Action on behalf of justice and participation in the transformation of the world fully appears to us a constitutive dimension of the preaching of the Gospel, or in other words, of the Church's mission for the redemption of the human race and its liberation from every oppressive situation.[515]

This commitment to justice is a call to embody the Gospel values of mercy and solidarity. For the Christian, this means putting love of God and love of neighbour into action in their lives, in thought, word and action. Christ exemplifies throughout his life recognition of the inherent dignity of every person, especially those marginalised in society. Jesus' parables stress God's love is unconditional and to become closer to God, people are called to be in right relationship with others through love and forgiveness, with a preferential option for the marginalised. The Good Samaritan (Luke 10:25–37) and the Unforgiving Servant (Matthew 18: 21–35) are such examples.

The Christian is called to embody this self-forgetting love by modelling right relationships with self, others, God and the world. In this way, justice represents a vital aspect of what it means to be Christian, putting the Good News into action to form communities of self-giving love and mercy. Pope Francis stresses that justice must be an integral element of contemporary

514 Grace argues that the concept of social justice, brought into formal discourse by Pope Pius XI's encyclical *Quadragesimo Anno* (1931), has been further developed and elaborated in the spirit of Vatican II, seen in documents such as Pope Paul VI's 1967 encyclical, *Populorum Progressio*. See Gerald Grace, 'First and Foremost the Church Offers its Educational Service to the Poor' Class. Inequality and Catholic Schooling in Contemporary Contexts' in *Gerald Grace, Faith, Mission and Challenge in Catholic Education: The Selected Works of Gerald Grace* (NY: RoutledgeFarmer, 2016), 68.

515 World Synod of Bishops, *Justice in the World,* (1971) Par 6. <https://www.cctwincities.org/wp-content/uploads/2015/10/Justicia-in-Mundo.pdf>. Accessed on 19 April 2021.

Christian faith, particularly in light of contemporary extremism, xenophobia and hatred.[516]

Catholic education demands of its schools a radical commitment to justice through a preferential love for those who are poor, excluded or voiceless. Church literature has defined this dedication as a central regulative principle for the development of Catholic schools.[517] This means that an authentic vision of Catholic education forms students to an awareness about structural inequalities in society and the initiative to work with others to challenge and eliminate them. McKinney has consistently stressed the prophetic vision of the preferential option for the poor, citing the Scriptural basis for this commitment, not least in light of the profound challenges presented by the COVID-19 pandemic.[518]

Jesus is the revelation of God's self-giving love for all, both the rich and the poor. Kieran and Hession note that Christ's life is devoted to the reign

516 Pope Francis, *Fratelli Tutti* (Dublin: Veritas, 2020) Par 86. 'Faith and the humanism it inspires, must maintain a critical sense in the face of these tendencies, and prompt an immediate response whenever they rear their head. For this reason, it is important that catechesis and preaching speak more directly and clearly about the social meaning of existence, the fraternal dimension of spirituality, our conviction of the inalienable dignity of each person, and our reasons for loving and accepting all our brothers and sisters'. The encyclical will be referenced thereafter as *Fratelli Tutti.*

517 See *CS*, Par 58. 'First and foremost the Church offers its educational service to the poor, or those who are deprived of family help and affection, or those who are from the faith. Since education is an important means of impoverishing the social and economic condition of the individual and of peoples …'.

518 For further reading, see Stephen J. McKinney, 'The Roots of the Preferential Option for the Poor in Catholic Schools in Luke's Gospel', *International Studies in Catholic Education 10*(2) (2018) 220–32, Stephen J. McKinney, 'The Preferential Option for the Poor and Catholic Schools'. In Sean Whittle (Ed.), *Researching Catholic Education: Contemporary Perspectives* (Singapore: Springer, 2018) 95–112, Stephen J. McKinney, 'Affirming the Place of Scripture in the Catholic School', in Sean Whittle (Ed.), *Religious Education in Catholic Schools* (Oxford: Peter Lang, 2018) 173–92, Stephen J. McKinney, 'Covid-19: Food Insecurity, Digital Exclusion and Catholic Schools', *Journal of Religious Education 68*(3) (2020) 319–30 and Stephen J. McKinney, 'Covid-19, Child Poverty, Catholic Schools and the Insights of Gustavo Gutiérrez'. In Sean Whittle (Ed.), *Irish and British Reflections on Catholic Education* (Singapore: Springer, 2021).

of God, but this message is especially directed to those excluded and looked down on precisely because of their situation.

> Perhaps the most scandalous aspect of Jesus' life was that he revealed a distinct partiality for those who were weak, dependent and oppressed … He believed that the reign of God is open to all but not in the same way to all. It is addressed only to the poor … Jesus' deepest desire was to create a social-political situation in which people could be free and so fulfil God's wish that they might have live and live it to the full. His deepest concern was for the victims of sinful structures, prejudices and practices.[519]

The Catholic school is rooted in Jesus Christ, and this means that the life of the school, its curriculum, management and ethos constantly embody Jesus' desire for equality and fairness. The Catholic school as a community is also called to model right relationship with self, others, God and creation, which highlights each person's ability to contribute to the common good. It requires learners to be nurtured into mindfulness of the poor and voiceless in society and the capacity to challenge such structural inequalities. This option for the poor is central to the mission of the Church, to bring the good news of salvation to all people. This is a task that must then be at the heart of a Catholic school.

In recent writings, Pope Francis has critiqued the continuing inequalities between rich and poor[520] falls short of a Christian teaching on human dignity, as well as the need to recognise in light of the climate crisis, '… a true ecological approach always becomes a social approach; it must integrate questions of justice in debates on the environment, so as to hear the cry of the earth and the cry of the poor'.[521] In this sense, justice is an integral element of what it means to be a Catholic today, and a Catholic educational vision must reflect and embody this.

519 Anne Hession and Patricia Kieran, *Children, Catholicism & Religious Education* (Dublin: Veritas, 2005) 254–55.

520 *Fratelli Tutti*, Par 22. 'While one part of humanity lives in opulence, another sees its own dignity denied, scorned or trampled upon, and its fundamental rights discarded or violated. What does this tell us about the equality of rights grounded in innate human dignity?'

521 *Laudato Si'*, Par 49.

Catholicity

Groome argues that 'catholic', with its etymological roots in '*kata holou*' meaning 'embracing the whole', is best understood as inclusive rather than universal. 'Both Nazism and Communism had ambitions of universality, but in a dominating way'.[522] Rather, to be Catholic means to be embracing and inclusive of all, welcoming others into community. In this sense, Catholic can never mean an exclusivity that closes off the possibility of fellowship and solidarity with the other. Catholic means an openness to all, acknowledging diversity and a spirit of hospitality to the other. As Kieran notes, 'To be Catholic is to be called to live a life focused on inclusivity. It recognises the unity and dignity of all human life …'[523]

Vatican II marks a seismic development of this characteristic with regard to this inclusivity, with particular reference to those of different faith backgrounds. This is seen in the Conciliar document *Nostra Aetate* (hereafter *NA*), which according to Lane '… was the shortest document of the Council' yet '… may however, have the longest effect on the life of the Church'.[524]

This document highlights this new self-understanding of what it means to be catholic with respect to other religions. This is seen in statements such as:

- The Church rejects nothing of what is good and true in other religions.[525]
- Other religions 'often reflect a ray of that Truth which enlightens all'.[526]
- Christians are called to acknowledge 'the spiritual and moral truths found among non-Christians'.[527]

522 Thomas Groome, 'What Makes a School Catholic?', in Terence McLaughlin, Joseph O' Keefe and Bernadette O' Keeffe, eds, *The Contemporary Catholic School: Context, Identity and Diversity* (Oxfordshire: RoutledgeFarmer, 1996), 123.

523 Patricia Kieran, 'Invisibility and Inclusivity: Approaches to Religious Difference in Schools', in Anne Hession and Patricia Kieran, eds, *Exploring Religious Education: Catholic Religious Education in an Intercultural Europe* (Dublin: Veritas, 2008), 157.

524 Dermot A. Lane, *Stepping Stones to Other Religions: A Christian Theology of Inter-Religious Dialogue* (Dublin: Veritas, 2011), 19.

525 Vatican II, *Nostra Aetate* (1965), Par 2.

526 Ibid.

527 Ibid.

- 'The Church ... urges its sons and daughters to enter, with prudence and charity, into discussion and collaboration with members of other religions'.[528]

This call to openness and dialogue with others is at the heart of catholicity, encountering those other to the Christian faith with respect and hospitality. Such an approach is not to dilute a Christian's personal faith. On the contrary, through dialogue and a spirit of fellowship with other religions, Christian faith can be deepened and enriched in recognising the universality of God's salvific will in all religions.

A vision of Catholic education must be permeated by this spirit of inclusivity and openness, characterised by inter-faith dialogue. This is especially necessary in an increasingly diverse and multicultural Irish society. According to Coll, schools in particular play an important role in initiating interfaith dialogue in the public square as they are communities of early encounter and learning with others. 'Schools should, therefore, seek to help students to grow in awareness and respect for both the religious search and experience which are at work in different traditions'.[529] This is a continuation of *NA*'s teaching of dialogue with others. In order for a Catholic school to be catholic, an inclusive and welcoming community must be built up that recognises the good in each other, irrespective of creed, colour or background.

Lane argues that authentic inter-religious dialogue is a significant aspect of post-Conciliar Catholic self-identity, which has implications for the inclusivity envisioned by Catholic education. In particular, in recognising and respecting other religions in dialogue, the Christian is acknowledging the irreducibility of the other's faith perspective, refusing to view it through the lens of relativism.

> Religious Education will go out of its way to take difference seriously, to value otherness and welcome diversity as a source of richness. Within its perspective, religious education will see the 'Religious other' not as a threat but as a gift to be welcomed,

528 Ibid.

529 Niall Coll, 'The Path of Interfaith Dialogue: Catholic Theological Explorations and their Significance for Education', in Niall Coll, ed., *Ireland and Vatican II: Essays Theological, Pastoral and Educational* (Dublin: Columba Press, 2015), 325.

> not as an outsider but as a companion on the journey of faith, not as a rival but as a partner in promoting the values of the Reign of God in the world.[530]

This commitment to inclusivity means that Catholic education recognises the Spirit of God at work in other faith traditions while not patronising or undermining them, as Murray notes.[531] In the Catholic school, such a catholic concern represents an embodiment of Christ's openness to others and wish to be in right relationship with them. This means that each person in the school community is welcomed, valued and celebrated for their uniqueness. Such an approach presupposes that Catholic students are being nurtured in the Christian faith as the deeper the person's relationship to Christ is, the greater the possibility of spiritual enrichment in encountering the other in dialogue.

A Catholic vision of education challenges schools to build up communities that are places of authentic dialogue. This means that learners are encouraged to enter into open dialogue with other cultures and religions while upholding the centrality of Jesus Christ as the revelation of God's universal salvific will. Such an inclusivity can lead to a deepening of one's own Christian faith while recognising in the other the shared promotion of human rights and freedoms. Moreover, Pope Francis argues that such inclusivity involves both a clear sense of one's Christian identity and an empathetic orientation towards others, especially the poor,[532] particularly evidenced in his encyclical *Fratelli Tutti*:

530 Dermot Lane, '*Nostra Aetate* and Religious Education', in Anne Hession and Patricia Kieran, eds, *Exploring Religious Education: Catholic Religious Education in an Intercultural Europe* (Dublin: Veritas, 2008), 94. For further reading, see Dermot A. Lane, *Stepping Stones to Other Religions: A Christian Theology of Inter-Religious Dialogue* (Maryknoll, NY: Orbis Books, 2011).

531 Donal Murray, *A Special Concern- The Philosophy of Education: A Christian Perspective* (Dublin: Veritas, 1991), 20. "Christian education should recognise that nothing which is genuinely human should fail to find an echo in the heart of the follower of Christ and that all that is humanly good: the dignity, the solidarity, the freedom and the achievements will be found again, free from every flaw, in God's eternal kingdom."

532 See Pope Francis, *Evangelii Gaudium: The Joy of the Gospel* (Dublin: Veritas, 2013), Par 51. '... true openness means remaining firm in one's deepest convictions, and therefore being able to understand others'.

> It follows that we believers need to find occasions to speak with one another and to act together for the common good and the promotion of the poor. This has nothing to do with watering down or concealing our deepest convictions when we encounter others who think differently than ourselves … For the deeper, stronger and richer our own identity is, the more we will be capable of enriching others with our own proper contribution.[533]

By recognising God in the other and in other religious traditions, Catholic education enables learners to be reflections of God and embody right relationship with self, others, God and creation.

Criteria for a vision of Catholic education

Having investigated the foundations of a coherent Catholic educational vision throughout this chapter, criteria for our evaluative task can now be devised.

Catholic education is inspired by a theological anthropology

This criterion is selected as it has been observed in this chapter as a foundational element of Catholic education. This is seen in the emphasis placed upon it in all of the Church documents explored above, as well as the importance placed upon it by a litany of Catholic educational scholars including Thomas Groome, John Sullivan, Patricia Kieran and Anne Hession. All education presupposes a view of the human person. Catholic education is no different in this regard, however such a vision incorporates a distinctive view of the human person and human flourishing, seeing each person as made for God and for good. This theocentric anthropology thus encompasses a recognition of the divine at work in the person. In this regard, any authentic

533 *Fratelli Tutti*, Par 282.

vision of Catholic education must be underpinned by a theological anthropology, promoting the holistic development of the child. As Randles puts it:

> ... the Catholic school is called on to be outstanding with regard to the solid human, moral, scholastic and cultural formation of its pupils and with regard to an up-to-date preparation of young people for active and responsible participation in every area of social, economic, professional, and civic life.[534]

Catholic education is radically Christocentric

Like theological anthropology above, the centrality of Christ to the educational endeavour of the Catholic schools means that it is an essential criterion for our evaluation. This is demonstrated by the consistent importance placed on Christocentricity in the post-Conciliar documents, especially *GE*, *CS* and *EIDCS*. Stephen McKinney further demonstrates this point, arguing that the epistemology and ontology of the Catholic school is rooted in Jesus Christ.[535] There is an intimate connection between theological anthropology and Christocentricity as it is in the person of Jesus Christ are we invited to see what authentic humanity represents, in right relationship with self, God, others and Creation. Himes reaffirms this position, highlighting how being formed to be Christlike brings us into closer relationship with God. '... whatever humanises, divinises. ... whatever makes you more genuinely human, more authentically, richly, powerfully human, whatever calls into

534 Eileen Randles, 'The Ethos of the Catholic Primary School' in *Catholic Primary Schools Management Association Board of Management Handbook 2012*, 49. <https://education.dublindiocese.ie/wp-content/uploads/sites/5/2012/02/CPSMA_Handbook_2012.pdf>. Accessed on 15 February 2022.

535 God is the source of all knowledge, and '... being for the school community ... is being in, with and for Christ'. Stephen McKinney, 'A Rationale for Catholic Schools', in Leonardo Franchi and Stephen McKinney, eds, *A Companion to Catholic Education* (Herefordshire: Gracewing, 2011), 151.

play all the reaches of your intellect, your freedom, energy, your talents and creativity, makes you more like God'.[536]

Catholic education is permeated by a sacramental imagination

This criterion is included on the basis of the importance placed on sacramentality in the Catholic tradition by Thomas Groome, as well as the thought of John Sullivan and Michael Himes on encouraging students in Catholic education to become sacramental beholders.[537] For Sullivan, 'Every subject in the curriculum has the potential … to allow us to see some feature of the world as a way into appreciating at least part of God's nature, purpose, call and presence'.[538] Sacramentality must then be included as it opens each student to an education rooted in wonder and imagination, enabling an openness to mystery and an outlook that sees life as sacred and grace-filled. Moreover, it dissolves a presupposed secular/sacred binary in Catholic education, further highlighting the distinctiveness of the education envisioned in a Catholic school.

Catholic education shares in the Church's mission of evangelisation

Evangelisation is radically connected to a Catholic educational vision and, as such, it merits inclusion as a criterion. Given the secularisation and decreasing levels of religious practice and communal worship in Ireland, the Catholic school has become for many children the only place where they come to

536 Michael J. Himes, 'Living Conversation: Higher Education in a Catholic Context', *Conversations on Jesuit Higher Education 8* (1995), 22. For further reading on Himes' reflection on the Incarnation, see Michael J. Himes, *The Mystery of Faith: An Introduction to Catholicism* (Cincinnati OH, Saint Anthony Messenger Press, 2004), 19–28.

537 Michael J Himes, 'Living Conversion', *Conversations on Jesuit Higher Education, Fall* (1995), 21–7.

538 John Sullivan, 'Philosophy of Catholic Education', in Anne Hession and Patricia Kieran, eds, *Exploring Religious Education: Catholic Religious Education in an Intercultural Europe* (Dublin: Veritas, 2008), 30.

know and be formed in light of the Good News. Groome recognises the significance of evangelisation to Catholic education, also seen in the importance placed on it in *GE*. Moreover, Eileen Randles asks some concise and at times challenging questions on how Catholic schools live out their evangelising character:

> Does faith in God inform our days and inspire our thinking and speaking? Is the importance of Ritual recognised and honoured in our school? Do you see your school as an integral part of the parish and of the church's mission? Is belief in God a given to be treasured and nurtured by and within the school community?[539]

Evangelisation remains an essential aspect of what a Catholic school does, but this is not to be confused with reductive terms such as indoctrination, proselytism or apologetics.

Catholic education is committed to academic integrity and the autonomy of subjects

A Catholic educational vision is committed to academic excellence, and as such, it must be included as a criterion. The Catholic school is an educational site, and the intellectual development of the student is a vital component of the holistic development of the pupil. This criterion is given expression in *GE*, *CS* and *RDECS*, and has been reiterated by many Catholic educational scholars, including Thomas Groome, Mario D'Souza and Sean Whittle. Moreover, *Vision 08* stresses the complementarity of faith and reason, and

539 Eileen Randles, 'The Ethos of the Catholic Primary School' in *Catholic Primary Schools Management Association Board of Management Handbook 2012*, 54. <https://education.dublindiocese.ie/wp-content/uploads/sites/5/2012/02/CPSMA_Handbook_2012.pdf>. Accessed on 18 April 2025.

the importance of a rigorous and stimulating academic education.[540] In this sense, the autonomy of subjects are especially important in highlighting the standard of academic excellence that is demanded of a Catholic educational vision, which merits inclusion as a criterion.

Catholic education is committed to dialogue between faith and culture

A renewal of the relationship between the Church and the modern world is at the heart of the legacy of the Second Vatican Council. Accordingly, the relationship between faith and culture must also be at the heart of a Catholic educational vision, thus meriting inclusion as a criterion. This is evidenced by the emphasis placed on it across all of the post-Conciliar documents explored above, as well as being observed in the work of Thomas Groome, Patricia Kieran and Leonardo Franchi, the latter going so far as arguing that the emergence of intercultural dialogue being '... an overarching aim of Catholic schooling'.[541] The importance of this criterion is further demonstrated by the writings of Pope Francis on promoting a fraternal humanism, a person-centred education rooted in openness and solidarity.[542]

540 Irish Catholic Bishops' Conference. *Vision 08: A Vision for Catholic Education in Ireland – Pastoral Letter* (2008) 3. 'Catholic education has always placed a high value on reason, both intellectual and practical. In continuity with the earliest traditions of the Church, it regards education and the cultivation of intellectual life as precious in themselves. It sees the use of rational thought and scientific analysis as essential to the advancement of technology and human progress ... Faith and reason must be seen as vibrant partners in the human quest for understanding and ultimate fulfilment which is pursued in Catholic schools'.

541 Leonardo Franchi, 'Catholic Education and Intercultural Dialogue', *Logos: A Journal of Catholic Thought and Culture 19*(4) (2016), 117.

542 *Fratelli Tutti*, Par 86. 'Faith and the humanism it inspires, must maintain a critical sense in the face of these tendencies, and prompt an immediate response whenever they rear their head. For this reason, it is important that catechesis and preaching speak more directly and clearly about the social meaning of existence, the fraternal dimension of spirituality, our conviction of the inalienable dignity of each person, and our reasons for loving and accepting all our brothers and sisters'.

Catholic education is committed to social justice

Finally, the preferential option for the poor is observed as a profound aspect of the Church's mission, which is connected with the recognition of the innate human dignity each person possesses. As such, any Catholic educational vision must include a commitment to social justice as a criterion, given the radical self-giving nature of Christ's life, death and mission. Several educational scholars observed above identify social justice as essential to Catholic education, including Thomas Groome, Gerald Grace and Anne Hession. The theme of justice is also central to much of Pope Francis' writings, highlighting the importance of fairness, equality and solidarity with the poor in living out the Christian faith.[543]

543 *Laudato Si'*, Par 49.

CHAPTER 5

Evaluating the Compatibility of Mindfulness with a Catholic Vision of Education

This chapter will answer the question at the heart of this work: the compatibility of mindfulness with ethos in the Irish Catholic primary school. First, it will outline the importance of scaffolding as an instructive evaluative tool in this evaluative task. Second, it will evaluate the compatibility of mindfulness practices highlighted in the second chapter and identified in the Irish education system in the third chapter with a Catholic educational vision proposed in Chapter 4. These constitutive criteria of a Catholic educational vision are (1) Theological Anthropology; (2) Christocentricity; (3) Sacramentality; (4) Evangelisation; (5) Academic Integrity and Autonomy of Subjects; (6) Dialogue between Faith and Culture and (7) Social Justice. In doing so, we are able to assess the congruence of mindfulness with Catholic ethos, which is the lived expression of belief, practices and conduct of a Catholic educational vision.

Mindfulness and scaffolding

As was seen in the second chapter, mindfulness as non-judgemental awareness and attention to the present moment has been argued as a basic human capacity in no way synonymous with religious practices such as Christian prayer or Buddhist meditation.[544] However, without a well-defined and clearly understood context for learning and practicing mindfulness, any

544 Ellen J. Langer and Alison I. Piper, 'The Prevention of Mindlessness', *Journal of Personality and Social Psychology* 53 (1987), 280–7.

possible benefits of mindfulness risk reduction to a sort of vague 'be here now mentality'.[545] For the purposes of this evaluative task, Bishop et al.'s definition of mindfulness is used here.[546] This is to clarify what exactly is being evaluated to be compatible or incompatible with the ethos of the Catholic school. While programs such as Paws b and Weaving Wellbeing incorporate mindfulness into their content, this task assesses whether this basic concept of mindfulness could be applicable and suitable for Catholic primary schools, outside of any formal program.

Our second chapter outlined how different forms of mindfulness are supported by a contextual framework or scaffolding. There is a robust scaffolding for Buddhist mindfulness, placing mindfulness or *sati* (and with the Sanskrit term *smrti*, meaning 'that which is remembered') as an integral aspect of Buddhist teachings including the Noble Eightfold Path. Burnett summarises how mindfulness is contextualised and supported by this scaffolding:

> Mindfulness is the first of seven 'awakening factors'; it is one of the five 'faculties' and 'powers'; and Right Mindfulness ... is one of the eight 'limbs' of the Noble Eightfold Path, very much a cornerstone of early Buddhism. Each of these frameworks sits in turn within the broader soteriological context of the Buddhist path. Mindfulness helps the Buddhist along that path, enabling insight into 'the way things are' at a profound level: the nature and causes of 'suffering' (dukkha) ... and the uncomfortable reality that when we look for an underlying, permanent essence to what we spend our lives thinking of as 'I', 'me' and 'my', there isn't one (anatta).[547]

545 B. Alan Wallace, 'A Mindful Balance', *Tricycle, XVII(3)* (Spring 2008), 62.

546 Scott Bishop, Mark Lau, Shauna Shapiro, Linda Carlson, Nicole D. Anderson, James Carmody, Zindel V. Sega, Susan Abbey, Michael Speca, Drew Velting and Gerald Devins, 'Mindfulness: A Proposed Operational Definition,' *Clinical Psychology: Science and Practice 11* (2004), 3. 'Broadly conceptualised, mindfulness has been described as a kind of nonelaborative, non-judgmental, present-centred awareness in which each thought, feeling or sensation that arises in the attentional field is acknowledged and accepted as it is'.

547 Richard Burnett, Mindfulness in Schools: Learning Lessons from the Adults-Secular and Buddhist (October 2009), 28. <https://mindfulnessinschools.org/wp-content/uploads/2013/03/Mindfulness-in-schools-dissertation-Burnett.pdf>. Accessed on 20 May 2021.

In this sense, there is a clear contextual framework, language and understanding of the purpose of mindfulness in Buddhist wisdom traditions. Rather than a non-evaluative or morally neutral practice, mindfulness involves self-awareness informed by other Buddhist precepts such as the Noble Eightfold Path, entailing rules such as Right Action and Right Speech. This means that mindfulness or *sati* is supported by an ethical and moral scaffolding, meaning that it is never a non-evaluative disposition in Buddhist teachings. Rather, it is an integral element of a broader Buddhist soteriological framework.

Likewise, there was a less comprehensive but nonetheless coherent contextual framework or scaffolding for Mindfulness 1, the applications of mindfulness in the clinical or healthcare setting. Jon Kabat-Zinn's 8-week MBSR program presents a secularised and simplified form of Buddhist meditation aimed at reducing suffering and tension in the practitioner through the cultivation of a non-judgmental awareness of the present moment.

> Participants were asked to commit to daily practice of mindfulness exercises, mostly in the form of sitting or vipassana meditation (in which attention is focused upon your breath) and also in regular movement awareness and 'body scanning' exercises, taught in a series of weekly sessions. These exercises were intended to dispel physical and mental tension and to foster the relaxed state conducive to the pursuit of meditation.[548]

While MBSR faced critiques including the deracination of mindfulness from the traditional Buddhist ethical framework, there remained an ethical grounding or framework through the Hippocratic Oath and competency standards for teachers. Mindfulness 1 in this regard '... is protected ... to some extent, by a pre-existing professional ethos in the healthcare fields; they have also developed a certification process for their instructors'.[549] Moreover, MBCT (Mindfulness-Based Cognitive Therapy) which is another form of Mindfulness 1, is presented by its co-founder John Teasdale as being

548 Paul Moloney, 'Mindfulness: The Bottled Water of the Therapy Industry', in Ronald E. Purser, David Forbes and Adam Burke, eds, *Handbook of Mindfulness: Culture, Context and Social Engagement* (Basel: Springer Publishing, 2016), 269–70.

549 Mark R. Poirier, 'Mischief in the Marketplace for Mindfulness', in Robert Meikyo Rosenbaum and Barry Magid, eds, *What's Wrong with Mindfulness (And What Isn't): Zen Perspectives* (Somerville, MA: Wisdom Publications, 2016), 17.

operative within an explicit psychological therapeutic framework.[550] Here, mindfulness techniques are used to address patterns of thoughts, enabling the practitioner to notice these patterns and become aware of alternative ways of responding to them.

> MBCT has a model of the nature of the pathology that it is trying to focus on so it is actually quite focussed … there is a model of understanding, as with Buddhism, both of the nature of the problem and also how the techniques may fit into help it. It's a much narrower model than you get in Buddhism, but there is a model there.[551]

In this sense, the critiques of Mindfulnesses 2 and 3 relate to this lack of a coherent scaffolding or contextual framework. The absence of an explicit ethical framework, language or context means that mindfulness can be misappropriated into being a tool for self-satisfaction rather than self-transformation or the liberation of others in society from structural sources of suffering. This is not to deny the potentially life-giving benefits of mindfulness for mental and physical wellbeing. Rather, it is to highlight the importance of a robust scaffolding or contextual framework for mindfulness practice to ensure these life-giving benefits are realised, rather than for mindfulness to devolve into that '… vague be here now mentality'.[552]

Scaffolding is then an important conceptual tool in evaluating the compatibility of mindfulness with ethos in Irish Catholic primary schools. The seven constitutive criteria for a Catholic educational vision proposed earlier are the contextual framework or scaffolding that underpins the characteristic spirit and life of the Catholic primary school. For mindfulness to be compatible this Catholic ethos, it must be congruent with each of those criteria. Moreover, the criteria for a Catholic educational vision may provide a scaffolding or contextual framework, offering a theological language, purpose

550 See John Teasdale, *Mindfulness-Based Cognitive Therapy for Depression: A New Approach to Preventing Relapse* (New York: Guilford Press, 2002).

551 Richard Burnett, Mindfulness in Schools: Learning Lessons from the Adults-Secular and Buddhist (October 2009), 28. <https://mindfulnessinschools.org/wp-content/uploads/2013/03/Mindfulness-in-schools-dissertation-Burnett.pdf> (accessed on 20 May 2021) 29 (9). Interview with John Teasdale, 26 January 2009.

552 B. Alan Wallace, 'A Mindful Balance', *Tricycle XVII*(3) (Spring 2008), 62.

and guidelines for mindfulness practice in the Catholic school. With these considerations in mind, we now begin our evaluative task.

Catholic education is inspired by a theological anthropology

There are several areas of dialogue between mindfulness and a theocentric understanding of the human person which merit evaluation. These areas are presented under the headings of personhood, wellbeing and sin. Personhood has been chosen as first, it has been consistently affirmed as an important theme in Catholic education, and second, it is important to examine how mindfulness interacts with this understanding of each student as a person made for right relationship. Wellbeing is selected as it brings the benefits proposed in mindfulness into conversation with a Catholic understanding of flourishing and what it means to be fully human. Finally, sin is selected as it is a significant theme in theological anthropology, portraying human nature as broken and dependent on God's grace. This provides an important counterbalance against contemporary ideas of human self-sufficiency and independence.

Personhood

Every Catholic school is committed to an integral education for the holistic development of the child. This is a recognition of the multidimensionality of the human person that is made in the likeness and image of God. As mindfulness has been presented as an innate human faculty rather than a variation of Buddhist meditation, it does not contradict such a theological vision. As has been highlighted earlier, there is a growing body of research arguing that mindfulness offers many benefits to pupils, including improved socialisation and better academic performance, albeit there is a need for further rigorous research to validate some of these claims. Mindfulness in this sense may contribute to several dimensions of the human person, including the social and academic realms. The social aspect is particularly important as a Catholic theological anthropology understands the person as essentially social, being made in the *imago Dei*, a relationship of self-giving love, called to holiness and created for right relationship with others, creation and with

God. Thus, Catholic education's commitment to holistic education means that mindfulness can help enable children to develop their social skills and academic achievement, helping them to reach their full potential.

Not only is mindfulness compatible with a theocentric understanding of the human person, but also applying Catholic scaffolding to mindfulness can help Catholic schools promote and model right relationship with others. Jon Kabat-Zinn, a leading advocate of mindfulness, proposes that the loving kindness generated by a mindfulness practitioner could be shared with others.[553] While a laudable goal, there is no underlying ethical framework that would necessarily encourage them to do so. This creates the danger of mindfulness being reduced to an individualist activity that buffers the practitioner from structural sources of suffering and injustice.

Here, a theological anthropology provides such a framework, in that students in a Catholic school are seen as reflections of God, made for right relationship with self, God, others and creation. Integral to this is a recognition of each person's inherent human dignity, realised in community and revealed in the life and ministry of Jesus Christ. Mindfulness in a Catholic school could then be a resource for promoting loving kindness with others and themselves, especially those who are marginalised or excluded, supported by the framework of theological anthropology. Such a scaffolding would mean that for the Catholic school, there is a commitment to share loving kindness with all in society through thought, word and action as each person is made to show love and to receive love as a reflection of God.

Wellbeing

The theological anthropology of Catholic education commits to an integral education that nurtures each pupil to flourish, fully achieve their potential and experience success. This means that the Catholic school must be a place where students enjoy an atmosphere that promotes their full wellbeing. Resources evidenced to positively contribute to this educational vision should be welcomed. In this regard, the growing evidence of mindfulness practice as having positive effects on child wellbeing is a boon for Catholic

553 Jon Kabat-Zinn, *Wherever You Go, There You Are: Mindfulness Meditation for Everyday Life* (London: Piatkus, 1994), 166.

education, particularly at a time when challenges to child mental health and wellbeing in Ireland remain a concern.

Programmes such as Kabat-Zinn's MBSR are clinical approaches to help patients reduce their suffering. These programmes represent a secularised and psychologised transmission of Buddhist teachings focused on the cessation of suffering. Through the processes of Buddhist modernism, mindfulness is presented as accessible to everyone. In this sense, there should be little concern that mindfulness practices in schools are Buddhist meditative practices by another name. Likewise, school-based programmes like Weaving Wellbeing use mindfulness techniques to help lower anxiety and aid the student in regulating their attention to the present moment. This suffering or stress reducing orientation of mindfulness is compatible with the educational vision of the Catholic school as the holistic education of the student is at the heart of this educational endeavour meaning that children can flourish and reach their full potential.

However, a theological anthropological framework can ensure greater compatibility between Catholic ethos and mindfulness. First, categorisations of mindfulness as a spiritual activity or a psychological, secular technique remains unclear. As was explored earlier, Kabat-Zinn originally sought to offer universal access to mindfulness by omitting any reference to Buddhist or spirituality.[554] However, for a Catholic school, with its emphasis on holistic development, mindfulness could be an important resource for nurturing the spiritual development of the child. The human person, made in the *imago Dei* is called to holiness and to relationship with God, which can be fostered in prayer. In regulating attention to the present moment, mindfulness can help children prepare for prayer or invite a sacramental perspective, noticing God's presence in every moment of life as gift. This would invite students to look beyond the immanent frame of the post-secular, post-Christian context, making possible an experience of the transcendent in their lives.

Moreover, a theological anthropological scaffolding to mindfulness could encourage students to develop a critical awareness of those in society and around them who suffer. In this sense, Catholic education should nurture

554 As noted in our second chapter, Kabat-Zinn's stance on this has been critiqued for its opaqueness over mindfulness being a secular psychological activity, a spiritual practice with some metaphysical assumptions, or both.

children to be mindful not just of their own wellbeing but that of others, challenging reductive and individualist forms of mindfulness. Where there is suffering or inequality in society, students should be aided in seeing themselves as active instruments of grace, mindful of God's presence in their lives and seek to reduce suffering for others. This commitment to putting faith into action for the benefit of others then becomes an embodiment of Jesus' teachings on the Kingdom of God. In this sense, mindfulness can then be understood as *praeparatio evangelica*—a preparation to hear the Good News.

Sin

The 'graced nature' theological anthropology of Catholic education presents humanity as made for God and for good. This includes taking seriously the reality of sin and its reductive impact on human flourishing and the person's capacity to give and receive love.[555] Two points may be made on how mindfulness can contribute to how sin is to be confronted and understood in the Catholic school.

First, mindfulness as a contemplative activity can allow students to become consciously aware of behaviours and actions in their lives that have fallen short of what it means to be human. Catholic education offers a robust moral and ethical framework that presents the human person as possessing innate dignity, with the freedom and responsibility to contribute to the common good. As has been highlighted, contemporary mindfulness is commonly operative as a non-evaluative 'bare attention' outlook. This has been criticised in previous chapters for lacking an ethical framework for action. Catholic anthropology can go further there, inviting students to notice and

555 Theologian Ethna Regan summarises the corrosive effects of sin on the human person made in the *imago Dei*: 'Sin denies the goodness of creation and damages human embodiment. Sin undermines human dignity and de-sacralises human life. Sin distorts and potentially refuses communion with God. Sin weakens human sociality and wounds the primordial communion between persons. Sin abuses our responsibility for the flourishing of life, moving from a relational *imago Dei* to an inflated anthropocentrism that is marked by possession, consumption and destruction'. See Ethna Regan, 'Catholic Anthropology', in Anne Hession and Patricia Kieran, eds, *Exploring Theology: Making Sense of the Catholic Tradition* (Dublin: Veritas, 2007), 164.

respond to the moral valence of situations in life and become aware that their thoughts, words and actions can be humanising as well as dehumanising.

Catholic anthropology provides mindfulness with a basis for loving-kindness towards self and others, rooted in God's self-giving love, providing a potential corrective for the self-oriented forms of mindfulness. By practising self-kindness and gentleness, students are encouraged not to dislike or have a conception of low self-worth or value. Rather, in the Catholic school, students are invited to see themselves as made in the *imago Dei*, made for right relationship with themselves, others, creation and God. In this sense, students can become mindful of their capacity for good and the need to be consciously aware of the impact their actions and behaviour have towards themselves and others.

However, it is important to differentiate here between prayer and technique in regard to sin. While mindfulness can be a potentially humanising activity, it is not a means of salvation or forgiveness through human effort. Hans Urs von Balthasar argues that unlike guilt[556], sin requires a forgiveness that is entirely grace-dependent, offered by God and responded to by humanity.

> Technique can help man compensate for the losses in his spiritual journey which guilt indicates, it cannot help with sin which requires a forgiveness which depends upon an initiative taken by God to which man 'responds by conversion.[557]

In this sense, for mindfulness to be compatible with the anthropology of a Catholic educational vision, there must be a recognition that the human person is dependent on God in a relationship of creature and Creator. The psychological and contemplative activities of mindfulness can cultivate in students a sacramental perspective, an awareness of creation as engraced but this does not mean that techniques bring us back into right relationship with God. Catholic anthropology can then invite the student to see themselves not as individuals who are fully independent and autonomous from each other. Rather, they can see themselves as interdependent on others and dependent on

556 Balthasar argues that the situation of humanity without God's Revelation in Jesus Christ can be understood through the characteristics of Longing (Sehnsucht), Guilt and Death. Guilt here, distinct from sin is a sense of alienness from the wholeness or unity of Creation. It is not sin as sin requires a personal relationship with God. See Raymond Gawronski, *Word and Silence: Hans Urs von Balthasar and the Spiritual Encounter between East and West* (WA: Angelico Press, 2015), 16–27.

557 Ibid, 23.

God who makes forgiveness possible through unmerited grace. Mindfulness can then help students in the Catholic school to see themselves as being made for right relationship with God, Whose grace perfects their human nature.

Second, mindfulness, when underpinned by a Catholic theological anthropology, can enable students to see themselves as made for right relationship with others and creation. This means cultivating an outlook that recognises and challenges aspects of society that are sinful, damaging and undermine human dignity and the ability of others to flourish. This includes the corrosive effects on human flourishing by anthropocentrism, individualism and excessive consumerism. As was highlighted in the second chapter, one of the dangers of Mindfulness 2 is the manner in which contemporary mindfulness practices have been misappropriated to support rather than subvert social structures that generate injustice and suffering. In contrast to this, mindfulness in the Catholic school must be supported by a theological anthropology that affirms and celebrates the innate human dignity of all, especially those oppressed and voiceless. This means that mindfulness must then be other and Other-centred, cultivating an awareness in students that their own personal wellbeing is radically connected to the wellbeing of others, especially the poor.

However, Charles Taylor,[558] Nicholas Lash[559] and Tomáš Halík[560] are all wary of contemporary spiritualties in that they tend to be therapeutic

558 Charles Taylor, *A Secular Age* (Cambridge: Harvard University Press, Belknap Press, 2007), 635–6. 'The belief in untroubled happiness is not only a childish illusion, but also involves a truncation of human nature, turning our backs on much of what we are ... Hasn't Christian preaching always repeated that it is impossible to be fully happy as a sinful agent in a sinful world? Certainly, this illusion can't be laid at the foot of the Christian faith, however much contemporary Christians may be sucked into this common view of the "pursuit of happiness" today'.

559 Nicholas Lash, *The Beginning and End of Religion* (Cambridge, Cambridge University Press, 1996), 174. 'My mistrust ... of contemporary interest in "spirituality" arises from the suspicion that quite a lot of the material set out in bookstores under this description sells because it does not stretch or mind or challenge our behaviour. It tends to sooth rather than subvert our well-heeled complacency'.

560 Martin Koči and Pavel Roubík, 'Searching the Altar of an Unknown God: Tomáš Halík on Faith in a Secular Age', in Tomáš Halík and Pavel Hošek, eds, *A Czech Perspective on Faith in a Secular Age* (Czech Philosophical Studies V, Christian Philosophical Studies X, 2015), 117. 'Halík approaches fashionable spiritual streams with some suspicion. They characteristically neglect important moral topics in the name of superficial individualism. They sometimes do not really count on transcendence but rather promote a sort of inner spirituality of the self'.

rather than transformational practices. Moreover, the work of sociologists Christian Smith and Melinda Denton on the contemporary American religious landscape highlight the emergence of Moralistic Therapeutic Deism (MTD) as an important paradigm in understanding the spiritual lives of many today.[561] This phenomenon risks relativising the distinctiveness of a Catholic theological anthropology where wellbeing must go beyond therapeutics and be transformational in character, rooted in the self-giving and sacrificial love of God, embodied in Jesus Christ.

Our second and third chapters highlighted the growing body of research arguing for the physical and mental wellbeing benefits of mindfulness. These are to be welcomed as resources that helps the ability of students to flourish and succeed in Catholic schools is a boon. However, the theological anthropology of Catholic education calls for mindfulness to be more than just a therapeutic device. Rather, mindfulness as a contemplative outlook would give students the time and space to probe deeper into the interior life, to discern and interrogate their inner thoughts, feelings and sources of meaning. In this sense, mindfulness would enable students to address the reality of sin in their lives and recognise their interdependence on each other and dependence on God in addressing potentially dehumanising behaviours and actions towards themselves and others. In this way, mindfulness could be a humanising practice in Catholic schools, inviting students to flourish in all dimensions of their being and live life to the full, as Christ promises: 'I have come that they may have life and have it to the full'.[562]

561 Smith and Denton summarise Moralistic Therapeutic Deism under five key beliefs: '1. A God exists who created and orders the world and watches over human life on earth. 2. God wants people to be good, nice, and fair to each other, as taught in the Bible and by most world religions. 3. The central goal of life is to be happy and to feel good about oneself. 4. God does not need to be particularly involved in one's life except when he is needed to resolve a problem. 5. Good people go to heaven when they die'. See Christian Smith and Melinda Benton, *Soul Searching: The Religious and Spiritual Lives of American Teenagers* (New York: Oxford University Press, 2005).

562 John 10:10.

Catholic education is radically Christocentric

The question of compatibility between mindfulness and this criterion of a Catholic educational vision is addressed under the headings of prayer and community. First, prayer is chosen as it is the location where Catholics come to speak and listen to Christ, to deepen their relationship with Him. It is also important to compare and contrast mindfulness and Christian prayer, to recognise that each are distinctive activities that do not substitute one another. Second, community is chosen as Catholics are called to communal worship, to praise and love God as parts of the Body of Christ, the Church. This communal emphasis is brought into conversation with mindfulness, which as we have seen has been criticised at times for its individualism and lack of concern for societal transformation.

Prayer

As has been argued, mindfulness as a basic human faculty does not belong to categories such as Buddhism or Christianity. The secular practice of regulating attention to the present moment which has been evidenced to offer a range of cognitive and health benefits is thus compatible with Catholic education as it is a resource to help pupils developmentally. In this regard, mindfulness should not be perceived as Buddhist meditation, nor should it undermine Christian prayer in Catholic schools.[563]

However, mindfulness can never be synonymous with Christian prayer nor a substitute for it. Hans Urs von Balthasar allows for mindfulness exercises as 'mental hygiene', recognising that meditative practices derived from Eastern traditions offer value to the Christian who wants to share in the

563 This theme is stressed in the Irish Catholic Bishop's Conference's reflection on mindfulness. However, it also reemphasises that in a Christian context, Christian forms of meditation involve a transcendent axis as well as a horizontal one. This is a key distinction from Buddhist and secular forms of meditation. See Council for Catechetics, Irish Catholic Bishops' Conference, *A Reflection on Mindfulness: Rediscovering the Christian Tradition of Meditation and Contemplation* (Dublin: Veritas, 2018).

prayer of Jesus to the Father, rather than rely on positivistic notions of belief in the Incarnation.

> The non-Christian religions make a great contribution in keeping man honestly aware of his hunger for God and not settling for any simply pious solution, as those who would mouth 'positivistic' formulae would offer.[564]

For the Christian, this means that mindfulness can keep them aware of their inner hunger for God Who is accessible through Christ, the Way, the Truth and the Life. However, Balthasar stresses that Christian prayer is *anathema* to techniques, which is central to his criticism of the Desert Father Evagrius Ponticus.[565] Moreover, Pope Benedict XVI recognises the benefits of silent recollection in God's presence, while cautioning against the idea of techniques which puts human nature and independence over the unmerited grace of God. In this sense, techniques can never replace prayer as the locus for encountering God's love as gift.[566]

For Catholic education, mindfulness may then offer a valuable resource in preparing students for prayer. As Jesus Christ is understood as the foundation of the Catholic school, it is then charged with enabling students to develop a personal relationship with Christ, with prayer an important

564 Raymond Gawronski, *Word and Silence: Hans Urs von Balthasar and the Spiritual Encounter between East and West* (WA: Angelico Press, 2015), 276–7.

565 Ibid, 293–4. 'He often contrasts technique with prayer. Technique is a "means of power" which "wants to reach in a practical way a goal set by man': prayer is the opposite, it is an openness to receive what God wills. We have seen in Christian prayer, a preoccupation with technique as in Evagrius ... tends to lead 'to an all too refined self-observation and experimentation of oneself'.

566 Congregation for the Doctrine of the Faith, *Letter to the Bishops of the Catholic Church on Some Aspects of Christian Meditation* (Vatican City: 15 October 1989), Par 23. 'Without doubt, a Christian needs certain periods of retreat into solitude to be recollected and, in God's presence, rediscover his path. Nevertheless, given his character as a creature, and as a creature who knows that only in grace is he secure, his method of getting closer to God is not based on any technique in the strict sense of the word. That would contradict the spirit of childhood called for by the Gospel. Genuine Christian mysticism has nothing to do with technique: it is always a gift of God, and the one who benefits from it knows himself to be unworthy'. <Letter to the Bishops of the Catholic Church on some aspects of Christian Meditation – Orationis formas (vatican.va)>. Accessed on 23 May 2021.

aspect of this. Mindfulness in this sense can help students to become more attuned to the present moment, calming the mind before entering into prayer with Jesus. The Christocentric nature of the Catholic school means that opportunities for encounter with Jesus in school life, such as the sacraments, Scripture readings or liturgies can find in mindfulness a potentially valuable resource in helping students become fully aware to the present moment. This would help protect prayer from being ossified into a routine and somewhat superficial activity at the end of a religion lesson.

School programmes in Ireland such as Noel Keating's Christian Meditation[567] offer a Christian approach to meditation which nurtures students to become mindful of the Spirit of God within them.[568] This approach, while respecting the use of secular mindfulness in schools, highlights the rich Christian tradition of contemplative prayer, particularly the Desert Father John Cassian which has been popularised in past decades by the Benedictine monk John Main and notes that such approaches to prayer help practitioners discover fruits of the Spirit. These Christian contemplative practices share the immanent perspective of secular mindfulness practice to the here and now. However, they also possess a transcendent dimension, where the person is drawn to awareness of the loving presence of God in their lives.[569] Keating cites Paul's letter to the Ephesians as encapsulating the intention in Christian meditation.[570] In this sense, Christian contemplative practices

567 <http://www.christianmeditation.ie/?q=meditationwithchildren. Accessed on 10 February 2021.

568 'And hope does not put us to shame, because God's love has been poured out into our hearts through the Holy Spirit, who has been given to us'. Romans 5:5.

569 This theme is explored in detail in the reflection on mindfulness offered by the Irish Catholic Bishops' Conference. See Council for Catechetics, Irish Catholic Bishops' Conference, *A Reflection on Mindfulness: Rediscovering the Christian Tradition of Meditation and Contemplation* (Dublin: Veritas, 2018).

570 'With this in mind, then, I kneel in prayer to the Father from whom every family in heaven and earth takes its name, that out of the treasures of his glory he many grant you strength and power through his Spirit in your inner self, so that Christ may dwell in your hearts through faith. And then, planted in love and built on love, with all God's people you will have the strength to grasp the breadth and length, the height and depth, so that knowing the love of Christ, which is beyond knowledge, you may be filled with the utter fullness of God. Ephesians 3, 14–19.

are a calling for personal transformation to follow the path of Christ by embodying right relationship through love of God and love of neighbour in thought, words and actions.

Community

In terms of a Catholic educational vision, Christocentricity can first ameliorate the criticism of mindfulness as being in danger of becoming an individualistic practice with no concern for the suffering of others, shorn of any ethical basis to be mindful of others. Christians are called to have the mind of Christ in their lives and in their dealings with others.[571] The life and ministry of Jesus highlight his mindfulness towards others, especially those excluded or oppressed in society. Mindfulness in a Christian framework is then not a passive mental exercise but an active and self-giving disposition, committed to the promotion of social justice.

In this sense, mindfulness in a Christian context is always both other-centred and Other-centred. It is other-centred in the sense that loving kindness should be shared with all in the community as each person is loved by God. For a Catholic school, this would mean fostering a school community that reflects the God's Reign, where every person is welcomed, valued and included, in particular those who are poor or voiceless as Christ was especially mindful of them. The loving kindness generated by mindfulness must be shared and nurtured with others in the Catholic school community. Mindful commitment to the other also means putting this loving kindness into action, challenging aspects of culture and society that cause suffering and injustice for others. Mindfulness in the Catholic school then possesses an explicitly Christian ethical framework that actively seeks to share the loving kindness of God with the school community and beyond.

It is Other-centred in that the Christian is called to be mindful of God's loving presence in their lives. Reynolds argues that this is a unique contribution of the Christian faith to mindfulness: 'This sense of "otherness" I believe

571 'Each of you should look not only to your own interests, but also to the interests of others. Let this mind be in you which was also in Christ Jesus'. Philippians 2:4–5.

is the gift of Christianity to mindfulness: Who we are in relation to others and the great other who is God'.[572] Unlike secular or many Buddhist forms of meditation, any Christian conception of mindfulness has both immanent and transcendent perspectives. The transcendent aspect means that we break out of Charles Taylor's immanent frame and become mindful of God's presence in our lives and the loving relationship that we are offered through God's grace, revealed in the person of Jesus Christ. In this sense, any Christocentric approach to mindfulness cannot be individualistic as every human person is made in the likeness and image of God, with the capacity for right relationship, to love and to be loved. Unlike some self-centred, individualistic iterations of Mindfulness 2, a Christocentric approach mindfulness is always related to God and to others. For Catholic education, this means that mindfulness practice which can help generate loving kindness in the individual is recognised as a life-giving resource. However, the Catholic school is called to ensure that loving kindness is also Other-orientated and other-orientated, especially to those who are oppressed or voiceless.

Catholic education is permeated by a sacramental imagination

This criterion will be evaluated under the headings of imagination and discipleship. Imagination is chosen as it is recognised in this chapter by scholars such as Gallagher and Lane as being a subject of crisis in contemporary culture, which has profound implications for the Catholic faith.[573] It is important then to explore what are the possible interactions between mindfulness and imagination. Second, discipleship is chosen as it represents moving beyond the sense of empathy and loving kindness expounded by proponents of certain branches of mindfulness. Discipleship represents carrying

572 Stefan G. Reynolds, *Living with the Mind of Christ: Mindfulness in Christian Spirituality* (London: Darton, Longman & Todd, 2016), 41.

573 Amos Wilder, *Theopoetic: Theology and the Religious Imagination* (Philadelphia: Fortress Press, 1976), 2. 'When imagination fails, doctrine becomes ossified, witness and proclamation wooden, doxologies and litanies empty, consolations hollow, and ethics legalistic'.

the Cross of Christ, putting faith and good deeds into action towards the benefit of others. This provides a relevant conversation point.

Imagination

As was explored in the previous chapter, Catholic education promotes a sacramental perspective on life. According to Sullivan:

> A sacramental perspective views the world as a whole, as the theatre of God's grace. It does not restrict God's operation to special moments in church, to holy places or activities. Instead, it acknowledges that God can be encountered anywhere, anytime ... Catholic education should strive to invite students to see God's presence in all aspects of their experience.[574]

This perspective views the world as created, sustained and redeemed by God, that God mediates Godself across every facet of our experiences. God's grace is not limited to the sacraments, communal worship or in reading Scripture, but can be experienced anywhere and at any time. Mindfulness can contribute to this sacramental imagination offered by Catholic education in two ways.

First, mindfulness as a contemplative practice in Catholic education can cultivate in students an awareness of God's grace in their everyday experiences. It is an invitation to view the world as being grounded in God, each moment offering something of God's creative, loving presence. For Catholic students with little connection to their faith, this approach allows them to encounter grace in the ordinary aspects of life, rather than creating a false dichotomy between the sacred and the secular. Mindfulness as an innate human capacity can then aid students in seeing the holy in the ordinary rather than the holy as limited to something in a church or at a pilgrimage site. This does not demean these moments in Church life, instead it highlights that every human experience is rooted in God's unmerited grace. Without

574 John Sullivan, 'Philosophy of Catholic Education', in Anne Hession and Patricia Kieran, eds, *Exploring Religious Education: Catholic Religious Education in an Intercultural Europe* (Dublin: Veritas, 2008), 30.

this sense of sacredness of everyday life, the seven great sacraments of the Church risk being seen as sacred moments in an otherwise secular world.

For the curriculum taught in a Catholic school, mindfulness can aid in dissolving any proposed secular/sacred binary in Catholic education, particularly any interpretation of religious education as the sole component of learning that explores the Holy Mystery of God.[575] The contemplative practice of mindfulness in a Catholic school can aid students in helping them make sense of their whole lives in light of the sacramental perspective that God mediates Godself across all our experiences. This cultivation of a sacramental imagination in students invites them to make meaning in their lives while also learning to understand and appreciate God's presence in their lives, which includes an openness to transcendence outside of Taylor's immanent frame.

This imagination must be nurtured not just in religious education but across all curricular subjects. For teachers, this means instilling in children a sense of wonder and attentiveness in their everyday lives, being attuned to sensing God's presence in their every experience of reality. Other curricular subjects represent teaching opportunities to reflect on creation as engraced by God, be that literature, art or the sciences. This development of a sense of wonder and awe in God's presence across the syllabus of Catholic education can be aided through mindfulness. The practice of regulating attention to the present moment can aid students in becoming consciously aware of God's presence in every moment of creation. This attentiveness to God's presence is necessary for pupils to come to develop a personal relationship with God, ensuring compatibility of mindfulness with this element of a Catholic educational vision.

Second, mindfulness can assist in the promotion of a sacramental imagination in Catholic education, as opposed to what Pope Francis calls the 'technocratic imagination' which is the dominant worldview currently operative in Western culture.[576] This technocratic paradigm of relating to the

575 For further reading on this in higher education, see Karen E. Eifler and Thomas M. Landy, eds, *Becoming Beholders: Cultivating Sacramental Imagination and Actions in College Classrooms* (Collegeville, MI: Liturgical Press, 2004).

576 See Pope Francis, *Laudato Si': On Care for Our Common Home* (Dublin: Veritas, 2015), Par 101–36.

world is characterised by utilitarianism, materialism and anthropocentrism. Such an imagination has potentially grave implications for education as it can reduce it from the development of the human person to mere knowledge transmission for economic for materialist ends.[577] This technocratic imagination is rooted in an anthropology that sees creation as an infinite resource for human consumption, emptying it of any sense of the sacred. This desire for productivity and efficiency can also be seen in neoliberal agendas in education explored earlier. Education in many settings are at risk of instrumentalisation and managerialism, with an increased focus on academic output than students flourishing.

This technocratic imagination is *anathema* to a Catholic educational vision. Where mindfulness is used to buffer such an imagination, it is not compatible with such a vision. However, the theological anthropology undergirding Catholic education sees the person as made for right relationship with self, others, God and creation and thus provides mindfulness with an ethical framework. Gaillardetz argues that this theocentric understanding of the human person means that we are invited to attend to the engraced world around us and receiving it as gift. In this sense, there is no sacred/secular divide in the world. Instead, God's grace saturates our reality, and a sacramental imagination opens the person up to discovering themselves in the life of communion. 'If God is love, and grace is the presence of God in our midst, then grace is a word we give to what happens to us whenever we are drawn into communion with God and God's creation. Quite simply, the communion *is* the life of grace'.[578] This means that despite the many

577 As Antony Seldon writes, 'A liberal education has too often been replaced by an indoctrination of the young in the answers they need to memorise and regurgitate for exams. It is so all-pervasive that we simply do not see any longer what has happened, and the education establishment -teachers, academics, administrators and those in the quango penumbra- does not acknowledge the impoverishment rather than the flowering of the lives of our young people'. See Antony Seldon, 'Our Education System is Collapsing into a Form of Mass Indoctrination', *Independent* (23 October 2011). <https://www.independent.co.uk/voices/commentators/anthony-seldon-our-education-system-collapsing-form-mass-indoctrination-2028709.html>. Accessed on 24 December 2020.

578 Richard R. Gaillardetz, *Transforming Our Days: Spirituality, Community and Liturgy in a Technological Culture* (NY: Crossroad Publishing Company, 2000), 60.

scientific and technological advances enjoyed by humanity, an imagination that translates creation as a commodity of resources to be plundered must be challenged in Catholic schools.

Mindfulness could enable students to become more aware of the ways they relate to the world around them when supported by a sacramental scaffolding. The sacramental imagination stresses that all of creation is engraced, and that God meditates Godself across all our experiences. In this sense, mindfulness can foster in students a mindful disposition towards their own actions and behaviours that damage their relationship with others and with creation. This means that Catholic education promotes the sacramentality of life, that it is within the ordinariness that holiness can be found. In this way, pupils become more attuned to seeing God in all things.

Moreover, enabling students to become more mindful of the wonders of God's creation would enable students to transcend the buffered self that Charles Taylor speaks of in the opening chapter, offering students a transcendent frame for relating to the world. By being open to the sacramentality of life, students are invited to encounter God's grace in the life of right relationship rather than through an individualistic or self-centred viewpoint. As Gaillardetz argues:

> When we stand in awe of the wonders of God's creation … we experience a kind of self-forgetfulness that draws us beyond ourselves into communion with our larger world. In this movement we become, however imperfectly, personal beings-in-communion, we are living the life of communion.[579]

In cultivating such a sacramental outlook in students, mindfulness also invites them to see themselves as made in the likeness and image of God, made for right relationship with self. God, others and creation. Mindfulness in this regard can contribute to the social, spiritual and relational education of the student in the Catholic school while also demonstrating a compatibility with the operative anthropology within a Catholic educational vision.

579 Ibid, 56.

Discipleship

Groome argues that sacramental consciousness should not be understood as easily accessible and unchallenging. Rather, it calls on Christians to bring our faith perspective into every aspect of our life.

> There is nothing automatic about developing a sacramental consciousness; as the latter term implies, it requires intentional alertness on our part … Toward what we initiate and what simply comes our way in life, it encourages us to wonder what God might be up to, to imagine how God's Spirit is moving, and how best to respond.[580]

This is a call to holiness, to take up the cross of Christ and be active agents in bringing about God's Reign, entailing an open and other-centred disposition. For Hession, this invitation to follow Christ is at the heart of Catholic religious education.[581] Mindfulness seeks to ground the person in the present moment, be intentionally aware of the here and now. This means that Catholic students can become aware of God's presence in each and every moment as gift and become attuned to God's will, discerning what is God calling them to do in their lives as disciples of Jesus.

Mindfulness as a contemplative practice allows students the time and space to reflect on the inner life, to help learn about themselves and what gives their lives meaning. The sacramentality of Catholic education can deepen this practice by inviting students to see themselves as being called

580 Thomas Groome, *Faith for the Heart: A 'Catholic' Spirituality* (NY: Paulist Press, 2019), 216.

581 Anne Hession, *Catholic Religious Education in a Pluralist Environment* (Dublin: Veritas, 2015), 169. 'Catholic religious education invites children into a particular kind of personal transformation which can be termed "conversion" or "holiness". Holiness for a Christian is living in relationship with Jesus Christ in such a way that the person is rooted in love. Accepting the presence of God's Holy Spirit in each and every circumstance of life, such a person lives a life of justice and compassion, serving others and making a difference in society and the world. This is the *raison d'être* of the Catholic religious education curriculum from a theological perspective'.

by God '... to interpret their existence in the light of God's plan'.[582] This invitation into discipleship for students encourages them to be intentionally alert and responsive to God's grace at work, but also noticing and challenging what is not of God's Kingdom in their lives.

This sacramental perspective means a critical social consciousness, following Christ's teachings and being mindful of social and political structures that generate and sustain all forms of injustice, discrimination and hatred. Moreover, this sacramental framework offers mindfulness in Catholic schools a bulwark against some of the more insidious misappropriations of mindfulness highlighted earlier such as McMindfulness and mindfulness that supports rather than challenging structural sources of suffering and injustice. In this sense, mindfulness in Catholic education can be a step towards a call to discipleship; an other-centred outlook that notices and responds to circumstances and situations in the world around them in which God's Reign is inhibited.

Pope Francis warns that even those who hold and practice the Christian faith may still '... frequently fall into a lifestyle which leads to an attachment to financial security, or to a desire for human glory at all cost, rather than giving their lives to other in mission'.[583] In this sense, a sacramental mindfulness would enable students to notice and respond to God's call to serve others in a particular way, taking up the cross of discipleship and embodying the Good News in their interactions with others. In the Catholic school, this means promoting an understanding of the human person as essentially social, promoting a spirit of justice, mercy and fairness in all aspects of school life.

Moreover, the holistic education offered in the Catholic school enables students to develop their intellectual, social and moral capacities to contribute to the common good of society. They are educated to become reasoned and active citizens who recognise their interdependence on others

582 Congregation for Catholic Education, *Consecrated Persons and their Mission in Schools* (2002), Par 55. <https://www.vatican.va/roman_curia/congregations/ccatheduc/documents/rc_con_ccatheduc_doc_20021028_consecrated-persons_en.html>. Accessed on 31 May 2021.

583 Pope Francis, *Evangelii Gaudium: The Joy of the Gospel* (Dublin: Veritas, 2013), Par 80.

and their responsibility as disciples of Christ to bring about the Kingdom of God by challenging structures that inhibit others to flourish. This sacramental, mindful outlook corresponds to Catholic education's vision of each person being made for right relationship with self, God, others and creation.

Each student in the Catholic school is understood and valued as being made in the *imago Dei*, with the capacity for unconditional, self-giving love. In following Christ's teaching, Christians are called to being about the God's Reign through acts of love, charity and kindness, especially care towards the poorest and vulnerable in society. This means that for a Catholic educational vision, mindfulness must also other and Other-orientated, that students recognise that their personal wellbeing is radically connected to the wellbeing of others.

In this sense, mindfulness is not only compatible with a sacramental critical consciousness but also with the Catholic school's evangelising mission, inviting others to see and respond to God's invitation to right relationship and bring about the Kingdom of God. In cultivating such a consciousness, mindfulness enables students to probe the inner life, allowing space and time to notice God's grace at work in their lives and become aware of cultural mores and trends that are incongruent with Christ's teachings.

Catholic education shares in the Church's mission of evangelisation

The compatibility of mindfulness and this criterion of Catholic education can be evaluated under the headings of pre-evangelisation and evangelisation. First, pre-evangelisation is selected as it is a recognition of the challenges facing the Church in sharing its message of the Good News. The first chapter highlighted the changed conditions of religious belief and experience today, rendering belief in a transcendent source of life increasingly implausible. Pre-evangelisation represents the necessary first step in evangelisation, an awareness of the mere possibility of belief in God. Second, evangelisation is chosen as it highlights that continued challenge of sharing the faith in a post-secular and post-Christian context, and the role mindfulness may play in this.

Pre-evangelisation

As explored earlier, there have been several shifts in the conditions of religious belief and experience in the contemporary Western context. The plausibility of the Christian narrative is challenged by postmodernism, pluralisation and detraditionalisation such that Lieven Boeve argues we now live in a post-Christian and post-secular age. As a consequence, Catholic education faces significant challenges in fulfilling its commitment to evangelisation in the face of cultural unbelief and secularisation of the imagination. However, a spiritual hunger remains alive in many, with this search for authenticity gravitating towards contemporary spiritualties as opposed to explicitly religious narratives such as Christianity. Mindfulness has exploded into mainstream culture and discourse during this time where a growing population state that they are 'spiritual but not religious'.

For Catholic education, mindfulness offers a potentially profound resource in pre-evangelisation. Given the widespread cultural unbelief operative in contemporary society, many children who attend Catholic schools have little personal experience or encounter with the Catholic faith that they often have been baptised into. In many cases, the Catholic school is the only site where children learn of the Good News proclaimed by Jesus Christ, the revelation of God's unconditional love for all. Before evangelisation can be a reality for Catholic education, pre-evangelisation is necessary to attune pupil's awareness of an experience of the transcendent and vivify the possibility of belief in God. Pre-evangelisation as highlighted in Michael Paul Gallagher's work echoes Rahner's theology of mystagogy, that is, to be led into mystery.[584] For Rahner, mystagogy meant '... bringing the *fides quae* (the content of faith) into the closest possible unity with the *fides qua* (the conscious act of faith itself)'.[585] Gallagher shares Rahner's view

584 Gallagher biographer Thomas Casey outlines this term in both Rahner's and Gallagher's theologies: 'His (Rahner's) idea is simple: it is necessary to find and name some signs of God's presence in a person's experience before telling that person about the Good News'. Thomas G. Casey, *Wisdom at the Crossroads: The Life and Thought of Michael Paul Gallagher SJ* (New Jersey: Paulist Press, 2018), 56.

585 William V. Dych, 'Karl Rahner: An Interview', *America 123*(13) (October 31, 1970), 357–8.

that '... what is at stake today is not the content of the creed but the very ability to believe'[586] and as such, human experience becomes the primary place of encounter with God. This mystagogical approach is for Rahner a fundamental element of his theological method.[587] Pre-evangelisation is then awakening a deeper sensibility in people's imaginations, making possible an encounter between wonder and mystery and rendering plausible an alternative to Charles Taylor's immanent frame, that is, openness to relationship with the transcendent mystery of God.

The possibility of evangelisation in Catholic education in many cases cannot occur unless students acquire a spiritual as well as a religious literacy through pre-evangelisation. Mindfulness offers such a possibility as a contemplative practice, which is defined by Roth as '... the many ways human beings have found, across cultures and across time, to concentrate, broaden and deepen conscious awareness'.[588] Such practices enable students to become attentive to their thoughts and feelings, enabling them to make and discover meaning in their lives. Within a Christian framework, mindfulness as a contemplative practice can then enable children to deepen their attention to spiritual wavelengths at the level of the imagination, making possible experience of the transcendent.

586 For further reading on Gallagher's writings on unbelief, see Michael Paul Gallagher, *Help My Unbelief* (Chicago: Loyola University Press, 1988), Michael Paul Gallagher, *Struggles of Faith: Essays by Michael Paul Gallagher* (Dublin, Columba Press, 1990) and Michael Paul Gallagher, *Questions of Faith* (Dublin: Veritas, 1996).

587 See Hubert Biallowons and Paul Imhof, *Karl Rahner in Dialogue: Conversations and Interviews 1962–1985*, translated by Harvey D. Egan (MI: Crossroad Publishing, 1986), 328. 'For me in my theology the givenness of a genuine, original experience of God and his Spirit is of fundamental importance. This precedes logically (and not necessarily temporally) theological reflection and verbalization and is never adequately overtaken by this reflection. What Christian faith teaches is never communicated merely by a conceptual indoctrination from without, but is and can basically be experienced through the supernatural grace of God as a reality in us. That does not mean that the linguistic representation and interpretation of the religious experience is not something that has to occur within the Church under the supervision of her magisterium. But I believe, it is true, that an awakening, a mystagogy into this original, grace-filled religious experience is today of fundamental importance [...] It is no longer necessary to think that such a mystagogy takes place only in absolute isolation and interiority'.

588 Harold D. Roth, 'Against Cognitive Imperialism', *Religion East and West 8* (2008), 19.

Mindfulness in the Catholic school is robustly compatible with pre-evangelisation as it offers a resource which aside from wellbeing and cognitive benefits, can be a means of disrupting barriers to belief in students. By fostering in students a conscious awareness of the Divine in their lives, Catholic education is better placed to offer them a conception of human flourishing that sees each person as loved unconditionally by God. Moreover, by stimulating these spiritual sensitivities, pupils are invited into learning more about the Christian life, a path to living authentically through relationship with Jesus Christ, who is the Way, the Truth and the Life.

Mindfulness as a pre-evangelisation resource in Catholic schools would enable Catholic education to better contextualise itself in a post-Christian and post-secular age. The cultural unbelief that pervades much of contemporary society means that before any evangelical task can be meaningfully undertaken in the Catholic school, students need to develop a spiritual and religious literacy that makes experience of God plausible. This contemplative practice can act as a first step in students coming to see the Christian life offered by the Church as a credible source of meaning and authenticity.

Mindfulness and pre-evangelisation in the Catholic school are certainly compatible. Moreover, it can be argued that Catholic education desperately needs resources like mindfulness to interrupt secular social imaginaries, frames of understanding the world which preclude any transcendental conception of human flourishing. In this way, Catholic education can only then attempt to share in the Church's evangelising mission.

Evangelisation

The contemporary processes of postmodernism, detraditionalisation and pluralisation outlined in the opening chapter means that Catholic education faces a contextual challenge in responding to the current spiritual climate. Pope Francis articulates the evangelising task for our contemporary age:

> To evangelise, therefore, it is necessary to open ourselves once again to the horizon of God's Spirit, without being afraid of what he asks us or of where he leads us. Let us

> entrust ourselves to him! He will enable us to live out and bear witness to our faith, and will illuminate the heart of those we meet.[589]

Mindfulness within a Christian framework offers Catholic schools an opportunity to respond to this postmodern context by offering a spiritual way of life rooted in the life, death and resurrection of Jesus Christ. For a Catholic educational vision, mindfulness offers three distinctive opportunities for evangelisation; as a precursor to coming to know Jesus in prayer; an educational endeavour which offers a transcendental dimension to human flourishing; and as a vehicle for witness to the Christian life.

First, mindfulness can help students regulate their attention to be fully present in the moment, quietening the mind to allow prayer to happen. Rather than prayer being reduced to a superficial activity in the classroom, mindfulness can aid the Catholic student in bringing themselves to be fully attentive to God's loving presence in their lives. Through the prayer opportunities offered in religious education and during the day, mindfulness can be a resource to encourage to be fully present before coming and meet Jesus in prayer, by gently stilling the mind of distractions and noise. In this way, children are encouraged into deeper relationship with Christ, who is the revelation of God's salvific will for all.

Second, mindfulness as contemplative practice in a Catholic school can help students to make and discover meaning in light of the Gospel story. The contemporary interest in spirituality despite religious narratives being challenged highlights that the Church must recontextualise their mission by attending to the spiritual needs of pupils. While religious education remains an important aspect of learning about, from and into the Christian faith, mindfulness as contemplative practice can draw students into making meaning of the world in light of God's revelation in Jesus Christ. This approach would respect the quest for spiritual authenticity without undermining the particularity of the Christian narrative. Moreover, this Christian scaffolding to mindfulness can act as a corrective to some contemporary approaches to mindfulness or spirituality that as theologian Nicholas Lash, '... does not

589 Pope Francis, General Audience, 22 May 2013 <http://www.vatican.va/content/francesco/en/audiences/2013/documents/papa-francesco_20130522_udienza-generale.html>. Accessed on 20 February 2021.

stretch the mind or challenge our behaviour. It tends to soothe rather than subvert our well-heeled complacency'.[590] Mindfulness within a Catholic educational vision must then encourage improved wellbeing but also a vision of life that offers personal transformation in a Christian community.

Third, mindfulness within a Christian framework can be a resource in helping the school community to be an embodiment of the Good News, offering a transcendental conception of human flourishing at a time when Charles Taylor's immanent frame is increasingly influential in Irish society. At a time when education is increasingly challenged by instrumentalisation and managerialism, the evangelising task of Catholic schools' risks being undercut. A Catholic educational vision must interrupt these processes and secular social imaginaries by being first a site for a distinctive community rooted in the person of Jesus Christ. This means that the school community is committed to be an inclusive, welcoming site that is an extension of the teaching Church and embodiment of the Kingdom of God. The mission of evangelisation can be aided by mindfulness by helping the school community to be mindful of the virtues and Gospel values that vivify a Catholic ethos. In this sense, staff and students are called to be mindful of the poor, oppressed and voiceless, to be mindful of the common ground that exists between every person, irrespective of creed, class or colour. Moreover, being mindful of Jesus' life and ministry through prayer and reflection can help members of the school community to model a view of the human person as made for right relationship with self, others, God and creation. In this way, others can be encouraged to come to learn more about what Christian life is and come to know more about the promise of the Gospel.

Catholic education is committed to academic integrity and the autonomy of subjects

Mindfulness can be presented as engaging with this criterion of a Catholic educational vision under the headings of holistic education and

590 Nicholas Lash, *The Beginning and End of Religion* (Cambridge, Cambridge University Press, 1996), 174.

instrumentalisation. Holistic education is chosen as it recognises that academic excellence is sought as part of an integral understanding of the human person, appreciating the multidimensionality of human development. Instrumentalisation is chosen as it represents the emerging threat of an instrumentalist view of education as solely knowledge transfer and skill acquisition for the labour market. Mindfulness interacts with these headings to see where it can benefit or stymie the opportunities and challenges they present.

Holistic Education

As outlined in the previous chapter, academic integrity is paramount to any authentic offering of Catholic education. This means that each subject enjoys the academic autonomy to be taught according to the principles and methodologies appropriate to them. This is vitally important as the transmission of knowledge is an important function of the Catholic school.[591]

Mindfulness can contribute to this aspect of Catholic educational vision in two ways. First, as an aid to the cognitive and academic performance of pupils in Catholic schools and second, as a resource for improving student wellbeing and flourishing. In doing so, mindfulness can ultimately contribute to the holistic development of the human person offered by Catholic education.

First, as has been highlighted earlier, a growing body of research has highlighted the benefits of mindfulness practice for children in terms of socialisation, cognitive function and academic performance. By regulating attention to the present moment, students are enabled to be more engaged in their learning and achieve greater success. For Catholic schools, this resource

591 John Henry Newman argues in *The Idea of a University* for the compatibility of knowledge transmission and the Church's educational mission. See Frank M. Turner, ed., *The Idea of a University (Rethinking the Western Tradition)* (New Haven, Yale University Press, 1996), 128. 'Right Reason, that is, Reason rightly exercised, leads the mind to the Catholic Faith and plants it there, and teaches in all its religious speculations to act under its guidance'. And Ibid, 161. '... let her (the Church) do for Literature in one way what she does for Science in another; each has its imperfection, and she has her remedy for each. She fears no knowledge, but she purifies all; she represses no element of our nature, but cultivates the whole'.

would potentially be invaluable in helping to offer an educational vision that is academically rigorous and stimulating, fully respecting the autonomy of subjects in the pursuit of knowledge. The holistic education offered by Catholic education means that intellectual and academic development must be nurtured to enable students to become critical and constructive citizens that contribute to the common good. Mindfulness that is evidenced-based and supported by critical research in psychology and neuroscience to improve student functioning is then compatible with academic integrity as part of a holistic education.

However, with Christian scaffolding, mindfulness can go further in contributing to the holistic education offered by a Catholic school. The theological anthropology underpinning Catholic education encompasses the multidimensionality of the child, promoting a transcendental conception of human flourishing. Mindfulness as a contemplative practice can enable students to become consciously aware of their thoughts and feelings as they engage in the academic subjects offered in the Catholic school.

The genuine pursuit of truth envisioned by Catholic education promotes the development of the whole person is itself an opportunity to experience God's presence in creation, as God is the ultimate source of Truth itself. In this sense, Catholic education must encourage teachers to find teachable moments where such an encounter with the Holy Mystery is possible, be it the wonder of creation, the beauty found in the arts or in the affective nature of literature and poetry. This can be aided by mindfulness as a contemplative practice, enabling students to make and discover meaning in their learning. In this sense, the academic integrity of each subject is being honoured as part of an integral education that nurtures each aspect of human development. In this sense, mindfulness is compatible with the academic integrity of Catholic education, offering the potential to further contribute to the holistic development of the pupil.

Instrumentalisation

The interaction between mindfulness and this criterion of a Catholic educational vision is operative within an educational context that is increasingly characterised by instrumentalisation, performance and competitiveness. As was highlighted, this neoliberal paradigm creates a school culture that decontextualises and interprets stress as personal failure in the pursuit of efficiency and academic attainment. Mindfulness in this context can be appropriated to support rather than subvert the neoliberal status quo of generating productive economic units rather than human beings that can flourish and contribute to society.

In the third chapter, it was highlighted that while further critical research is needed, early indicators are that mindfulness offers several benefits to pupils, including cognitive functioning and academic attainment. Exercises and techniques that enable students to develop their critical thinking skills and enjoy academic success and achievement are to be welcomed in any Catholic school. Mindfulness in this regard can make an important contribution to the intellectual development of a Catholic educational vision, helping each child to reach their full potential. Moreover, resources that provide children with coping mechanisms to become more resilient to stress is a vital aspect of any educational model. However, if the purpose of these benefits is to buffer students from structural sources of suffering, inequality or injustice rather than challenge them, then it is legitimate to argue this is a problematic application of mindfulness incompatible with Catholic education.

Academic integrity in Catholic education is one dimension of a distinctive theological vision of what it means to be human and what constitutes human flourishing. The transmission of knowledge and the development of the intellectual faculties are components of an integral education promoting the holistic development of the child. In this sense, academic attainment is important but can never be the sole arbiter for deciding the value or success of a pupil's education. In a Catholic school, all children, irrespective of ability or educational need are viewed as having an innate human dignity made in the *imago Dei*, encouraged to discover their skills and talents and to experience success. This educational vision is not at odds with mindfulness, but with the instrumentalisation and compartmentalisation of education for a neoliberal agenda. However, mindfulness is compatible with the academic integrity of a Catholic educational vision in two ways.

First, the demonstrated benefits of mindfulness to students' wellbeing and cognitive development help pupils achieve success academically. The autonomy of subjects and academic integrity is at the heart of the work of the Catholic school, an important principle given the charges by some[592] that faith-based education is indoctrination.[593] In the Catholic school, students are offered an education which proposes a Christian understanding of the human person, helping them achieve their potential as active and contributing citizens of a common human family. Mindfulness is then compatible with this aim of Catholic education.

Second, as a contemplative practice mindfulness is compatible with the Catholic vision of the holistic development of the child, which includes academic development. The capacity for students to make and discover meaning and to interrogate their thoughts and feelings through mindfulness can enable them to become critical and prudent actors in society. In the Catholic educational context, the preferential option for the poor and oppressed and the innate human dignity of each person can be cultivated by mindfulness as a contemplative practice. In this sense, mindfulness becomes an other-centred practice, where the student becomes mindful that their wellbeing is radically connected to the wellbeing of others, especially the poor and excluded in society. This humanising practice can nurture in students a

592 These criticisms have been presented in different over past decades, including John Wilson, *Introduction to Moral Education* (England: Penguin Books, 1967), Richard Stanley Peters, *Ethics and Education* (London: Allen and Unwin, 1970), John White, *The Aims of Education Restated* (London: Routledge, 1982) and Paul Hirst, 'Christian Education: A Contradiction in Terms', in Jeff Astley and Leslie Frances, eds, *Critical Perspectives on Christian Education* (Leominster: Gracewing, 1992).

593 Richard Pring challenges the charge that religious instruction or education is indoctrination, arguing "... though lacking the sort of verification which characterises empirical knowledge, religious beliefs can be reasonable, based as they are on long and critical traditions in making sense of experience of different kinds. Such critical traditions arise from doubts which need to be (and have constantly been) addressed in the light of further evidence and argument. Such reasonableness may not entail absolute certainty, as indeed such certainty escapes even scientific claims to knowledge where such knowledge grows through criticism of what previously was accepted as true. There is a need therefore to distinguish verification (in the strict and empirical sense) from belief held on 'appropriate evidence' (as in political and social sciences) which opens up a much wider range of reasonable beliefs, as in the evaluation of the arts, in moral deliberations, and in political and social studies." Richard Pring, *Challenges for Religious Education, Is There a Disconnect Between Faith and Reason?* (NY: Taylor & Francis, 2020), 119.

mindfulness that encourages them to put themselves at the service of others for the common good.[594]

By enabling students to be mindful of the world around them, Catholic education can cultivate pupils that are not passive recipients of information but informed citizens that challenge societal sources of suffering and injustice, especially sources that effect the most vulnerable in society. Such an approach must be at the heart of the ethos of the Catholic school. Mindfulness at its best means that the academic integrity of Catholic education is oriented towards awareness and care for others, with the students' gifts and intellect put at the service of others in society, especially those most in need.

Catholic education is committed to dialogue between faith and culture

This criterion will be evaluated under the headings of post-Christian and post-secular context, and interfaith and intercultural dialogue. The first heading is relevant as it provides an opportunity to explore how mindfulness can interact with Catholic education in a context that is characterised by the processes of detraditionalisation, secularisation and postmodernism. It allows us to assess how mindfulness may be a resource to the manner in which Catholic education communicates its message today. Second, intercultural dialogue is chosen as it is highlighted by Franchi as an overarching aim of Catholic education today.[595] It is necessary to explore what role mindfulness can play in this.

Post-Christian and post-secular context

As was explored in the opening chapter, the contemporary Western context has been characterised by pluralisation, detraditionalisation and postmodernism. Moreover, the secularisation thesis as proposed by prominent

594 For further reading see Martha Craven Nussbaum, *Cultivating Humanity: A Classical Defense of Reform in Liberal Education* (Cambridge, MA: Harvard University Press, 1997).

595 Leonardo Franchi, 'Catholic Education and Intercultural Dialogue', *Logos: A Journal of Catholic Thought and Culture 19*(4) (2016), 117.

sociologists of religion such as Berger and Cox has failed, highlighting the altered conditions of religious belief and experience operative today. What has resulted is a climate where religious identity has become more reflexive, religious grand narratives are viewed with greater suspicion and an increasing interest in spirituality has emerged.

This presents the Christian faith with a profound contextual challenge in responding to these present post-Christian, post-secular conditions. Catholic education, particularly in the Catholic school, is a significant site for faith to enter into creative, constructive dialogue with contemporary culture. Mindfulness can be a valuable resource here in two ways.

First, mindfulness in Catholic education can help to address the growing cultural phenomenon of 'somethingism', a worldview that is described as spiritual but not religious.[596] This spiritual grey area does not discount belief in God or in an Ultimate Reality that transcends human categories. To use Tomáš Halík's term, there are spiritual seekers, suspicious of religious narratives but searching for an authenticity in life that is not found solely in materialistic perspectives. Mindfulness as a contemplative practice allows pupils growing up in this context to first develop a greater awareness of their thoughts and feelings and of the world around them. This examination of the inner life enables students to reflect on what is meaningful or authentic within their lives. This ability to pause, ponder and be present in the moment is especially important given the growing influence of smartphone use, social media and screen time in children's lives today. The capacity to simply be

596 This 'something-ism' echoes the phenomenon of 'Sheilaism', as described by sociologist of religion Robert Bellah. The term stems from the description of a young nurse named Sheila of her spiritual outlook. 'I believe in God. I'm not a religious fanatic. I can't remember the last time I went to church. My faith has carried me a long way. It's Sheilaism. Just my own little voice … It's just try to love yourself and be gentle with yourself. You know, I guess, take care of each other. I think He would want us to take care of each other'. Robert N. Bellah, Richard Madsen, William M. Sullivan, Ann Swidler and Steven M. Tipton, *Habits of the Heart: Individualism and Commitment in American Life* (CA: University of California Press, 1985), 221. This radically individualistic religion emphasises personal spirituality rather than a community of believers, not necessarily connected to doctrines, sacred texts or building relationship with a deity.

present and attentive in the face of such constant stimulation and distraction is a potentially life-giving resource for Catholic schools.

Mindfulness practice can also respond to the hunger for authentic experience felt by many seekers. For many students who have a negligible relationship with the faith they have been baptised into, mindfulness in Catholic education can become a resource for pre-evangelisation. By beginning with silent awareness of their thoughts and feelings, pupils can become better attuned to the possibility of an experience that is radically authentic and life-giving. A Christian scaffolding reveals this experience as having its source in the Ultimate Reality that is God. In this sense, mindfulness can enable the Christian faith to respond to the spiritual hunger for authenticity in the contemporary context. Catholic education offers a site for such opportunity.

Second, mindfulness can be a helpful resource in Catholic education's commitment to faith, life and culture being synthesised, or as Sullivan puts it, 'Catholic education as ongoing translation'.[597] In a post-Christian, post-secular context, Catholic education is tasked with being a constructive and critical dialogue partner with contemporary culture, rejecting elements that frustrate the transmission of the Gospel message while accepting those that are congruent with it.

Sacks offers an overview of the cultural climate change of recent decades, presenting several trends in Western society that are in tension with a Christian conception of human flourishing. These include the emergence of a corrosive brand of populist politics, fake news and alternative facts which have led to cynicism and mistrust in political discourse and public institutions.[598] Moreover, Sacks offers a deeper diagnosis of this cultural climate crisis, including growing economic inequalities between rich and poor, an upsurge in depression, anxiety and attempted and actual suicides and the climate emergency. Sacks references the prediction of sociologist

597 John Sullivan, 'Catholic Education as Ongoing Translation', *International Studies in Catholic Education*, 4(2) (2012), 200–7.

598 Sacks cites Bill Emmett's description of the West as 'Demoralised, decadent, deflating, demographically challenged, divided, disintegrating, dysfunctional, declining'. See Jonathan Sacks, *Morality: Restoring the Common Good in Divided Times* (London: Hodder & Stoughton, 2020), 5–6.

Émile Durkheim in highlighting the lack of an *anomie*, a shared moral code, in contemporary society.[599,600] In this regard, the lack of a shared language or framework for morality has led to several trends that run counter to the message of the Gospel and to a reductive understanding of what it means to be human.

These include what D'Souza calls '... the frantic pace and the instrumentalist ideology that marks and disfigures modern living'.[601] Despite the many benefits of technology and innovation, contemporary culture is marked by a relentless drive for infinite progress, profit and productivity. In this pursuit for growth and efficiency, economies and societies become disconnected, destroying the human webs and networks of connections and interdependence, tearing the relations, values and norms that bind people together.[602] An individualist mindset can develop, buffered by modern culture's celebration of consumerism, autonomy and relativism. Any sense of responsibility or duty towards the common good is offset by a hunger for self-satisfaction and a desire for more things and products.

Such developments are *anathema* to what authentic human flourishing in the Christian tradition. Rather than independent, self-serving individuals, the Christian faith calls people to see themselves as interdependent and made for right relationship with self, others, God and creation. Mindfulness can assist Catholic education in this regard. By nurturing a contemplative outlook in pupils, they can be encouraged to notice their capacity for goodness, love and right relationship, supported by a robust Christian ethical and moral framework. This would provide a protection against mindfulness being appropriated to serve the purposes of neoliberal educational agendas. Rather than utilise mindfulness for instrumentalist educational goals, which would set academic output and results as a measure of student success and flourishing, mindfulness in a Catholic school must also be self

599 Ibid, 18.

600 Halík offers a similar argument in Chapter 1 on how religion as a common language or framework of meaning no longer binds communities together as it did in the past.

601 Mario D'Souza, *A Catholic Philosophy of Education: The Church and Two Philosophers* (Quebec: McGill-Queen's University Press, 2016), 186.

602 See Raghuram Rajan, *The Third Pillar: How Markets and the State Leave Community Behind* (NY: Penguin, 2019).

and other-orientated. This means that students realise their uniqueness and gifts as persons but also recognise that their own wellbeing is radically connected to others in society, especially the poor and voiceless. It also means becoming mindful of their relationship with Creation, recognising the harm done to the planet and environment through human action and greed, and the disproportionate consequences this anthropocentrism has on the poorest and vulnerable in society.[603]

Mindfulness in the Catholic school can enable students to develop a contemplative outlook, helping them to make sense of the Gospel message in their lives while also noticing and challenging trends in contemporary culture that inhibit human flourishing. In this way, mindfulness can be compatible with Catholic education's commitment to be a constructive and critical dialogue partner with society.

Interfaith and intercultural dialogue

Mindfulness can play an important part in the promotion of interfaith and intercultural dialogue. As was highlighted in the previous chapter, among the fruits of Vatican II was the Church's recognition of the need for authentic interreligious dialogue. Given the gamut of faith and belief perspectives in the contemporary postmodern context, Catholic education offers a singular opportunity for the Christian faith to engage in open and constructive dialogue with other faiths.

Mindfulness can assist Catholic education in being a process that forms students in a culture of open and inclusive dialogue with others. This means that Catholic education is open to encounter with other faith and belief perspectives. However, this commitment cannot mean the erasure of the

603 Dermot Lane provides an overview of Pope Francis' critique of anthropocentrism in *Laudato Si'*. 'The modern self-understanding of the human is at the centre of the ecological crisis. It is primarily human beings who have to change their self-understanding if there is to be a more balanced and integrated relationship between the human and ecology'. Dermot A. Lane, *Theology and Ecology in Dialogue: The Wisdom of Laudato Si'* (Dublin: Messenger Publications, 2020), 36.

otherness and particularity of the Christian tradition.[604] A Catholic educational vision puts the person at the heart of intellectual, moral and civic education while cultivating relationships that form community. As was highlighted by Lane in the previous chapter, interreligious and intercultural dialogue is not an adjunct to Catholic education. Rather, in light of *Nostra Aetate* and subsequent Church publications, it is an overarching aspect of what it means to be Catholic in the twenty-first century.[605] For such dialogue, students need to be truly mindful of others, consciously aware of their innate human dignity, regardless of colour, creed or social background. In this way, dialogue goes beyond information exchange or tolerance. Rather, authentic intercultural dialogue in Catholic education calls students to become mindful of universal values such as freedom and democracy that they share with others as part of a human family, learning from each other in the pursuit of the common good. Pope Francis argues:

604 Lieven Boeve has written extensively on the Catholic Dialogue School model in Flanders. Central to this model is the conviction that authentic encounter with otherness and Otherness is a central aspect of the Christian narrative. In this sense, Christian faith cannot be diluted into vague terms such as 'Christian values' or fall into 'something-ism'. See Lieven Boeve, 'Faith in Dialogue: The Christian Voice in the Catholic Dialogue School', *International Studies in Catholic Education 11*(1) (2019), 45. 'As a voice in the dialogue, the Christian narrative can make a difference. What constitutes being a Christian today, is not in the first place what people seem to have in common, what unites them, but also – and especially – what makes them different, what introduces O/otherness. Christian faith is not just about believing in "something more" or sticking to "meaningful values", helping people to deal with their experiences of contingency, insecurity, loss of meaning. Rather it is about surrendering oneself to somebody who asks more from people: the recognition of A/another who seeks to encounter people in history'.

605 Pope Francis highlights the significance of this for education and religious dialogue. See Pope Francis with Dominique Wolton, *A Future of Faith, The Path of Change in Politics and Society* (New York: St. Martin's Essentials, 2018), 19. 'In the education of children, of young people … each one has their own identity … concerning interreligious dialogue; it must exist, but one cannot establish a sincere dialogue between religions if one does not take one's own identity as a starting point! I have my identity, and I speak with mine. We come closer to one another, we find points in common, things we don't agree on, but on those points in common we forge ahead for the good of all, we do charitable works, we perform educational actions, together, lots of things'.

> In the education of children, of young people ... each one has their own identity ... concerning interreligious dialogue; it must exist, but one cannot establish a sincere dialogue between religions if one does not take one's own identity as a starting point! I have my identity, and I speak with mine. We come closer to one another, we find points in common, things we don't agree on, but on those points in common we forge ahead for the good of all, we do charitable works, we perform educational actions, together, lots of things.[606]

A Catholic educational vision thus demands that such intercultural and interreligious dialogue has a commitment to action. This means that students work together in solidarity to promote a fraternal humanism in society, promoting an authentic conception of human flourishing and identifying and challenging aspects of life that oppress or silence the most vulnerable and excluded in society. It also means challenging elements of culture that diminish human flourishing, such as excessive materialism, moral relativism and consumerism.

Second, mindfulness can assist in Catholic education's commitment to translating Gospel values into contemporary culture. Within a Christian framework, mindfulness must go beyond personal wellbeing and be both other-centred and Other-centred. Such a conception of mindfulness that is rooted in a Christian conception of human flourishing is robustly compatible with Catholic education. In this sense, students in the Catholic school are called to be mindful of their interdependence on others as part of a shared community, working together for the common good. This means that behaviours, actions and relationships in schools are viewed through the prism of a fraternal humanism, based on respect, mutuality and openness.

In terms of interfaith and intercultural dialogue, mindfulness can aid Catholic education in fostering a fraternal humanism, fostering open and constructive dialogue with others, irrespective of creed, colour or social status. This means that students are encouraged to be mindful of the innate dignity each person shares as part of the human family, working together with different faith perspectives and beliefs towards the common good. It also means being especially mindful of the poor and excluded, challenging cultural forces that inhibit the wellbeing of others, such as excessive

606 Ibid.

consumerism and moral relativism. In particular, the humanising vision of Catholic education means that solidarity in community leads to action. This would assist in countering the individualistic trend seen in some forms of mindfulness.

In terms of the ecological crisis, the poorest and most vulnerable have been disproportionately harmed by the actions of richer, developed countries.[607] Catholic education must nurture students that are mindful of their own actions and behaviours, and as reflections of God that are made for right relationship. It also means being mindful of the human dignity of all people, working in open and constructive interreligious dialogue with others to improve the wellbeing of society, particularly the wellbeing of the poor and voiceless. Moreover, this means that students recognise their roles as interdependent stewards of Creation, which is the common home for all people, challenging cultural forces such as excessive materialism, individualism and greed which frustrate the realisation of the common good. In this sense, a Catholic educational vision calls for intercultural dialogue that is truly mindful of the other and not just the self, acting as a constructive and critical partner in society.

Catholic education is committed to social justice

The compatibility of mindfulness with this aspect of Catholic education is evaluated under the headings of love of God and love of neighbour, and fraternal humanism. The first heading is chosen as it examines how mindfulness, which has faced criticism for an individualistic stance, interacts with the other-centred outlook of the Golden Rule.[608] The second heading corresponds to Pope Francis' call for a humanising education; a renewed vision

607 Nazrul Islam and John Winkel, 'Climate Change and Social Inequality', *UN Department of Economic and Social Affairs (DESA) Working Papers, No. 152* (NY: United Nations, 2017). <https://www.un.org/esa/desa/papers/2017/wp152_2017.pdf>. Accessed on 2 March 2021.

608 Matt 22:34–40. 'Jesus said unto him, Thou shalt love the Lord thy God with all thy heart, and with all thy soul, and with all thy mind. This is the first and great commandment. And the second is like unto it, Thou shalt love thy neighbour as thyself. On these two commandments hang all the law and the prophets'.

of community as a framework of relationships, and how mindfulness can interact with this fraternal humanism.

Love of God and love of neighbour

As was highlighted in the previous chapter, the commitment to social justice is a defining characteristic of not just Catholic education but Catholicism itself. This means that a Catholic school must embody Christ's Golden Rule: 'Love the Lord your God with all your heart and with all your soul and with all your mind and with all your strength ... Love your neighbour as yourself. There is no commandment greater than these'.[609] There are several areas in which mindfulness can contribute to this decree in relation to Catholic education.

First, mindfulness can be a valuable resource in reaffirming the human dignity and worth of each person in the school community, as well as all people. The theological anthropology underpinning Catholic education views the person as created in God's likeness and image, made for holiness and right relationship with self, others, creation and God. Mindfulness in a Catholic educational context could assist here in giving opportunities to students in a Catholic school to reflect and contemplate their own profound human dignity, their capacity for goodness and their lives as worthwhile and significant. Catholic education envisions the holistic development of students, nurturing their talents and abilities to be embodiments of right relationship in the world and as positively contributing to the common good of society. In this sense mindfulness can help students become mindful of their potential as responsible, engaged citizens whose lives have ultimate meaning.

Second, Catholic education can be aided by mindfulness as a means to realising and acting upon Christ's command to love our neighbour as ourselves. As stated in previous chapters, mindfulness is found to generate loving kindness in the practitioner, reducing personal stress and suffering. However, as seen earlier, some forms of mindfulness have been appropriated to privatise stress and buffer the practitioner from the sufferings of others or

609 Mark 12:30–31.

the structures in society that support such stress. Moreover, MBSR founder Jon Kabat-Zinn's claims that loving-kindness generated in mindfulness will naturally transmit to other people is problematic in that there is no axiomatic ethical framework to support such a claim in secular psychological mindfulness. Mindfulness in a Catholic educational context offers an instructive resource that can engender loving kindness in the self but also in the other, providing an ethical framework that stresses personal and collective wellbeing.

Christ's teachings are permeated by a preferential option to the poor and oppressed in society. Jesus recognises the profound dignity of those marginalised and voiceless, those that God especially favours. Mindfulness in Catholic education can foster in students not just concern for personal wellbeing but also the wellbeing of others, especially the poorest. This commitment to participate in the public square and promote the common good, with a preferential option towards the most vulnerable and excluded in society, is at the heart of Catholic social teaching. In this sense, there is a public significance to the Catholic faith which cannot be relegated to the private sphere, as argued by Himes and Himes.[610] Christ's proclamation of the Kingdom of God provides an ethical framework whereby students are called to be mindful of the wellbeing of others, especially those who suffer due to injustice, inequality and hatred in society. Living a holy life means that our relationships with others are agapic and self-giving, as we are made for right relationship with self, others, creation and God. Christian-scaffolded mindfulness can then become a means of generating loving-kindness of ourselves but also to others.[611] This is then can a humanising practice as it brings the practitioner closer to what is authentic human flourishing in the Catholic tradition. Moreover, in being a humanising practice, it becomes a divinising practice in that it brings us into closer relationship with God.

For the Catholic school, whose foundation is the person of Jesus Christ, Christian-scaffolded mindfulness is an important resource in placing a commitment to social justice at the heart of school life. By being mindful of

610 Michael J. Himes & Kenneth R. Himes, *Fullness of Faith: The Public Significance of Theology* (NJ: Paulist Press, 1993).

611 Loving-kindness finds in the Hebrew tradition the theologically compatible concept of *chesed*.

others, the school community is reminded to position Gospel values of mercy, charity and justice in every school policy, plan and management decision. It means that the Catholic school is an embodiment of right relationship in its teaching, learning and relationships between students, staff, parents and the community. Moreover, it means that students are not just encouraged to be mindful of the poor and marginalised but encouraged to challenge aspects of society that inhibit fairness and equality for others. Pope Francis has consistently criticised these aspects of a 'globalisation of indifference' operative in contemporary culture, instead proposing a culture of encounter[612] rooted in care towards all members of our common home, especially the poorest in the world.[613] Mindfulness in a Catholic educational context can then nurture students into a conscious awareness of their interdependence upon others and creation as part of an ecology of relationships.

Students are offered a holistic education to aid them in contributing to the common good of society, meaning they develop a critical consciousness of the wellbeing of others and interrupting sources of suffering and inequality for them. For the Catholic school, charity and justice for others are vital components of school life, and mindfulness encourages students to notice the wellbeing of others as well as their own. In this way, Catholic education aids pupils in becoming embodiments of right relationship and active agents in translating God's grace into transformative change in society.

612 Pope Francis, *Fratelli Tutti* (Dublin: Veritas, 2020), Par 216. 'To speak of a "culture of encounter" means that we, as a people, should be passionate about meeting others, seeking points of contact, building bridges, planning a project that includes everyone. This becomes an aspiration and a style of life'.

613 See Pope Francis, *Laudato Si': On Care for Our Common Home* (Dublin: Veritas, 2015), Par 231 'When we feel that God is calling us to intervene with others in these social dynamics, we should realise that this too is part of our spirituality, which is an exercise of charity and, as such, matures and sanctifies us ... Thus a community can break out of the indifference induced by consumerism. These actions cultivate a shared identity, with a story which can be remembered and handed on. In this way, the world, and the quality of life of the poorest, are cared for, with a sense of solidarity which is at the same time aware that we live in a common home which God has entrusted to us'.

Fraternal humanism

In the previous chapter, we explored the Church educational document *Educating to Fraternal Humanism: Building a 'Civilisation of Love' 50 Years after Popolorum Progressio (2017)* which highlighted Pope Francis' call for education that nurtures fraternal humanism. This is a humanising education which views the human person as being '… in a framework of relationships that make up a living community, which is interdependent and bound to a common destiny. This is fraternal humanism'.[614] Mindfulness offers several opportunities to strengthen this person-centred educational vision. First, mindfulness can assist Catholic education by fostering in students an attentiveness to the dignity of all people in society. Pope Francis writes of the corrosive effects of excessive consumerism on the quality of human relationships.

> Consumerist individualism has led to great injustice. Other persons come to be viewed simply as obstacles to our own serene existence … this is even more the case in times of crisis, catastrophe and hardship … we are tempted to think in terms of the old saying 'every man for himself'.[615]

Mindfulness is a basic human capacity that can be nurtured to recognise and attend to our own personal wellbeing but also the wellbeing of others. A Catholic educational vision is rooted in the conviction that as reflections of God, we are made for right relationship and share a common dignity. This means that for Catholic education, mindfulness can improve personal wellbeing but must also enable the practitioner to see others as members of a human fraternity.

Examples of Mindfulness 2 have been observed earlier which risk buffering practitioners from structural sources of suffering in others. These modes of mindfulness fail to recognise our nature as social and relational beings made for love. Mindfulness in the Catholic school would then cater for wellbeing as both a personal and collective goal. By generating loving kindness for ourselves and others, Catholic education can use mindfulness to

614 Congregation for Catholic Education, *Educating to Fraternal Humanism* (2017), Par 8.

615 Pope Francis, *Fratelli Tutti* (Dublin: Veritas, 2020), Par 222.

cultivate in students a concerned disposition for others, especially the poor, that challenges the cultural mores of consumerist individualism.

Second, mindfulness can aid Catholic education in nurturing the moral and social potential of students to engage in a culture of dialogue with others. The Catholic school as rooted in Jesus Christ envisions a school community that is welcoming and inclusive to all. This means that pupils are called to be mindful of the Catholic worldview that permeates their education but also the perspectives and principles of other faiths and cultures. This means that Catholic education champions a culture of encounter with others, grounded in openness, communion and solidarity. In this way, students become mindful of shared human values with other cultures and faiths, and consciously aware of societal forces that inhibit the human dignity of others. By focusing on what unites us rather than what divides or separates us, students are encouraged to work together with others for the common good.

Fraternal humanism stresses the recognition of the dignity of all members of the human family. Catholic education can be helped by mindfulness in that it calls students to work with others to challenge sources of injustice and inequality globally that prevent others from flourishing. Thus, a mindful Catholic education notices and responds to the needs of others by promoting a view of the human person as interdependent and interconnected and part of a common family. This means that mindfulness can assist in reinforcing Catholic education's commitment to social justice and educating to a fraternal humanism.

Finally, mindfulness can strengthen the development of kindness in students in Catholic schools, in their thoughts, words and actions. This cultivation of kindness enables pupils to become active citizens that can bring out transformative change in society and contribute to the common good. Pope Francis cites Saint Paul's description of kindness as a fruit of the Spirit.[616] 'Individuals who possess this quality help make other people's lives more bearable, especially by sharing the weight of their problems, needs and fears'.[617]

Kindness is a disposition that implies a concern or care towards another person and their wellbeing. A Christian-scaffolded mindfulness offers an

616 'The Greek word *chrestótes* denotes an attitude that is gentle, pleasant and supportive'. Ibid, 223.
617 Ibid.

explicit ethical framework that sees the other as a reflection of God, possessing an intrinsic human dignity and as made for right relationship. This means that the kindness generated in mindfulness practice extends from the individual to the other, fostering a sense of community and solidarity as part of the human family. This means that Catholic education offers a holistic education that nurtures students to be kind in their relationship to the world.

Kindness as a fruit of the Spirit highlights that students can become creative catalysts of God's grace, the Holy Spirit working through them to help bring about the Kingdom of God. Mindfulness in Catholic education can then become a vehicle for the Spirit of God in the world, enabling students to embody right relationship in their thoughts, words and actions. For Catholic education, the life-giving benefits of mindfulness can then be a source of living authentically and flourishing for the student, the school community and ultimately the common good. In this sense, mindfulness is compatible with Catholic education's commitment to social justice.

Mindfulness and a Catholic educational vision

Having evaluated the compatibility of mindfulness and each characteristic of the Catholic educational vision proposed earlier, several remarks can be made. First, it has been established that mindfulness is not an exclusive property of the Buddhist wisdom tradition nor any religious tradition. It is a universal human capacity to notice the present moment, consciousness awareness of now. Proponents of secular mindfulness such as Jon Kabat-Zinn have engaged in detraditionalising and recontextualising the practice from Eastern wisdom traditions. In other words, they have changed the contextual framework that mindfulness was operative in. In terms of Catholic education, mindfulness is compatible with ethos when it fits into the contextual framework that is the educational vision of the Catholic school.

Second, the evaluation of the relationship of mindfulness with each component of a Catholic educational vision found that there is broad compatibility present. Each characteristic can be aided by mindfulness to be more fully realised in the Catholic school. Moreover, the contextual framework of

Catholic education means that mindfulness is provided with a theological language and moral framework which can help to ground it as both a contemplative practice and a means of maintaining positive student wellbeing.

In terms of a *theological anthropology*, mindfulness can help the Catholic school present a more humanising education, where the student is encouraged to be mindful of their own wellbeing, the wellbeing of others and their capacity for right relationship with God. Mindfulness can help foster the holistic development of the person envisioned in Catholic education. It means that the child recognises their own human dignity, their potential to contribute to transformative change in society and that their life has ultimate meaning. This Catholic anthropology invites students to develop a sacramental perspective, seeing the world as engraced. Moreover, far from being a passive and non-evaluative exercise, mindfulness in the Catholic school must be active and challenge aspects of culture that deny the human dignity of others and inhibit human flourishing. This means bringing the Christian conception of human flourishing into conversation with contemporary culture, with a special commitment to the needs of the poor.

From a *Christological* perspective, mindfulness can assist children in calming the mind before prayer, making authentic prayer possible rather than a superficial, routine activity. A mindful disposition towards others is also essential in the Catholic school's mission of recognising dignity in community, irrespective of background, creed or class. This embodying of the Good News is part of the Catholic school's evangelising task, inviting others to relationship with Jesus and to see how a community of self-giving love is a microcosm of the Kingdom of God.

In terms of *sacramentality*, mindfulness has profound potential for application in Catholic education. The intentional awareness of the student to the present moment offers the possibility of inculcating a sacramental perspective, where the world is viewed as engraced, and God's presence is to be felt across the entire spectrum of human experience. This also means that a preferential option for the poor must be operative, recognising the societal forces that frustrate human flourishing in others. This is a call to be mindful of personal but also collective wellbeing.

Mindfulness can be a significant boon to the *evangelising task* of the Catholic school. Given the post-secular and post-Christian climate that schools operate in, mindfulness can be a resource for pre-evangelisation. By helping students to attune their awareness to the present moment, the possibility of experiencing the transcendent becomes possible. Given the oft negligible connection students have to their Catholic faith, mindfulness can aid children in noticing in the silence the presence of God, perhaps for the first time.

Mindfulness is also compatible with Catholic education's commitment to *academic integrity*. As an aid to the cognitive and academic performance of pupils in Catholic schools, mindfulness reinforces the rich, intellectually stimulating education offered. As a resource for improving student wellbeing and flourishing, mindfulness can help students to reach their full potential and experience success, robustly compatible with the holistic education of the Catholic school.

In mindfulness, Catholic education's commitment to fostering *dialogue between faith and culture* has a compatible resource. As a means of responding to the contemporary post-secular and post-Christian conditions for faith, mindfulness offers Catholic education a resource that can address the spiritual hunger felt by many. Mindfulness can also assist in facilitating intercultural dialogue in the Catholic school, where students are called to notice and affirm the dignity of the other, working together to challenge cultural forces that inhibit human flourishing in society.

Finally, mindfulness is compatible with the *social justice* demanded of Catholic education. This means that students are mindful of the wellbeing of others and that there is a commitment to challenging societal injustice and inequality that harms the flourishing of the poor and vulnerable. Mindfulness can bolster Catholic education's vision of each person as made for right relationship and as possessing innate dignity. Catholic education can embody the fraternal humanism called for by Pope Francis by nurturing a vision of the human person as interdependent and interconnected.

Mindfulness is compatible with the ethos of Catholic primary schools

This chapter was an evaluative exercise in establishing whether mindfulness is compatible with a Catholic vision of education, which is at the heart of this work. First, this chapter argued that scaffolding was an appropriate evaluative resource in examining the compatibility of mindfulness with ethos in the Catholic primary school. It was highlighted that mindfulness is a basic human capacity that transcends labels such as Christian, Buddhist or secular. Moreover, it was argued that Christian scaffolding could be applied to mindfulness practice to ensure greater compatibility with the Catholic educational vision underpinning the Irish Catholic primary school. This would also alleviate concerns that mindfulness being a Buddhist meditative practice which would be incoherent with Catholic ethos.

Following this, the evaluative exercise was outlined, with mindfulness being brought into critical conversation with the seven characteristics of a Catholic educational vision developed in the previous chapter. These characteristics of theological anthropology, Christocentricity, sacramentality, evangelisation, academic integrity, dialogue between faith and culture, and social justice served as the evaluative criteria in assessing the compatibility of mindfulness with the theological vision grounding the Irish Catholic primary school. Each of these were found to be coherent with the practice of mindfulness as a contemplative practice that enables children to notice their inner thoughts, feelings and the sources of meaning in their lives. Moreover, in several instances a Christian scaffolding was suggested to deepen the compatibility of mindfulness with a Catholic educational vision. This would lead to the overall conclusion that mindfulness is compatible with the ethos of the Irish Catholic primary schools.

CHAPTER 6

Conclusions, Findings and Recommendations

This concluding chapter will present the conclusions, findings and recommendations which are a distillation of the work built upon in each preceding chapter. The guiding questions of these chapters have been:

(i) What are the contemporary conditions of religious belief and experience that contextualise this research question? (Chapter 1)

(ii) What are the origins, Buddhist etymology, history and contemporary understandings of mindfulness, and what kinds of mindfulness are operative in our contemporary context? (Chapter 2)

(iii) How is mindfulness operative within Irish educational policy and curricular reform at both primary and post-primary levels, and what is the relationship between mindfulness and wellbeing? (Chapter 3)

(iv) What criteria for a Catholic educational vision can be derived from the Church's post-Conciliar teaching on Catholic education and in contemporary academic discourse on Catholic education? (Chapter 4)

(v) Using the criteria derived above, what is the compatibility of mindfulness with a Catholic educational vision? (Chapter 5).

This final chapter will first present the conclusions drawn from each chapter. It will then present the findings of this work along with recommendations for how mindfulness can be operative in the Irish Catholic primary school whilst enjoying significant compatibility with the school's ethos. This will mean recognising both the opportunities and challenges that exist in ensuring that mindfulness might be not just compatible with the Catholic ethos but in fact can be a valuable resource to a Catholic educational vision.

Conclusions

Chapter 1—The contemporary conditions of religious belief and experience have contributed to the growth in popularity of mindfulness

As the first chapter indicated, there has been a religious climate change over recent decades. This is perhaps best articulated by Charles Taylor's thesis in *A Secular Age*, which presents a radically transformed context for religion today, where the essential secularising change lies on the level of the social imaginary. For the first time, religious belief is not only questioned but increasingly contested by an immanent frame of viewing the world. Belief in God becomes more implausible to many and for the first time, a conception of human flourishing with no transcendental aspect is possible. These altered conditions are further explored through the insights of Lieven Boeve, Tomáš Halík, Michael Paul Gallagher and Grace Davie, which offer an interdisciplinary approach to understanding how religious belief is felt and experienced today.

However, despite the predictions of sociologists of religion and zero-sum secularisation theories, religious belief and experience in the contemporary Western context have changed, not ended. The emergence of postmodernism, with its suspicion of grand narratives, objective truth claims and institutions of power in society, has challenged the transmission of religious beliefs, practices and participation in communal worship from one generation to the next. The continuing decrease in Irish citizens who identify as Catholic, attend Mass or participate in the liturgical life of the Church is a microcosm of this broader phenomenon of institutional religion being challenged by new narratives.

This pluralised, detraditionalised and individualised context has led to a diverse marketplace of religious and spiritual worldviews, including New Age spiritualities and practices derived from Eastern wisdom traditions, including Buddhism. Aspects of these traditions, including mindfulness and meditation, have become increasingly attractive alternatives to the doctrines, communal worship and transcendental or supernatural elements of traditional religious narratives. For the growing demographic who identify as spiritual but not religious, practices like mindfulness offer an experiential source of meaning or fullness. This cohort, subscribing to 'something-ism' and holding vague beliefs in God, an afterlife, or a higher spiritual power, searches for a fullness or authenticity to their lives beyond the flatness of postmodern life. The contemporary interest in spirituality and mindfulness over doctrinal adherence and communal worship in a religious tradition signifies this hunger for meaning or otherness. Mindfulness in this sense is a contemporary post-secular resource that is for many a humanising and spiritually affirming practice. Moreover, it is a phenomenon that fits with theologian Lieven Boeve's categorisation of our contemporary context being both post-Christian and post-secular. In this way, the contemporary conditions of religious beliefs and experience have provided fertile soil for the seeds of mindfulness to blossom in our contemporary context, which in Ireland includes Catholic primary schools.

Chapter 2—Mindfulness has evolved beyond its traditional Buddhist context

As indicated in Chapter 2, while mindfulness traces its roots back to the Buddhist wisdom tradition, the ability to regulate one's attention to the present moment and notice thoughts and feelings should be seen as a human faculty rather than as an exclusive element of a religion or wisdom tradition. However, this does not and should not undermine the significance of mindfulness to the Buddhist tradition. Moreover, in order to better understand what is mindfulness and why it is practiced today, it is important to appreciate how mindfulness has evolved from a central tenet of Buddhist teaching to a contemporary Western phenomenon.

In its traditional Buddhist context, Right Mindfulness is integral to the Noble Eightfold Path, a central tenet of Buddhism which presents an ethical and moral framework of behaviour and practices central to following the path of the Buddha. Importantly, mindfulness in this framework relates to actively noticing the moral valence of situations and responding accordingly, implying the difference between right mindfulness and wrong mindfulness. This means that far from being a passive, non-evaluative or 'bare attention' stance, Right Mindfulness is active and ethically motivated by Buddhist teachings towards the reduction of suffering or *dhukka* in the world. This, in turn, is oriented towards the broader Buddhist soteriological goal of Nirvana, which is the ultimate cessation of suffering.

The migration of mindfulness from Eastern practice to Western phenomenon can be best understood through the process of Buddhist modernism. This multi-faceted process of detraditionalisation, secularisation and recontextualisation reveals how mindfulness gradually became detached from its original place as an integral element of Buddhist teaching and practice. Through the work of influential Buddhist teachers Mahāsī Sayādaw and Nyanaponika Thera, this new form of non-evaluative or 'bare attention' mindfulness emerged, removed of its explicitly religious or transcendental language and concepts such as karma and reincarnation. Mindfulness became both the essence of Buddha's teaching and a practice that did not require any adherence to traditional Buddhist tenets or teachings. In this way, Buddhist modernism helps to account for how a non-theistic spiritual practice from the East adapted to the increasingly secular conditions in the West, recontextualising mindfulness into the popular phenomenon it is today across many facets of society.

Chapter 2 also demonstrated that mindfulness is a complex term which has several iterations in the contemporary Western context. Despite the exponential growth of interest in mindfulness, there is an elasticity to the meanings and understandings of mindfulness in the contemporary Western context. Bishop et al.'s definition of mindfulness as a non-evaluative, non-judgemental, present-centred awareness and acceptance of thoughts, sensations and feelings as they arise offers a relatively inclusive understanding of the term in this regard. However, as Buddhist scholar Rupert Gethin argued, there are three distinctive strands of mindfulness operative in our contemporary context.

Mindfulness 1 relates to the secular psychological model, best exemplified by Jon Kabat-Zinn's MBSR (Mindfulness-based Stress Reduction) program. This participant-centred behavioural medicine program highlights how this iteration of mindfulness has become a clinical resource for pain reduction and healing for patients, using mindfulness techniques such as body scans and breathing exercises as part of treatment. Buddhist terminology and religious concepts are absent in Mindfulness 1 in order to present mindfulness as a method of healing accessible to those of all faiths and none. In this sense, Mindfulness 1 is an indicator of the processes of Buddhist modernism, where mindfulness has been secularised, detraditionalised and recontextualised to adapt to its new cultural environment. A growing body of research indicates the benefits of Mindfulness 1 in areas including physical wellbeing, mental health, addiction treatment and cognitive functioning. In this sense, Mindfulness 1 has provided an important, evidence-based resource in treating pain, suffering and illness and in this regard, is to be welcomed in improving quality of life for so many.

Mindfulness 2 represents the commercialised, privatised version of mindfulness, observed in the masses of mindfulness products on the market, such as apps and books. This commercial mindfulness focuses on immanent goals, including stress reduction, improving performance and physical and mental wellbeing. This development has been broadly positive as resources that are evidenced to improve the quality of life for people are to be welcomed, particularly in light of the devastating effects of the COVID-19 pandemic for countless people, not least children. However, without any ethical or moral framework, Mindfulness 2 is at risk of misappropriation by companies and businesses. Marketed as a panacea or a quick-fix solution to stress, this mutated form of Mindfulness 2 risks privatising stress and buffering the practitioner from noticing and responding to structural sources of suffering in society or the suffering of others. In terms of education, mindfulness can be reduced to serving a neoliberal agenda. In this case, instead of being a humanising and transformational practice, mindfulness becomes an instrument to optimise efficiency, performance and ultimately student grades. In this sense, it risks contributing to a deficient vision of human flourishing.

Finally, Mindfulness 3 is the post-secular spirituality iteration of mindfulness today. Mindfulness 3 is broadly decoupled from the religious or metaphysical assumptions of its traditional Buddhist framework while also acting as a response to the spiritual needs of many in our contemporary context. In this sense, it encapsulates a spiritual practice that fits with the post-secular, post-Christian context of today, where many identify as spiritual but not religious. Mindfulness 3 is then a continuation of Buddhist modernism, where the original practice has become radically deracinated from its traditional Buddhist context, with its religious or metaphysical tenets. This creates a spiritual grey area, where some practice mindfulness without any reference to the teachings of the Buddha, with others arguing that mindfulness is itself the heart of those teachings.

Chapter 3—Mindfulness has become increasingly significant in the Irish education system through the vehicle of wellbeing

The contemporary explosion of interest in mindfulness has coincided with the emergence of wellbeing promotion at the heart of current educational discourse. In the Irish context, wellbeing has become a significant element of educational policy, planning and curricular reform, as evidenced by reports and documents from the Department of Education, as well as the National Council for Curriculum and Assessment and the National Educational Psychological Service. This focus on wellbeing has, if anything, intensified in light of the COVID-19 pandemic and its debilitating effects on children's education and development. It is likely that mindfulness practice will grow in schools through the vehicle of wellbeing promotion.

These practices are supported by an increasing body of literature detailing the benefits of mindfulness in schools, including improved physical and mental wellbeing, socialisation and academic performance. However, there remains a paucity of critical papers in this area, which means it is possible that the zeal in sharing the good news of mindfulness in schools has overtaken the evidence supporting it. While mindfulness may indeed offer many positive and welcome benefits to students' wellbeing, it is clear that critiques of mindfulness in education remain few. This is an important issue as critical research and studies would help to ground mindfulness practices and programmes in schools in best practice, ensuring better outcomes for pupils.

Finally, programmes such as Paws b and Weaving Wellbeing have also introduced secular mindfulness practices into schools in Ireland. For Catholic schools, this should be welcomed as resources that are shown to improve student wellbeing are to be welcomed. Moreover, several educationalists have indicated the profound educational potential of mindfulness as a contemplative activity, enabling students to explore and interrogate their inner thoughts, feelings and sources of meaning, which again should be welcome in the Catholic school. However, these programmes need to be reinforced by more rigorous research using robust methods such as randomisation, controls and larger sample sizes. This would ground such programmes in best practice and help to deliver on stated outcomes and objectives.

Chapter 4—A robust Catholic educational vision for schools can be drawn from post-Conciliar teaching on Catholic education

In order to evaluate the compatibility of mindfulness and Catholic ethos in schools, criteria were developed by examining influential documents in Catholic education over recent decades. These documents included *Gravissimum Educationis (1965)*, *The Catholic School (1977)*, *The Religious Dimension of Education in a Catholic School (1988)*, *Educating to Intercultural Dialogue in Catholic Schools: Living in Harmony for a Civilisation of Love (2013)* and *Educating to Fraternal Humanism: Building a 'Civilisation of Love' 50 Years after Popolorum Progressio (2017)*. These present a development in the self-understanding of Catholic education, inspired by the spirit of openness that characterised Vatican II. The Irish Church educational documents *Vision 08: A Vision for Catholic Education in Ireland (2008)* and *Share the Good News: The National Directory for Catechesis (2011)* were also explored. The themes outlined here are further developed through the use of theologian Thomas Groome's work on the characteristics of Catholicism and Catholic education, in dialogue with other influential scholars in Catholic education, such as John Sullivan and Stephen McKinney.

Given the variety of settings which Catholic education is operative, it is impossible to present *the* definitive Catholic educational vision. However, through interrogating the sources above, a vision that correlates with the characteristic spirit of the Irish Catholic primary school is possible, constituted of seven interrelated and interconnected characteristics. First, a Catholic educational vision is underpinned by a theological anthropology. This means that each person is seen as being made in the likeness and image of God, made for right relationship with self, others, God and creation and possessing an innate human dignity. This graced nature anthropology is at the heart of the holistic development of the child in the Catholic school, presenting a distinctive Christian vision of human flourishing.

Second, this educational vision is radically Christocentric, as the person of Jesus Christ is foundational to the life and work of the Catholic school. Through his life and ministry, Jesus Christ, as the human *par excellence*, offers the school a definitive vision of what it means to be human. To strive towards such an ideal requires the Catholic school to cultivate its identity and ethos through Word, worship, welfare and witness, where students are given opportunities to come to know and love Jesus in prayer.

Third, this vision is sacramental, meaning that students are encouraged to view the world as engraced, dissolving false notions of a sacred/secular binary. Catholic schools invite students to view the world through this sacramental lens, 'seeing' grace at work in their lives. Such a perspective must permeate the entire curriculum of the Catholic school, with opportunities across many subjects for students to experience the infinite number of moments of wonder and awe of God's presence in the world.

Fourth, a Catholic vision of education shares in the evangelising mission of the Church. This call to conversion means that every Catholic is inspired to be authentic witnesses to the Christian faith in their lives, encouraging others to experience the Good News proclaimed by Jesus Christ. Evangelisation is an ongoing process, encouraging every Catholic in the school community to be witnesses to their faith in freedom, through words and actions to others, embodying the Gospel values of charity, love and justice.

Fifth, this vision is committed to academic integrity and the autonomy of subjects. The Catholic school provides an education that is committed to transmitting knowledge to pupils, forming them into proactive citizens who can contribute to the common good. Students are to be nurtured into becoming critical and creative partners in society, meaning that the intellectual realm of their development is vital. Academic subjects enjoy the academic autonomy to be taught according to the principles and methodologies appropriate to them, as this embodies the genuine pursuit of truth at the heart of Catholic education.

Sixth, a Catholic educational vision is committed to being a place of dialogue between faith and culture. Following the spirit of Vatican II, Catholic education is tasked with the ongoing translation of Christian faith in contemporary culture. This means working with secular culture to recognise what values they share that contribute to the common good, such as freedom, democracy and justice, while rejecting aspects of culture that inhibit human flourishing, including ethical relativism, excessive consumerism and anthropocentrism. The Catholic school must be a community that reflects the Kingdom of God; an inclusive, loving place where the poor, excluded and voiceless are given special care.

Finally, social justice must be at the heart of any Catholic educational vision. Catholic education is inspired by Jesus' preferential love for the poor, excluded and voiceless in society and recognises that each person, irrespective of creed, class, or background, has profound human dignity and is made in the likeness and image of God. For this reason, Catholic schools must especially care for those most marginalised in society. In the processes, this becomes an embodiment of the Kingdom of God, a community rooted in love, generosity and equality.

Chapter 5—Mindfulness is compatible with a Catholic educational vision

Having established evaluative criteria for our research criteria, this chapter found that mindfulness is compatible with the educational vision at the heart of the Catholic school, which is expressed and lived out in the school's ethos. The educational vision of the Irish Catholic primary school has, in mindfulness, a resource that is potentially invaluable in supporting and vivifying the patterns of belief, conduct and practice that embody this vision of life, which is Catholic ethos. In order to better understand this conclusion, which is the basis of our research question, the findings will now indicate how mindfulness is compatible with Catholic ethos, along with the opportunities and challenges this presents.

Findings

Mindfulness is compatible with the Catholic ethos when it contributes to the holistic development of the student

As was argued in Chapters 2 and 3, there is an increasing body of evidence that mindfulness offers many benefits to practitioners, including lower anxiety, enhanced physical and mental wellbeing and improved cognitive function. Moreover, despite the need for critical papers on mindfulness and education, and more rigorous large-scale studies on the impact of mindfulness in schools, there is a growing consensus that mindfulness offers similar benefits to pupils. This means that mindfulness is a potentially invaluable resource to Catholic schools in caring for and nurturing students' wellbeing after the debilitating effects of the COVID-19 pandemic and subsequent lockdowns.

When mindfulness is a humanising activity that lowers wellbeing and enables pupils to flourish, it is compatible with the Catholic ethos. The Catholic educational vision of the school is underpinned by a theological anthropology that sees the pupil as made for God and for good, their nature being perfected through God's grace. The student is seen as made in the *imago Dei*, made for right relationship, and as possessing an innate human dignity, and as such, any activity in the Catholic school that humanises the pupils also divinises them. That is a practice that enables the student to become more genuinely human, developing their freedom, talents, creativity and capacity for relationships, making them more authentic reflections of God. When mindfulness supports this effort at the holistic development of the pupil and the distinctive vision of human flourishing, it is compatible with the Catholic ethos.

However, while mindfulness may improve student's academic performance, this should never be the sole focus of the practice in the Catholic school. Just as the intellectual development of the student is not the definitive measure of human flourishing, nor can academic output be the overarching metric of a pupil's value or success. In this sense, mindfulness may help the Catholic school's commitment to academic integrity and excellence while resisting any effort to instrumentalise mindfulness to optimise grades and test scores over the holistic development of the student.

Mindfulness is compatible with Catholic ethos when it aids preparation for prayer

Despite the variance in the strands of mindfulness operative in the contemporary West as explored in Chapter 2, a shared characteristic is their deracination from their traditional Buddhist context. Put simply, mindfulness as practiced in Irish Catholic primary schools is a secular activity which has been decoupled from Buddhism. This means that concerns over mindfulness acting as a Trojan horse for Buddhism in Catholic schools should be alleviated. Moreover, the capacity for mindfulness to cultivate regulated attention to the present moment means it can be an invaluable resource to the Catholic school's commitment to helping each child foster a personal relationship with Christ through prayer.

When mindfulness calms students' minds of noise and distractions, a space for authentic prayer is made possible. Rather than a cursory rattling off of prayers during the school day, students are invited to be present in the moment, aware of themselves and mindful that in prayer, they come to know and love Jesus more fully. When practiced this way, mindfulness is compatible with the Catholic ethos as it supports the Christocentric nature of the school, where Christ is the exemplar of human flourishing and his teachings and ministry as the basis for conduct, behaviour and witness in the school.

However, mindfulness is compatible in this sense precisely because it is preparation for prayer, *not* a replacement for prayer. No technique, including mindfulness, can in itself deepen a person's relationship with God, as it is by God's unmerited grace that this relationship is nourished and realised, rather than by human initiative or mastery. Any effort to replace authentic prayer with mindfulness must then be resisted. In this sense, mindfulness is compatible with Catholic school ethos only when it gently brings students to a place of stillness and quiet, inviting them into a loving relationship with Christ, who is the revelation of God's salvific will. It is a resource that helps students become more prayerful, rather than prayer itself.

Mindfulness is compatible with Catholic ethos when it is practiced as a contemplative activity

As was evidenced in Chapter 3, there is a growing call among several educationalists that mindfulness offers a profound educational potential, enabling students to develop a greater awareness of their thoughts, feelings and sources of meaning. Where mindfulness offers such a transformative potential for students and engendering of a contemplative outlook, it is compatible with Catholic ethos.

As students grow and develop in a post-COVID environment punctuated by social media use, smartphones and heightened anxiety, they face new challenges to their wellbeing and their ability to concentrate on the here and now. Put simply, it has become harder for children to just be in the present moment. The sacramentality of Catholic education invites students to see the present moment as engraced, revealing God's creative action in the world. In this sense, mindfulness can offer Catholic schools a means of offering students a means to notice God's presence in the moment through calming the mind of distractions. This can cultivate a contemplative outlook more attuned to the beauty and mystery of the world, a sacramental perspective which is at the heart of the Catholic ethos.

While the therapeutic benefits of mindfulness, if supported by evidence are welcome in the Catholic school, as a contemplative activity, it can also be transformative. By giving students the time and space to explore their inner world, mindfulness can cater to the spiritual needs of pupils, especially those with little connection to their Christian faith. While mindfulness is not a replacement for prayer, it generates a space for students to become more self-aware of the importance of the inner life of spirituality. Spiritual development is an important element of the holistic education of the child in Catholic school, enabling the student to flourish and find meaning and authenticity in their lives. Where mindfulness contributes to this endeavour, it is compatible with the Catholic ethos.

Mindfulness is compatible with the Catholic ethos when it acts as praeparatio evangelica

In Chapter 1, Charles Taylor argues that the immanent frame is common to us all in the West today. By this, he means that we operate within a secularised social imaginary, where belief in God has become increasingly implausible and meaningless and where human flourishing can be understood without any reference to the transcendent. This presents unique challenges to Irish Catholic primary schools, where, despite having a significant Catholic student population, many students have little connection to the faith they are baptised into, outside of religious education and sacramental preparation.

Mindfulness as a contemplative practice is compatible with Catholic school ethos when it challenges this secular social imaginary and enflames the imagination into seeing the world as having a transcendent or religious dimension. Therefore, before evangelisation can be a reality in the Catholic school, pre-evangelisation is necessary to attune pupils' awareness of an experience of the transcendent and enliven the possibility of belief in God. Mindfulness is compatible with the Catholic ethos when it is a resource for interrupting the immanent frames of students, inviting students to find and name some signs or echoes of God's presence in their experience.

The cultural unbelief that Michael Gallagher describes in Chapter 1 pervades much of contemporary society, including in Catholic schools and this means that students need to develop a sacramental perspective that makes the experience of God plausible. Mindfulness is compatible with the Catholic ethos in this regard when it dissolves any proposed secular/sacred binary. Mindfulness can then be a first step for students coming to see the Christian life offered by the Church as a credible source of meaning and authenticity, rooted in God's unconditional love and embodied in Jesus Christ.

Beyond a question of compatibility, it can be argued that Catholic education needs resources precisely like mindfulness to interrupt frames of understanding the world which preclude any transcendental conception of human flourishing. In this way, Catholic school ethos is only then in a position to share in the evangelising task of the Church.

Mindfulness is compatible with the Catholic ethos when it is other-oriented

Among the critiques of mindfulness offered in Chapter 2 was the danger of mindfulness mutating into a self-centred, ethically neutral instrument to support rather than subvert structural sources of suffering in society. Such an application of mindfulness would be *anathema* to the Catholic ethos of a school.

Mindfulness can be an important resource for wellbeing promotion, but in a Catholic school, a commitment to social justice means mindfulness is compatible with the Catholic ethos when it is ethically oriented towards the needs of others. In this sense, while mindfulness can be personally therapeutic for the pupil, there is a need to recognise that one's own wellbeing is radically connected to the wellbeing of others, especially the poorest and marginalised in society. The Catholic school is a microcosm of the Kingdom of God and mindfulness can contribute to this vision of human flourishing by inviting students to see the innate dignity in each person.

For mindfulness to be compatible with Catholic school ethos it must also be active rather than passive. This means that students are called not just to notice the voiceless and oppressed but to challenge and reject elements of society that reinforce and perpetuate the suffering and injustices they endure. Mindfulness in the Catholic school can never be individualist as to ignore the needs and suffering of the poorest in society is to fall short of Christ's teachings on the Kingdom of God and to diminish the theocentric understanding of the human person which is at the heart of Catholic education.

This means that mindfulness is only compatible with Catholic ethos when it is committed to both individual and collective wellbeing, concerned with enabling each person to flourish, irrespective of class, ethnicity or creed. When mindfulness achieves this, it is an invaluable, humanising resource for Catholic schools.

Mindfulness is compatible with Catholic ethos when it is committed to the common good

As was highlighted in Chapters 4 and 5, educational documents during the pontificate of Pope Francis speak of fraternal humanism, the concept that humans belong to a web of relationships, interconnected and interdependent upon each other and the world around us to flourish. This idea is rooted in a conception of human flourishing that sees the person as made for right relationship and committed to the common good. Mindfulness is compatible with this commitment and anthropology when it enables students in the Catholic school to become critical and constructive citizens in society, working towards this distinctive Christian anthropology.

This means that mindfulness as a contemplative activity goes beyond passive neutrality and allows students to explore their inner life, noticing their thoughts, feelings and sources of meaning. Rather, for compatibility, mindfulness in the Catholic school can invite students to work with the prevailing culture towards important social goals of freedom, care for the poor and democracy. However, this also means that students become mindful of the need to reject corrosive aspects of culture that inhibit human flourishing, such as anthropocentrism, greed and ethical relativism. The vision of life in a Catholic school means the continuing translation of Gospel values into contemporary culture, and where mindfulness cultivates a constructive, critical outlook, it is compatible with the Catholic ethos.

Moreover, this also means that mindfulness cannot serve an instrumentalist educational agenda, which presents human development and success solely through the lens of academic output. Mindfulness can assist Catholic schools in resisting this damaging trend in education by contributing to the holistic development of the person, which is at the heart of the school's Catholic ethos. This is possible through mindfulness, nurturing a contemplative outlook in pupils, encouraging them to notice their talents, capacity for goodness, love and right relationship, and the contribution they can make to the common good. Where mindfulness achieves this, it is a significant boon for the characteristic spirit of Irish Catholic schools being lived out.

Recommendations

At this juncture, conclusions and findings have been established based on an evaluation of the compatibility of mindfulness and ethos in the Irish Catholic primary school. These have provided insights into how and when mindfulness is congruent with the Catholic school's characteristic spirit, offering an answer to the research question at the heart of this project. However, in order for this research to meaningfully contribute to contemporary discourse on mindfulness and Catholic primary schools, as well as Catholic education more generally, several recommendations are offered.

Catholic primary schools should see mindfulness as a potentially life-giving resource compatible with the Catholic ethos

Mindfulness can offer Catholic primary schools a humanising resource which can contribute to student wellbeing, socialisation and academic performance. Given the profound disruption to children's development and education due to the COVID-19 pandemic, resources that help to lower anxiety and enable children to flourish are needed now more than ever. Moreover, in an age of smartphones, social media and distraction, resources that enables students to be attentive to the present moment is a boon to the Catholic school. As has been demonstrated, there is much in mindfulness that resonates with a Catholic educational vision and its lived expression in the Catholic ethos of the primary school. For these reasons, Catholic schools should see mindfulness as a potential in their educational mission.

Further research on mindfulness in Catholic education is necessary

While a growing body of research highlights the benefits of mindfulness in education, there remains a paucity of critical papers in the field. This means that an overoptimistic narrative can develop, which overplays the benefits of mindfulness or fails to address any issues or negative effects of mindfulness. Moreover, several studies have been found to suffer from several limitations, including small sample size, no control group or lack of randomisation. This absence of rigorous research methods undermines the results of such studies. Pupils in Catholic schools should have mindfulness resources supported by robust studies and evidence to provide any benefits that are promoted. Further research in this area, such as large-scale qualitative and quantitative methods, would be recommended in this regard. In particular, exploring any link between mindfulness and spiritual wellbeing could be an important contribution to the field.

Continuous professional development for teachers on Christian contemplative prayer is necessary

The contemporary popularity of mindfulness in education speaks to a deeper spiritual need for forms of contemplative practices for students.

In the Catholic tradition, there have been many approaches to contemplative or meditative prayer, including the Hesychast tradition, Desert Fathers such as Evagrius and John Cassian, Teresa of Ávila and Ignatius of Loyola, up to contemporary movements such as John Main's Christian Meditation and Thomas Keating's Centering Prayer.

For Catholic schools, there should be continuous professional development (CPD) courses developed and made available to teachers who wish to offer Catholic approaches to mindfulness or contemplative prayer. Dr Noel Keating's work in promoting John Main's form of Christian Meditation in Irish primary schools is contributing to this area. However, patrons of Catholic education should fund and develop courses in mindfulness within the Christian tradition and contemplative prayer for teachers to offer Catholic schools resources that contribute to the holistic development of pupils while also drawing upon the rich spiritual tradition of the Church. Moreover, such courses would also provide opportunities for Catholic teachers to learn about such contemplative practices for their own continuing faith formation and spiritual development as well as professional development.

Catholic school communities should engage in self-evaluation of their Catholic ethos

In order to assess how mindfulness would contribute to Catholic ethos, Irish Catholic primary schools should self-evaluate what is distinctive about their characteristic spirit. This would lead each Catholic school to a better self-understanding of the particularity of their ethos, and how they live out this ethos in a unique way. In terms of mindfulness, this would mean that schools could identify how mindfulness would make a meaningful contribution to the life of the school, be that as preparation for prayer, a mode of improving student wellbeing or offering a sacramental perspective to students.

The Catholic Education Service has developed an ethos self-reflection process, for Irish Catholic primary and post-primary schools in this area. In order to help each Catholic school community assess how mindfulness would best fit into their distinctive living out of Catholic ethos, dioceses should actively promote this process to all Catholic primary schools.

Closing comments

This work has sought to bridge a gap in current research. Although in recent years there have been some studies on the relationship between Christian spirituality and mindfulness,[618] there has been only a single journal article on how mindfulness is operative within Irish Catholic schools.[619] Despite the contemporary explosion in popularity of mindfulness in Irish schools, of which the majority are under Catholic patronage, there has never been a significant theological study undertaken in this area. In this sense, this work makes an original and distinctive contribution to Catholic educational research both nationally and internationally, particularly in regard to Catholic schooling. It fills a lacuna of knowledge in relation to how mindfulness is to be understood within Irish Catholic primary schools and how it is compatible with the school's characteristic spirit. Given the debilitating effects of the COVID-19 pandemic and subsequent lockdown on the well-being of so many Irish children, this research provides an opportunity to address the implications of mindfulness practice in Irish education and its possible benefits to wellbeing and child development. Moreover, it makes an original contribution to research into the resources a Catholic educational vision offers to each child in order for them to flourish and reach their full potential.

The conclusions, findings and recommendations of this thesis make an original contribution to patrons and managerial bodies in Catholic education who may see mindfulness as incompatible with the ethos of Catholic schools, or who understand contemporary mindfulness practice as a spiritual practice belonging to Buddhism. It may prompt them to consider whether mindfulness practice can contribute to the Catholic educational vision of these schools, in terms of pre-evangelisation or as a contemplative practice that can improve wellbeing. Likewise, they may consider whether resources

618 See Stefan G. Reynolds, *Living with the Mind of Christ: Mindfulness in Christian Spirituality* (London: Darton, Longman & Todd, 2016) and Peter Tyler, *Christian Mindfulness: Theology and Practice* (London: SCM Press, 2018).

619 Stefan G. Reynolds, 'Mindfulness, Yoga and Schools: An Opportunity or a Problem?', *The Furrow* (December 2019).

in the Catholic faith tradition could also be drawn upon or devised to promote Christian contemplative or silent prayer. For Catholic educational practitioners, it may encourage them to explore how mindfulness practice contributes to the holistic development of the child and how it would contribute to their distinctive Catholic school ethos.

At a time of change, crisis and conflict, resources that enable each person to notice the presence of God in their lives, present to the Holy Mystery at the ground of their being, are to be welcomed wholeheartedly. In the Catholic school, mindfulness may be yet another gift that enables Christ's proclamation that he has come that we may have life in abundance, a means of flourishing and being more fully and authentically human.

Bibliography

Books

Bäckström, Anders, Edgardh, Nina and Pettersson, Per, *Religious Change in Northern Europe: The Case of Sweden* (Stockholm: Verbum, 2004).

Bellah, Robert N., Madsen, Richard, Sullivan, William M., Swidler, Ann and Tipton, Steven M, *Habits of the Heart: Individualism and Commitment in American Life* (CA: University of California Press, 1985).

Berger, Peter, *The Desecularization of the World: Resurgent Religion and Global Politics* (Grand Rapids: Eerdmans, 1999).

Biallowons, Hubert and Imhof, Paul, *Karl Rahner in Dialogue: Conversations and Interviews 1962–1985*, translated by Egan, Harvey D. (MI: Crossroad Publishing, 1986).

Blanchard, Shaun and Bullivant, Stephen, *Vatican II: A Very Short Introduction* (Oxford: Oxford University Press, 2023).

Boeve, Lieven. *God Interrupts History: Theology in a Time of Upheaval* (NY: Continuum, 2007).

Boeve, Lieven. *Interrupting Tradition: An Essay on Christian Faith in a Postmodern Context* (Louvain: Peeters Press, 2003).

Boeve, Lieven. *Lyotard and Theology* (London: Bloomsbury, 2014).

Boyce, Barry, *The Mindfulness Revolution: Leading Psychologists, Scientists, Artists, and Spiritual Teachers on the Power of Mindfulness in Daily Life* (Boston, MA: Shambala, 2011).

Bruce, Steve. *God Is Dead: Secularization in the West, Religion in the Modern World* (Malden, MA: Blackwell, 2002).

Bullivant, Stephen. *Faith and Unbelief: Faith Going Deeper* (London: Canterbury Press Norwich, 2013).

Carrette, Jeremy R., and King, Richard. *Selling Spirituality: The Silent Takeover of Religion* (New York: Routledge, 2005).

Carter, Stephen L., *The Culture of Disbelief: How American Law and Politics Trivialize Religious Devotion* (New York: Basic Books, 1993).

Carus, Paul. *The Gospel of Buddha: According to Old Records* (LaSalle, IL: Open Court Publications, 2004).

Casey, Thomas G. *Wisdom at the Crossroads: The Life and Thought of Michael Paul Gallagher SJ* (New Jersey: Paulist Press, 2018).
Chaskalson, Michael. *The Mindful Workplace* (Oxford: Wiley-Blackwell, 2011).
Chomsky, Noam. *Profit Over People: Neoliberalism and Global Order* (New York: Seven Stories Press, 1999).
Davids, Thomas W. R, *Buddhist Suttas* (Oxford: Clarendon, 1881).
Davie, Grace, *Religion in Britain: A Persistent Paradox, 2nd Edition* (Oxford: Blackwell Press, 2015).
Davie, Grace, *Religion in Modern Europe: A Memory Mutates* (New York: Oxford University Press, 2000).
Davie, Grace, *The Sociology of Religion: A Critical Agenda* (London: SAGE Publications, 2013).
D'Souza, Mario, *A Catholic Philosophy of Education: The Church and Two Philosophers* (Quebec: McGill-Queen's University Press, 2016).
Eifler, Karen E. and Landy, Thomas M., eds, *Becoming Beholders: Cultivating Sacramental Imagination and Actions in College Classrooms* (Collegeville, MI: Liturgical Press, 2004).
Eliot, Thomas Stearns., *On Poetry and Poets* (London: Faber & Faber, 1957).
Ergas, Oren, *Reconstructing 'Education' Through Mindful Attention: Positioning the Mind at the Center of Curriculum and Pedagogy* (London: Palgrave, 2017).
Farias, Miguel and Wikholm, Catherine, *The Buddha Pill: Can Meditation Change You?* (London: Watkins, 2015).
Flannery, Austin, ed., *Vatican Council II: The Basic Sixteen Documents* (Dublin: Dominican Publications, 1996).
Forbes, David, *Mindfulness and Its Discontents: Education, Self and Social Transformation* (Nova Scotia: Fernwood Publishing, 2019).
Freire, Paulo. *Pedagogy of the Oppressed* (New York: Continuum, 1970).
Gaillardetz, Richard R., *Transforming Our Days: Spirituality, Community and Liturgy in a Technological Culture* (NY: Crossroad Publishing Company, 2000).
Gallagher, Michael P., *Clashing Symbols: An Introduction to Faith and Culture* (New York: Paulist Press, 2003).
Gallagher, Michael P., *Help My Unbelief* (Chicago: Loyola University Press, 1988).
Gallagher, Michael P., *Questions of Faith* (Dublin: Veritas, 1996).
Gallagher, Michael P., *Struggles of Faith: Essays by Michael Paul Gallagher* (Dublin, Columba Press, 1990).
Gawronski, Raymond, *Word and Silence: Hans Urs von Balthasar and the Spiritual Encounter between East and West* (WA: Angelico Press, 2015).
Gray, John, *Seven Types of Atheism* (London: Penguin Books, 2019).
Greeley, Andrew, *Religion in Europe at the End of the Second Millennium: A Sociological Profile* (London: Transaction, 2003).
Gribben, Crawford, *The Fall of Christian Ireland* (Oxford: Oxford University Press, 2021).

Groome, Thomas, *Educating for Life: A Spiritual Vision for Every Teacher and Parent* (Allen, Texas: Thomas More, 1998).
Groome, Thomas, *Faith for the Heart: A 'Catholic' Spirituality* (NY: Paulist Press, 2019).
Groome, Thomas, *What Makes Us Catholic: Eight Gifts for Life* (NY: HarperCollins, 2002).
Grün, Anselm, Halík, Tomáš and Nonhoff, Winfried, *Is God Absent? Faith, Atheism and Our Search for Meaning* (NJ: Paulist Press, 2016).
Halík, Tomáš, *From the Underground Church to Freedom* (Notre Dame, Indiana: University of Notre Dame Press, 2019).
Halík, Tomáš, *I Want You to Be: On the God of Love* (Indiana: Notre Dame Press, 2016).
Halík, Tomáš, *Night of the Confessor: Christian Faith in an Age of Uncertainty* (New York: Image Books, 2012).
Halík, Tomáš, *Patience with God: The Story of Zacchaeus Continuing in Us* (New York: Doubleday, 2009).
Halík, Tomáš, *The Afternoon of Christianity: The Courage to Change* (Notre Dame, Indiana: University of Notre Dame Press, 2024).
Hanh, Thich N., *The Heart of the Buddha's Teaching: Transforming Suffering into Peace, Joy and Liberation* (New York: Harmony Books, 2015).
Hanh, Thich N. and Levitt, Peter, *The Heart of Understanding: Commentaries on the Prajñaparamita Heart Sutra* (Berkley: Parallax Press, 1988).
Harvey, Peter, *An Introduction to Buddhism: Teachings, History and Practices. 1st Edition* (Cambridge: Cambridge University Press, 1990).
Harvey, Peter, *An Introduction to Buddhism: Teachings, History and Practices. 2nd Edition* (Cambridge: Cambridge University Press, 2013).
Hastings, Adrian, *A History of English Christianity 1920–1990* (London: SCM Press, 1991).
Hession, Anne, *Catholic Primary Religious Education in a Pluralist Environment* (Dublin: Veritas, 2015).
Hession, Anne and Kieran, Patricia, *Children, Catholicism and Religious Education* (Dublin: Veritas, 2005).
Himes, Michael J. and Himes, Kenneth R, *Fullness of Faith: The Public Significance of Theology* (NJ: Paulist Press, 1993).
Himes, Michael J., *The Mystery of Faith: An Introduction to Catholicism* (Cincinnati, OH, Saint Anthony Messenger Press, 2004).
Jones, David A. and Barrie, Stephen, *Thinking Christian Ethos: The Meaning of Catholic Education* (Oxford: Catholic Truth Society, 2015).
Kabat-Zinn, Jon, *Coming to Our Senses: Healing Ourselves and the World Through Mindfulness* (New York: Hachete, 2006).
Kabat-Zinn, Jon, *Full Catastrophe Living: Using the Wisdom of Your Body and Mind to Face Stress, Pain and Illness* (New York: Bantam Dell, 2000).

Kabat-Zinn, Jon, *Wherever You Go, There You Are: Mindfulness Meditation for Everyday Life* (London: Patikis, 1994).

Kavanagh, Patrick, *The Great Hunger* (London: Penguin, 2018).

Kearney, Richard and Zimmerman, Jens, *Reimagining the Sacred: Richard Kearney Debates God* (NY: Columbia University Press, 2016).

Keating, Noel, *Meditation with Children: A Resource for Teachers and Parents* (Dublin: Veritas, 2017).

Keown, Damien, *Buddhism: A Very Short Introduction* (Oxford: Oxford University Press, 2013).

Lane, Dermot A., *Catholic Education in the Light of Vatican II and Laudato Si'* (Dublin: Veritas, 2015).

Lane, Dermot A., *Challenges Facing Religious Education in Contemporary Ireland* (Dublin: Veritas, 2008).

Lane, Dermot A., *Religion and Education: Reimagining the Relationship* (Dublin: Veritas, 2013).

Lane, Dermot A., *Stepping Stones to Other Religions: A Christian Theology of Inter-Religious Dialogue* (Dublin: Veritas, 2011).

Lane, Dermot A., *Theology and Ecology in Dialogue: The Wisdom of Laudato Si'* (Dublin: Messenger Publications, 2020).

Lash, Nicholas, *The Beginning and End of Religion* (Cambridge, Cambridge University Press, 1996).

McEvoy, James E., *Leaving Christendom for Good: Church-World Dialogue in a Secular Age* (Maryland: Lexington Books/Rowman and Littlefield, 2014).

McIntyre, Alister, *After Virtue, 3rd Edition* (NY: Bloomsbury, 2011).

McKinney, Stephen and Sullivan, John, *Education in Catholic Perspective* (Surrey: Ashgate, 2013).

McMahan, David L., *The Making of Modern Buddhism* (Oxford: Oxford University Press, 2008).

McMahan, David L. *Rethinking Meditation: Buddhist Meditative Practice in Ancient and Modern Worlds* (Oxford: Oxford University Press, 2023).

Mulcahy, Caitríona, *Does the Weaving Well-being programme (WW) Affect the Academic Achievement and Engagement of Irish Primary School Students?* PhD Thesis, Mary Immaculate College PhD Thesis, 2023.

Murray, Donal, *A Special Concern – The Philosophy of Education: A Christian Perspective* (Dublin: Veritas, 1991).

Nussbaum, Martha C., *Cultivating Humanity: A Classical Defense of Reform in Liberal Education* (Cambridge, MA: Harvard University Press, 1997).

O' Malley, John W., *What Happened at Vatican II?* (MA: Harvard University Press, 2010).

Pope Francis and Wolton, Dominique, *A Future of Faith: The Path of Change in Politics and Society* (New York: St. Martin's Essentials, 2018).

Pring, Richard, *Challenges for Religious Education: Is There a Disconnect Between Faith and Reason?* (NY: Taylor & Francis, 2020).
Purser, Ronald E., *McMindfulness: How Mindfulness Became the New Capitalist Spirituality* (London: Repeater, 2019).
Rāhula, Walpolo, *What the Buddha Taught* (NY: Grove Press, 1974).
Rahner, Karl, *The Christian Commitment; Essays in Pastoral Theology,* edited by Hastings, Cecily (NY: Sheed & Ward, 1963).
Rajan, Raghuram, *The Third Pillar: How Markets and the State Leave Community Behind* (NY: Penguin, 2019).
Ratzinger, Joseph, *Theological Highlights of Vatican II* (NJ: Paulist Press, 2009).
Reynolds, Stefan G, *Living with the Mind of Christ: Mindfulness in Christian Spirituality* (London: Darton, Longman & Todd, 2016).
Roy, Olivier, *Secularism Confronts Islam* (New York: Columbia University Press, 2007).
Sacks, Jonathan, *Morality: Restoring the Common Good in Divided Times* (London: Hodder & Stoughton, 2020).
Schonert-Reichl, Kimberley A. and Roeser, Robert W., *Handbook of Mindfulness in Education: Integrating Theory and Research into Practice* (New York: Springer, 2016).
Segal, Zindel W., Williams, Mark and Teasdale, John, *Mindfulness-Based Cognitive Therapy for Depression: A New Approach to Preventing Relapse* (New York: Guilford Press, 2002).
Seligman, Martin E., *Flourish: A Visionary New Understanding of Wellbeing and Happiness* (NY: Free Press, 2011).
Seligman, Martin E. and Peterson, Christopher, *Character Strengths and Virtues: A Handbook and Classification* (Oxford, Oxford University Press, 2004).
Sheldrake, Philip, *Spirituality: A Very Short Introduction* (Oxford: Oxford University Press, 2012).
Smith, Christian and Benton, Melinda, *Soul Searching: The Religious and Spiritual Lives of American Teenagers* (New York: Oxford University Press, 2005).
Smith, James K.A., *How (Not) to Be Secular: Reading Charles Taylor* (Grand Rapids: Eerdmans, 2014).
Stanley Peters, Richard, *Ethics and Education* (London: Allen and Unwin, 1970).
Stock, Marcus, *Christ at the Centre: Why the Church Provides Catholic Schools* (Oxford: Catholic Truth Society, 2012).
Sullivan, John, *Catholic Education: Distinctive and Inclusive.* PhD Thesis, Institute of Education, University of London, 1998.
Taylor, Charles, *A Secular Age* (Cambridge: Harvard University Press, Belknap Press, 2007).
Taylor, Charles, *Modern Social Imaginaries* (Durham, Duke University Press, 2004).

Teasdale, John, *Mindfulness-Based Cognitive Therapy for Depression: A New Approach to Preventing Relapse* (New York, Guilford Press, 2002).
Thaye, Lama J., *Wisdom in Exile: Buddhism and Modern Times* (Bristol: Ganesha Press, 2017).
Thera, Nyanponika, *The Heart of Buddhist Meditation: The Buddha's Way of Mindfulness* (San Francisco, CA: Weiser Books, 2014).
Thomas, George, *Evaluating the Impact of the Paws b Mindfulness Programme on Mainstream Primary School Aged Pupils' Suppressing and Sustaining Attention Skills, and their Academic Proxy Measures*, PhD Thesis, University of Manchester, 2015.
Thompson, Katherine, *Christ-Centred Mindfulness: Connections to Self and God* (Sydney: Acorn Press, 2018).
Turner, Denys, *The Darkness of God: Negativity in Christian Mysticism* (Cambridge: CUP, 1995).
Turner, Frank M, *The Idea of a University (Rethinking the Western Tradition)* (New Haven: Yale University Press, 1996).
Tyler, Peter, *Christian Mindfulness: Theology and Practice* (London, SCM Press, 2018).
Vattimo, Gianni, *After Christianity* (New York: Columbia University Press, 2002).
Vattimo, Gianni, *Belief* (Cambridge: Polity Press, 1996).
Wexler, Philip and Hotam, Yotam, *New Social Foundations for Education: Education in 'Post-Secular' Society* (NY: Peter Lang, 2015).
Whittle, Sean, *A Theory of Catholic Education* (London: Bloomsbury, 2015).
White, John, *The Aims of Education Restated* (London: Routledge, 1982).
Wilder, Amos, *Theopoetic: Theology and the Religious Imagination* (Philadelphia: Fortress Press, 1976).
Williams, J., Mark G. and Kabat-Zinn, Jon, *Mindfulness: Diverse Perspectives on its Meaning, Origins and Applications* (Abingdon: Routledge, 2013).
Wilson, John, *Introduction to Moral Education* (England: Penguin Books, 1967).

Chapters in books

Abbey, Ruth, 'The Missing Question Mark', in Ian Leask, ed., *The Taylor Effect: Responding to a Secular Age* (Newcastle: Cambridge Scholars Publishing, 2010), 8–25.
Batchelor, Stephen, 'The Everyday Sublime', in Manu Bazzano, ed., *After Mindfulness: New Perspectives on Psychology and Meditation* (London: Palgrave McMillan, 2014), 37–48.

Boeve, Lieven, 'Thinking Sacramental Presence in a Postmodern Context: A Playground for Theological Renewal', in Boeve, Lieven Boeve and Leijssen, Lambert, eds, *Sacramental Presence in a Postmodern Context* (Leuven: Leuven University Press, 2001), 3–29.

Brown, Candy G., 'Can "Secular" Mindfulness Be Separated from Religion?' in Purser, Ronald E., Forbes, David and Burke, Adam, eds, *Handbook of Mindfulness: Culture, Context and Social Engagement* (Basel: Springer Publishing, 2016), 75–94.

Brugués, Jean-Louis, 'La Declaracion *Gravissimum Educationis* del Concilio Vaticano II', in Vide, Vicente Vide and Villar, José R., eds, *El Concilio Vaticano II: Una Perspectiva Teologica* (Madrid: Sao Paulo, 2013), 525–43.

Byrne, Gareth, 'The National Directory of Catechesis in Ireland: An Outworking of the Council', in edited by Coll, Niall, ed., *Ireland and Vatican II: Essays Theological, Pastoral and Educational* (Dublin: Columba Press, 2015), 298–314.

Coll, Niall, 'The Path of Interfaith Dialogue: Catholic Theological Explorations and their Significance for Education', in Coll, Niall, ed., *Ireland and Vatican II: Essays Theological, Pastoral and Educational* (Dublin: Columba Press, 2015), 299–315.

Conway, Eamonn, 'Vatican II on Christian Education: A Guide Through Today's 'Educational Emergency?', in Coll, Niall, ed., *Ireland and Vatican II: Essays Theological, Pastoral and Educational* (Dublin: Columba Press, 2015), 253–73.

Costello, Stephen, "Beyond Flourishing: 'Fullness' and 'Conversion' in Taylor and Lonergan", in Leask, Ian, ed., *The Taylor Effect: Responding to a Secular Age* (Newcastle: Cambridge Scholars Publishing, 2010), 8–25.

Cox, Harvey, 'The Myth of the Twentieth Century: The Rise and Fall of Secularization', in Baum, Gregory, ed., *The Twentieth Century: A Theological Overview* (New York: Orbis, 1999), 135–43.

Evans, David, 'Faith and Reason: The Route to Wisdom', in McKinney, Stephen and Sullivan John, eds, *Education in a Catholic Perspective* (NY: Routledge, 2013).

Forbes, David, 'Critical Integral Contemplative Education', in Purser, Ronald E., Forbes, David and Burke, Adam, eds, *Handbook of Mindfulness: Culture, Context and Social Engagement* (Basel: Springer Publishing, 2016), 355–68.

Gooch, Alex, 'Mindfulness as a Secular Spirituality', In Manu Bazzano, ed., *After Mindfulness: New Perspectives on Psychology and Meditation* (London: Palgrave McMillan, 2014), 101–11.

Grace, Gerald, 'First and Foremost the Church Offers its Educational Service to the Poor' Class. Inequality and Catholic Schooling in Contemporary Contexts, in Grace, Gerald, ed., *Gerald Grace, Faith, Mission and Challenge in Catholic Education: The Selected Works of Gerald Grace* (NY: RoutledgeFarmer, 2016), 65–84.

Groome, Thomas, 'What Makes a School Catholic?', in McLaughlin, Terence, O' Keefe, Joseph and O' Keeffe, Bernadette, eds, *The Contemporary Catholic School: Context, Identity and Diversity* (Oxfordshire: RoutledgeFarmer, 1996), 107–23.

Halifax, Joan, 'The Third Body: Buddhism, Shamanism and Deep Ecology', in Badiner, Alan H., ed., *Dharma Gaia: A Harvest of Essays in Buddhism and Ecology* (Berkley: Parallax Press, 1990), 20–38.

Halík, Tomáš, 'Europe between Laicity and Christianity', in Halík, Tomáš and Hošek, Pavel, eds, *A Czech Perspective on Faith in a Secular Age* (Washington: Council for Research and Values in Philosophy 2015), 53–60.

Hanh, Thich N., 'The Sun in My Heart', in Kaza, Stephanie and Kraft, Kenneth, eds, *Dharma Rain: Sources of Buddhist Environmentalism* (Boston: Shambala, 2000), 83–91.

Hession, Anne, '"Come and See": The Process of Catechesis', in Hession, Anne and Kieran, Patricia, eds, *Exploring Religious Education: Catholic Religious Education in an Intercultural Europe* (Dublin: Veritas, 2008), 199–211.

Hirst, Paul, 'Christian Education: A Contradiction in Terms', in Astley, J. and Frances, Leslie, eds, *Critical Perspectives on Christian Education* (Leominster: Gracewing, 1992), 6–11.

Hogan, Pádraig, "Inheritances of Learning and the 'Unquiet Frontiers of Modernity'", in Leask, Ian, ed., *The Taylor Effect: Responding to a Secular Age* (Newcastle: Cambridge Scholars Publishing, 2010), 39–52.

Hošek, Pavel, 'Towards a Kenotic Hermeneutics of Contemporary Czech Culture', in Halík, Tomáš and Hošek, Pavel, eds, *A Czech Perspective on Faith in a Secular Age* (Washington: Council for Research and Values in Philosophy 2015), 1–12.

Hwang, Yoon Suk and Kearney, Patrick, 'A Genealogy of Mindfulness', in Hwang, Yook Suk and Kearney, Patrick, eds, *A Mindfulness Intervention for Children with Autism Spectrum Disorder: Mindfulness in Behavioural Health* (Cham: Springer International Publishing, 2015), 5–21.

Kieran, Patricia, 'Invisibility and Inclusivity: Approaches to Religious Difference in Schools', in Hession, Anne and Kieran, Patricia, eds, *Exploring Religious Education: Catholic Religious Education in an Intercultural Europe* (Dublin: Veritas, 2008), 151–67.

Kilbride, Thomas, 'Understanding the Church Today', in Franchi, Leonardo and McKinney, Stephen, eds, *A Companion to Catholic Education* (Herefordshire: Gracewing, 2011), 56–74.

Koči, Martin and Roubík, Pavel, 'Searching the Altar of an Unknown God: Tomáš Halík on Faith in a Secular Age', in edited by Halík, Tomáš and Hošek, Pavel, eds, *A Czech Perspective on Faith in a Secular Age* (Washington: Council for Research and Values in Philosophy 2015), 95–124.

Lane, Dermot A., 'Nostra Aetate and Religious Education', in Hession, Anne and Kieran, Patricia, eds, *Exploring Religious Education: Catholic Religious Education in an Intercultural Europe* (Dublin: Veritas, 2008), 83–96.

Leahy, Brendan, 'Tradition', in Hession, Anne and Kieran Patricia, eds, *Exploring Theology: Making Sense of the Catholic Tradition* (Dublin: Veritas, 2007), 90–8.

Loy, David, 'The Challenge of Mindful Engagement', in Purser, Ronald E., Forbes, David and Burke, Adam, eds, *Handbook of Mindfulness: Culture, Context and Social Engagement* (Basel: Springer Publishing, 2016), 15–26.

Magid, Barry and Poirier, Marc R., 'The Three Shaky Pillars of Western Buddhism', in edited by Rosenbaum, Robert Meikyo and Magid, Barry, eds, *What's Wrong with Mindfulness (And What Isn't): Zen Perspectives* (Somerville, MA: Wisdom Publications, 2016), 39–52.

McClelland, V. Alan, 'Wholeness Faith and the Distinctiveness of the Catholic School, in edited by McLaughlin, Terence, O' Keefe, Joseph and O' Keeffe, Bernadette, eds, *The Contemporary Catholic School: Context, Identity and Diversity* (Oxfordshire: RoutledgeFarmer, 1996), 155–61.

McCombs, Barbera L., 'The Learner-Centered Psychological Principles: A Framework for Balancing Academic Achievement and Social-Emotional Learning Outcomes', in edited by Zins, Joseph E., Bloodworth, Michelle, Weissberg, Roger and Walberg, Herbert, eds, *Building Academic Success in Social and Emotional Learning* (New York: Teachers College Press, 2004), 23–9.

McLaughlin, Terence, 'The Distinctiveness of Catholic Education', in McLaughlin, Terence, O' Keefe, Joseph and O' Keeffe, Bernadette, eds, *The Contemporary Catholic School: Context, Identity and Diversity* (Oxfordshire: RoutledgeFarmer, 1996), 136–54.

McKinney, Stephen J., 'Affirming the Place of Scripture in the Catholic School', in Sean Whittle, ed., *Religious Education in Catholic Schools* (Oxford: Peter Lang, 2018), 173–92.

McKinney, Stephen J., 'Covid-19, Child Poverty, Catholic Schools and the Insights of Gustavo Gutiérrez', in Sean Whittle, ed., *Irish and British Reflections on Catholic Education* (Singapore: Springer, 2021), 29–40.

McKinney, Stephen J., 'The Preferential Option for the Poor and Catholic Schools', in Sean Whittle, ed., *Researching Catholic Education: Contemporary Perspectives* (Singapore: Springer, 2018), 95–112.

McKinney, Stephen, J., 'A Rationale for Catholic Schools', in Franchi, Leonardo and McKinney, Stephen, eds, *A Companion to Catholic Education* (Herefordshire: Gracewing, 2011), 147–61.

Moloney, Paul, 'Mindfulness: The Bottled Water of the Therapy Industry', in Purser, Ronald E., Forbes, David and Burke, Adam, eds, *Handbook of Mindfulness: Culture, Context and Social Engagement* (Basel: Springer Publishing, 2016), 269–92.

Morris, Andrew B., 'Selected Official Church Documents and Statements', in Morris, Andrew B., ed., *Catholic Education: Universal Principles, Locally Applied* (Newcastle: Cambridge Publishing, 2012), 11–25.

Poirier, Marc R., 'Mischief in the Marketplace for Mindfulness', in Rosenbaum, Robert M. and Magid, Barry, eds, *What's Wrong with Mindfulness (And What Isn't): Zen Perspectives* (Somerville, MA: Wisdom Publications, 2016), 13–28.

Pohlschneider, Johannes, 'Declaration on Christian Education', in Vorgrimler, Herbert, ed., *Commentary on the Documents of Vatican II* (NY: Herder & Herder, 1967–1969), 1–2.

Regan, Ethna, 'Catholic Anthropology', in Hession, Anne and Kieran Patricia, eds, *Exploring Theology: Making Sense of the Catholic Tradition* (Dublin: Veritas, 2007), 161–170.

Rosenbaum, Robert Meikyo, '"I" Doesn't Mind', in Rosenbaum, Robert Meikyo and Magid, Barry, eds, *What's Wrong with Mindfulness (And What Isn't): Zen Perspectives* (Somerville, MA: Wisdom Publications, 2016), 29–38.

Scharf, Robert, 'Epilogue', in Rosenbaum, Robert M. and Magid, Barry, eds, *What's Wrong with Mindfulness (And What Isn't): Zen Perspectives* (Somerville, MA: Wisdom Publications, 2016), 139–152.

Senauke, Alan Hozan, 'One Body, Whole Life: Mindfulness and Zen', in Rosenbaum, Robert M. and Magid, Barry, eds, *What's Wrong with Mindfulness (And What Isn't): Zen Perspectives* (Somerville, MA: Wisdom Publications, 2016), 69–80.

Sheridan, John-Paul, 'Catholic Teacher Formation in the Republic of Ireland', in Franchi, Leonardo and Rymarz, Richard, eds, *Formation of Teachers for Catholic Schools: Challenges and Opportunities in a New Era* (Singapore: Springer, 2022), 55–66.

Shields, James Mark, The Scope and Limits of Secular Buddhism: Watanabe Kaikyoku and the Japanese New Buddhist 'Discovery of Society', in Havnevik, Hanna, Hüsken, Ute, Teeuwen, Mark, Tikhonov, Vladimir and Wellens Koen, eds, *Buddhist Modernities: Re-Inventing Tradition in the Globalizing World* (NY: Routledge, 2017), 15–32.

Stanley, Steven. 'Sīla and Sati: An Exploration of Ethics and Mindfulness in Pāli Buddhism and their Implications for Secular Mindfulness-Based Applications', in Shonin, Edo, Van Gordon, William and Singh, Nirbay N., eds, *Buddhist Foundations of Mindfulness* (Berlin: Springer, 2015), 89–113.

Sullivan, John, 'Philosophy of Catholic Education', in Hession, Anne and Kieran, Patricia, eds, *Exploring Religious Education: Catholic Religious Education in an Intercultural Europe* (Dublin: Veritas, 2008), 27–34.

Wood, W. Jay, 'Christian Theories of Virtue', in Nancy E. Snow, ed., *The Oxford Handbook of Virtue* (Oxford: Oxford Press, 2018), 281–300.

Church documents

Congregation for Catholic Education. *Consecrated Persons and their Mission in Schools*, 2002.

Congregation for Catholic Education. *Educating to Intercultural Dialogue in Catholic Schools: Living in Harmony for a Civilisation of Love*, 2013.

Congregation for Catholic Education. *Educating to Fraternal Humanism: Building a 'Civilisation of Love' 50 Years after Populorum Progressio*, 2017.

Congregation for Catholic Education. *The Catholic School*, 1977.

Congregation for Catholic Education. *The Identity of the Catholic School for a Culture of Dialogue*, 2022.

Congregation for Catholic Education. *The Religious Dimension of Education in a Catholic School*, 1988.

Congregation for the Doctrine of the Faith. *Letter to the Bishops of the Catholic Church on Some Aspects of Christian Meditation*, 1989.

Council for Catechetics, Irish Catholic Bishops' Conference. *A Reflection on Mindfulness: Rediscovering the Christian Tradition of Meditation and Contemplation* (Dublin: Veritas, 2018).

Irish Catholic Bishops' Conference. *Share the Good News: National Directory for Catechesis in Ireland* (Dublin: Veritas, 2014).

Irish Catholic Bishops' Conference. *Vision 08: A Vision for Catholic Education in Ireland-Pastoral Letter*, May 12, 2008. <https://www.catholicbishops.ie/wp-content/uploads/images/stories/cco_publications/Education/vision08pastoralletter.pdf> Accessed on 10 April 2021.

Pope Francis. *Evangelii Gaudium: The Joy of the Gospel*. Dublin: Veritas, 2013.

Pope Francis. *Fratelli Tutti*. Dublin: Veritas, 2020.

Pope Francis. General Audience, 22 May 2013. <http://www.vatican.va/content/francesco/en/audiences/2013/documents/papa-francesco_20130522_udienza-generale.html>. Accessed on 20 February 2021.

Pope Francis. *Laudato Si': On Care for Our Common Home*. Dublin: Veritas, 2015.

Pope Francis. *Message for the Launch of the Global Compact on Education*. Rome: Vatican, 2019.

Vatican II. *Dei Verbum (Dogmatic Constitution on Divine Revelation)*, 1965.

Vatican II. *Gravissimum Educationis (Declaration on Christian Education)*, 1965.

Vatican II. *Nostra Aetate (Declaration on the Church's Relations with non-Christian Religions)*, 1965.

World Synod of Bishops. *Justice in the World*. (1971) <https://www.cctwincities.org/wp-content/uploads/2015/10/Justicia-in-Mundo.pdf>. Accessed on 19 April 2021.

Journal articles

Albrecht, Nicole J., Albrecht, Patricia M. and Cohen, Marc, 'Mindfully Teaching in the Classroom: A Literature Review', *Australian Journal of Teacher Education, 37*(12) (2012), 1–14.

Alsubaie, Merfat A., 'Hidden Curriculum as One of Current Issue of Curriculum. *Journal of Education and Practice 6*(33) (2015), 125–8.

Amundsen, Richard, Riby, Leight M., Hamilton, Calum, Hope, Melanie and McGann, Deborah, 'Mindfulness in Primary School Children as a Route to Enhanced Life Satisfaction, Positive Outlook and Effective Emotion Regulation', *BMC Psychology 8(8)* (2020), 71.

Bakosh, Laura S., Snow, Renee M., Tobias, Jutta M., Houlihan, Janice L. and Barbosa-Leiker, Celestina, 'Maximizing Mindful Learning: Mindful Awareness Intervention Improves Elementary School Students' Quarterly Grades', *Mindfulness 7*(1) (2016), 59–67.

Berthold, Anne and Ruch, Willibald, 'Satisfaction with Life and Character Strengths of Non-Religious and Religious People: It's Practicing One's Religion That Makes the Difference', *Frontiers in Psychology 5* (2014), 876.

Bodhi, Bhikku, 'What Does Mindfulness Really Mean? A Canonical Perspective', *Contemporary Buddhism 12*(1) (2011), 19–39.

Boeve, Lieven, 'Faith in Dialogue: The Christian Voice in the Catholic Dialogue School', *International Studies in Catholic Education 11*(1) (2019), 37–50.

Boeve, Lieven, 'Interrupting Christian Identity Construction: Catholic Dialogue Schools and Negative Theology', *Religions 13*(2) (2022), 170.

Boeve, Lieven, 'Religion after Detraditionalization: Christian Faith in a Post-Secular Europe', *Irish Theological Quarterly 70*(2) (2005), 99–122.

Boeve, Lieven, 'Religious Education in a Post-secular and Post-Christian Context', *Journal of Beliefs and Values: Studies in Religion and Education 33*(2) (2012), 143–56.

Boeve, Lieven, 'The Shortest Definition of Religion: Interruption', *Communio Viatorum 46* (2004), 299–322.

Bishop, Scott, Lau, Mark, Shapiro, Shauna, Carlson, Linda, Anderson, Nicole D., Carmody, James, Sega, Zindel V., Abbey, Susan, Speca, Michael, Velting, Drew and Devins, Gerald, 'Mindfulness: A Proposed Operational Definition', *Clinical Psychology: Science and Practice 11*(3) (2004), 230–41.

Black, David S. and Fernando, Randima, 'Mindfulness Training and Classroom Behaviour Among Lower-Income and Ethnic Minority Elementary School Children', *Journal of Child and Family Studies 23* (2014), 1242–6.

Bonell, Chris, Humphrey, Neil, Fletcher, Adam, Moore, Laurence, Anderson, Rob and Campbell, Rona, 'Why Schools Should Promote Students' Health and Wellbeing', *The British Medical Journal Clinical Research 348*(May 13:2) (2014), g3078.

Boeve, Lieven, 'Faith in Dialogue: The Christian Voice in the Catholic Dialogue School', *International Studies in Catholic Education 11*(1) (2019), 37–50.

Broderick, Patricia C. and Metz, Stacie, 'Learning to BREATHE: A Pilot Trial of a Mindfulness Curriculum for Adolescents. Advances', *School Mental Health Promotion 2* (2009), 35–46.

Brunwasser, Steven M. and Gillham, Jane E., 'A Meta-Analytic Review of the Penn Resiliency Programme'. Presented at the Society for Prevention Research, San Francisco, CA (2008).

Carroll, Thomas, 'Mindfulness as *Praeparatio Evangelica* in the Irish Catholic School', *Irish Theological Quarterly 88*(4) (2023), 323–39.

Carroll, Thomas, 'Mindfulness in Catholic Primary Schools: An Irish Perspective', *Religions 14*(11) (2023), 1348.

Chen, Ying and VanderWeele, Tyler J., 'Associations of Religious Upbringing with Subsequent Health and Well-Being From Adolescence to Young Adulthood: An Outcome-Wide Analysis', *American Journal of Epidemiology 187*(11) (2018), 2355–64.

Chiesa, Alberto and Serretti, Alessandro, 'Mindfulness Based Cognitive Therapy for Psychiatric Disorders: A Systematic Review and Meta-analysis', *Psychiatry Research 187*(3) (2011), 441–53.

Ciarrochi, Joseph, Atkins, Paul W. B., Hayes, Louise L., Sahdra, Baljinder K. and Parker, Philip, 'Contextual Positive Psychology: Policy Recommendations for Implementing Positive Psychology into Schools', *Frontiers in Psychology 7* (2016), 1561.

Conway, Eamonn and Finegan, Thomas, 'Public Funding and Divestment of Public Schools', *Melita Theologica 66*(1) (2016), 47–68.

Coronado-Montoya, Stephanie, Levis, Alexander W., Kwakkenbos, Linda, Steele, Russell J., Turner, Erick H. and Thombs, Brett D, 'Reporting of Positive Results in Randomized Controlled Trials of Mindfulness-based Mental Health Interventions', *PLOS ONE 11*(4) (2016).

Cotterill, Aden, 'Tomáš Halík: A Theology for the Post-Secular', *Theological Studies 85*(1) (2024), 78–95.

Crompton, Katie, Kaklamanou, Daphne, Fasulo, Allesandra and Somogyi, Eszter, 'The Effects of a School-Based Mindfulness Programme (Paws b) on Empathy and Prosocial Behaviour: A Randomised Controlled Trial', *Mindfulness 15*(3) (2024).

Curtin, Margaret, O' Shea, Maria and Hayes, Claire, 'The Impact and Lived Experience of Covid-19 Restrictions for Vulnerable Children and Families in a Low-Income Irish Community', *Child Care in Practice 29*(4) (2023), 470–86.

Davie, Grace, 'Religion in 21st Century Europe: Framing the Debate', *Irish Theological Quarterly 78*(3) (2013), 279–93.

Dewey, John, 'My Pedagogic Creed', *School Journal 54*(3) (1897), 77–80.

Dobkin, Patricia L. and Zhao, Qinki, 'Increased Mindfulness – The Active Component of the Mindfulness-based Stress Reduction Program?', *Complementary Therapies in Clinical Practice 17*(1) (2011), 22–7.

Dreyfus, Georges, 'Is Mindfulness Present-centred and Non-judgmental? A Discussion of the Cognitive Dimensions of Mindfulness', *Contemporary Buddhism 12*(1) (2011), 41–54.

Durlak, Joseph A., Weissberg, Roger P., Dymnicki, Allison B., Taylor, Rebecca D. and Schellinger, Kriston B., 'The Impact of Enhancing Students' Social and Emotional Learning: A Meta-Analysis of School-Based Universal Interventions', *Child Development 82*(1) (2011), 405–32.

Dych, William V., 'Karl Rahner: An Interview', *America 123*(13) (October 31, 1970), 357–8.

Ergas, Oren and Hadar, Linor L., 'Mindfulness in and as Education: A Map of a Developing Academic Discourse from 2002 to 2017', *Review of Education 7*(3) (2019), 757–97.

Franchi, Leonardo, 'Catholic Education and Intercultural Dialogue', *Logos: A Journal of Catholic Thought and Culture 19*(4) (2016), 117–39.

Gallagher, Michael P., 'Imagination Gone Secular?', *The Furrow 57*(11) (2006), 589–93.

Gallagher, Michael P., 'Secularization and New Forms of Faith', *Studies, An Irish Quarterly Review, Spring* (1985), 12–25.

Gallagher, Michael P., 'What Are We doing When We Do Theology?', *Landas: Journal of Loyola School of Theology 28* (2014), 1–12.

Gillet-Swan, Jenna and Sargeant, Jonathan, 'Wellbeing as a Process of Accrual: Beyond Subjectivity and Beyond the Moment', *Social Indicators Research 121*(1) (2015), 135–48.

Glendenning, Tony and Bruce, Steve, 'New Ways of Believing or Belonging: Is Religion Giving Way to Spirituality?', *The British Journal of Sociology 57*(3) (2006), 399–414.

Godzieba, Anthony J., 'The Catholic Sacramental Imagination and the Access/Excess of Grace', *New Theology Review 21*(3) (August 2008), 14–26.

Goyal, Madhav, Singh, Sonal, Sibinga, Erica, Gould, Neda F., Rowland-Seymour, Anastasia, Sharma, Ritu, Berger, Zackary, Sleicher, Dana, Maron, David D., Shihab, Hasan M., Ranasinghe, Padmini, Linn, Shauna, Saha, Shonali, Bass, Eric B. and Haythornthwaite, Jennifer, 'Meditation Programs for Psychological Stress and Well-being: A Systematic Review and Meta-analysis', *JAMA Internal Medicine 174*(3) (2014), 357–68.

Greenfield, Emily A. and Marks, Nadine F., 'Religious Social Identity as an Explanatory Factor for Associations Between More Frequent Formal Religious Participation and Psychological Well-Being', *The International Journal for the Psychology of Religion 17*(3) (2007), 245–59.

Gunawardena Harshi, Voukelatos Alexander, Nair Sham, Cross Shane and Hickie, Ian B., 'Efficacy and Effectiveness of Universal School-Based Wellbeing Interventions in Australia: A Systematic Review', *International Journal of Environmental Research and Public Health 20(15)* (2023), 6508.

Haldane, John, 'Philosophy and Catholic Education', *The Sower 16*(3) (1995), 30–1.

Harrington, Anne and Dunne, John, 'Mindfulness Meditation: Frames and Choices', *American Psychologist*, 1-27. <http://nrs.harvard.edu/urn-3:HUL.InstRepos:10718406> Accessed on 18 November 2019.

Hayes, Stephen C., 'Acceptance and Commitment Therapy, Relational Frame Theory and the Third Wave of Behavioural Therapies', *Behaviour Therapy 35*(4) (2004), 639–55.

Heinz, Manuela, Davison, Kevin and Keane, Elaine, 'I Will Do It but Religion Is a Very Personal Thing': Teacher Education Applicants' Attitudes Towards Teaching Religion in Ireland, *European Journal of Teacher Education 41* (2018), 232–45.

Himes, Michael J., 'Living Conversation: Higher Education in a Catholic Context', *Conversations on Jesuit Higher Education*, Fall (1995), 21–7.

Hülsheger, Ute R., Alberts, Hugo J. E. M., Feinholdt, Alina and Lang, J. W. B., 'Benefits of Mindfulness at Work: The Role of Mindfulness in Emotion Regulation, Emotional Exhaustion, and Job Satisfaction', *Journal of Applied Psychology 98*(2) (2013), 310–25.

Huppert, Felicia A. and Johnson, Daniel M., 'A Controlled Trial of Mindfulness Training in Schools: The Importance of Practice for an Impact on Well-being', *The Journal of Positive Psychology 5*(4) (2010), 264–74.

Hyland, Terry, 'The Limits of Mindfulness: Emerging Issues for Education', *British Journal of Educational Studies, 64*(1) (2016), 97–117.

Ivey, Gavin, 'The Mindfulness Status of Psychoanalytic Psychotherapy', *Psychoanalytic Psychotherapy 29*(4) (2015), 382–98.

Kabat-Zinn, Jon, 'An Outpatient Program in Behavioral Medicine for Chronic Pain Patients Based on the Practice of Mindfulness Meditation: Theoretical Considerations and Preliminary Results', *General Hospital Psychiatry 4*(1) (1982), 33–47.

Kabat-Zinn, Jon, 'Mindfulness-Based Interventions in Context: Past, Present and Future', *Clinical Psychology: Science and Practice 10*(2) (2003), 144–56.

Kabat-Zinn, Jon, 'Some Reflections on the Origins of MBSR, Skilful Means and the Trouble with Maps', *Contemporary Buddhism 12*(1) (2011), 183–97.

Kabat-Zinn, Jon, Lipworth, Leslie and Burney, Robert, 'The Clinical Use of Mindfulness Meditation for the Self-regulation of Chronic Pain', *Journal of Behavioural Medicine 8*(2) (1985), 163–90.

Keng, Shian-Ling, Smoski J., Moria J. and Robins, Clive J., 'Effects of Mindfulness on Psychological Health: A Review of Empirical Studies', *Clinical Psychology Review 31*(6) (2011), 1041–56.

Kieran, Patricia, and Mullaly, Aiveen, 'Beyond Belief? Pre-service Teachers' Perspectives on Teaching RE in Ireland', *Journal of Religious Education 69* (2021), 423–37.

Killoran, Isobel, 'Mindfulness in Education: Using and Teaching Mindfulness in Schools', *Childhood Education 93*(2) (2017), 99.

Kirmayer, Laurence J. 'Mindfulness in Cultural Context', *Transcultural Psychiatry 52*(4) (2015), 447–69.

Klein, Luiz F., Richard Philippe and Wodon, Quentin, 'Pope Francis' Vision for Education and the Call for a Global Compact on Education', *The Review of Faith and International Affairs 21* (2023), 7–14.

Kuyken, Willem, Weare, Katherine, Ukoumunne, Obioha C., Vicary, Rachael, Motton, Nicola, Burnett, Richard, Cullen, Chris, Hennelly, Sarah and Huppert, Felicia, 'Effectiveness of the Mindfulness in Schools Programme: Non-Randomised Controlled Feasibility Study', *British Journal of Psychiatry 203*(2) (2013), 126–31.

Lambert, Yves, 'A Turning Point in Religious Evolution in Europe', *Journal of Contemporary Religion 19* (2004), 29–45.

Langer, Ellen J., 'A Mindful Education', *Educational Psychologist 28*(1) (2003), 43–50.

Langer, Ellen J. and Piper, Alison I., 'The Prevention of Mindlessness', *Journal of Personality and Social Psychology 53* (1987), 280–7.

Mani, Madhaven, Kavanagh, David J., Hides, Leanne and Stoyanov, Stoyan R., 'Review and Evaluation of Mindfulness-Based iPhone Apps', *JMIR mHealth and uHealth, 3*(3) *e82* (2015).

Marini, Guillermo and Galioto, Carmelo, 'The Way of Beauty' in Catholic Schools: Keys of Understanding and Pedagogical Orientations', *International Studies in Catholic Education 16*(2) (2023), 208–23.

McKinney, Stephen J., 'The Roots of the Preferential Option for the Poor in Catholic Schools in Luke's Gospel', *International Studies in Catholic Education 10*(2) (2018), 220–32.

McGrath, Alister E., 'On the Threshold of Mystery: Tomáš Halík on Cultural Witness in an Age of Uncertainty and Change', *Religions* 14 (2023), 399.

McIntyre, Alastair, 'The End of Education: The Fragmentation of the American University', *Commonweal 133*(18) (2006), 10–14.

Meehan, Amalee, 'Religion as a Source of Well-Being: Implications for Second-Level School Programs in Ireland and Beyond', *Religious Education 115*(5) (2020), 507–21.

Meehan, Amalee, 'Wellbeing in the Irish Junior Cycle: The Potential of Religious Education', *Irish Educational Studies 38*(4) (2019), 501–518.

Monteiro, Lynette, Musten, Frank and Compson Jane F., 'Traditional and Contemporary Mindfulness: Finding the Middle Path in the Tangle of Concerns', *Mindfulness 6*(1) (2014), 1–13.

Noddings, Nel, 'A Morally Defensible Mission for Schools in the Twenty First Century', *The Phi Delta Kappan 76* (1995), 365–68.

Nohilly, Margaret and Tynan, Fionnuala, 'The Evolution of Wellbeing in Educational Policy in Ireland', *International Journal of Wellbeing 12*(1) (2022), 42–53.

O'Donnell, Aislinn, 'Contemplative Pedagogy and Mindfulness: Developing Creative Attention in an Age of Distraction', *Journal of Philosophy of Education 49*(2) (2015), 187–202.

O' Sullivan, Katriona, Clark, Serena, McGrane, Amy, Rock, Nicole, Burke, Lydia, Boyle, Neasa, Joksimovic, Natasha and Marshall, Kevin, 'A Qualitative Study of Child and Adolescent Mental Health during the COVID-19 Pandemic in Ireland', *International Journal of Environmental Research and Public Health 18*(3) (2021), 1062.

Palermo, Francisco, Hanish, Laura D., Martin, Carol L., Fabes, Richard A. and Reisier, Mark, 'Preschoolers' Academic Readiness: What Role does the Teacher–Child Relationship Play?', *Early Childhood Research Quarterly 22*(4) (2007), 407–22.

Palmer, Parker, 'Teaching with Heart and Soul: Reflections on Spirituality in Teacher Education', *Journal of Teacher Education 54* (2003), 376–85.

Reynolds, Steffan Gillow, 'Mindfulness, Yoga and Schools: An Opportunity or a Problem?', *The Furrow* (December 2019), 678–83.

Rosen, Gerald M. and Davison, Gerald C., 'Psychology Should List Empirically Supported Principles of Change (ESPs) and not Credential Trademarked Therapies or Other Treatment Packages', *Behavioral Modification 27* (2003), 300–12.

Roth, Harold D., 'Against Cognitive Imperialism: A Call for a Non-Ethnographic Approach to Cognitive Science and Religious Studies', *Religion East and West 8* (2008), 1–26.

Scharf, Robert, 'Is Mindfulness Buddhist? (and Why it Matters)', *Transcultural Psychiatry 52*(4) (2015), 470–84.

Scharf, Robert, 'Buddhist Modernism and the Rhetoric of Meditative Experience', *Numen 42*(3) (1995), 228–83.

Schmidt, Andreas T., 'The Ethics and Politics of Mindfulness-Based Interventions', *Journal of Medical Ethics 0* (2016), 1–5.

Schonert-Reichl, Kimberley A. and Lawlor, Molly S., 'The Effects of a Mindfulness-Based Education Program on Pre-and Early Adolescents' Well-being and Social and Emotional Competence', *Mindfulness 1*(3) (2010), 137–51.

Seligman, Martin E. and Csikszentmihalyi, Mihaly, 'Positive Psychology: An Introduction', *American Psychologist 55*(1) (2000), 5–14.

Seligman, Martin E., Ernst, Randall M., Gillham, Jane E., Reivich, Karen J. and Linkin, Mark, 'Positive Education: Positive Psychology and Classroom Interventions', *Oxford Review of Education 35* (2009), 293–311.

Seligman, Martin E. and Sheena Sethi, 'Optimism and Fundamentalism', *Psychological Science 4*(4) (1993), 256–9.

Senauke, Alan and Gates, Barbera, 'The Thousand Year View: An Interview with Jon Kabat-Zinn', *Inquiring Mind 30*(2) Spring 2014.

Shonin, Edo and Van Gordon, William, 'Thupten Jingpa on Compassion and Mindfulness', *Mindfulness 7* (2016), 279–283.

Sohn, Samantha, Rees, Philippa, Wildridge, Bethany, Kalk, Nicola J. and Carter, Ben, 'Prevalence of Problematic Smartphone Usage and Associated Mental Health Outcomes amongst Children and Young People: a Systematic Review, Meta-analysis and GRADE of the Evidence', *BMC Psychiatry 19 Article Number 356* (2019).

Starkey, Caroline, 'British Buddhism, Secular Mindfulness and the Politics of Sustainability', *Religion 54* (2023), 179–202.

Sullivan, John, 'Catholic Education as Ongoing Translation', *International Studies in Catholic Education 4*(2) (2012), 200–7.

Thomas, George and Atkinson, Cathy, 'Measuring the Effectiveness of a Mindfulness-Based Intervention for Children's Attentional Functioning', *Educational & Child Psychology 33*(1) (2016), 51–64.

Wimmer, Lena F. and Dorjee, Dusana, 'Towards Determinants and Effects of Long-Term Mindfulness Training in Pre-Adolescence: A Cross-Sectional Study Using Event-Related Potentials', *Journal of Cognitive Education and Psychology 19* (2020), 65–83.

Van Cappellen, Peter, Toth-Gauthier, Maria, Saraglou, Vassilis and Fredrikson, Barbara L., 'Religion and Well-Being: The Mediating Role of Positive Emotions', *Journal of Happiness Studies 17* (2016), 485–505.

VanderWeele, Tyler J., 'Religious Communities and Human Flourishing', Current Directions, *Psychological Science 26*(5) (October 2017), 476–81.

Vickery, Charlotte E. and Dorjee, Dusanna, 'Mindfulness Training in Primary Schools Decreases Negative Affect and Increases Meta-Cognition in Children', *Frontiers in Psychology 6* (2016), 2025.

Voas, David and Crockett, Alasdair, 'Religion in Britain. Neither Believing nor Belonging', *Sociology 39*(1) (2005), 11–28.

Vörös, Sebastjan, 'Mindfulness De- or Recontextualized? Traditional Buddhist and Contemporary Perspectives', *Taiwan Journal of East Asian Studies 13*(1) (2016), 1–34.

Wallace, B. Alan, 'A Mindful Balance', *Tricycle XVII*(3) (Spring 2008), 60–63, 100.

Waters, Lea, 'A Review of School-Based Positive Psychology Interventions', *The Australian Educational and Developmental Psychologist 28*(2) (2011), 75–90.

Weare, Katherine, 'Developing Mindfulness with Children and Young People: A Review of the Evidence and Policy Context', *Journal of Children's Services 8*(2) (2013), 141–53.

Wong, Penelope, 'Dissenting Voices of and About Mindfulness: What Can We Learn?' *Journal for the Liberal Arts and Sciences 24*(2) (2021), 64–76.

Zenner, Charlotte, Herrnleben-Kurz, Solveig and Walach, Harald, 'Mindfulness-Based Interventions in Schools – A Systematic Review and Meta-Analysis', *Frontiers in Psychology* 5 (2014), 603–16.

Zgierska, Aleksandra, Rabago, David, Chawla, Neharika, Kushner, Kenneth, Koehler, Robert and Marlatt, Allan, 'Mindfulness Meditation for Substance Use Disorders: A Systematic Review', *Substance Abuse 30* (2009), 266–94.

Žižek, Slavoj, 'From Western Marxism to Western Buddhism', *Cabinet 2* (Spring 2001).

News articles

Chaykowski, Kathleen, 'Meet Headspace: The App That Made Meditation a $250 Million Business'. *Forbes*, 8 January 2017. <https://www.forbes.com/sites/kathleenchaykowski/2017/01/08/meet-headspace-the-app-that-made-meditation-a-250-million-business/#21efbc911f1b>. Accessed on 22 March 2020.

Gelles, David, 'The Mind Business. *UK Financial Times*, 25–26 August 2012'. <https://www.ft.com/content/d9cb7940-ebea-11e1-985a-00144feab49a>. Accessed on 28 November 2019.

Kabat-Zinn, Jon, 'Mindfulness has Huge Health Benefits- But McMindfulness is no Panacea'. *The Guardian*, 20 October 2015. <https://www.theguardian.com/commentisfree/2015/oct/20/mindfulness-mental-health-potential-benefits-uk>. Accessed on 28 November 2019.

Kluger, Jeffrey, 'The Coronavirus Seems to Spare Most Kids from Illness, but Its Effect on Their Mental Health Is Deepening'. *TIME Magazine*, 23 July 2020. <https://time.com/5870478/children-mental-health-coronavirus>. Accessed on 4 August 2020.

Landeau, Elizabeth. 'Can Mindfulness Help Manage Pain and Mental Illness?' *CNN Edition*, 16 November 2010. <https://edition.cnn.com/2010/HEALTH/11/16/mindfulness.therapy.meditation/index.html>. Accessed on 24 March 2021.

Manning, John, "'Weaving well-being' Fiona Forman and Mick Rock talk to John Manning about the ground-breaking school programme they developed to teach the power of positivity". *Fingal Independent*, 29 April 2017. <https://www.independent.ie/regionals/fingalindependent/lifestyle/weaving-well-being-35649138.html>. Accessed on 15 September 2020.

McBride, Michelle, 'Breathing Bells and Mind Jars: Mindfulness Comes to School'. *Irish Times*, 17 January 2017. <https://www.irishtimes.com/news/education/breathing-bells-and-mind-jars-mindfulness-comes-to-school-1.2933176>. Accessed on 12 August 2020.

Naughton, Celine, 'How Mindfulness is Teaching Children to Cope in School', *Irish Independent*, 12 April 2016. <https://www.independent.ie/life/health-wellbeing/how-mindfulness-is-teaching-children-to-cope-in-school-34618690.html>. Accessed on 25 March 2021.

Pickert, Kate, 'The Mindful Revolution', *TIME Magazine*, 3 February 2014. <http://content.time.com/time/subscriber/article/0,33009,2163560,00.html>. Accessed on 4 November 2019.

Seldon, Anthony, 'Our Education System is Collapsing into a Form of Mass Indoctrination', *Independent*, 23 October 2011. <https://www.independent.co.uk/voices/commentators/anthony-seldon-our-education-system-collapsing-form-mass-indoctrination-2028709.html>. Accessed on 24 December 2020.

Reports and policy documents

Andrews, Arlene B., Ben-Arieh, Asher, Carlson, Maya, Damon, William, Dweck, Carol, Earls, Felton, Garcia-Coll, Cynthia, Gold, Robert, Halfon, Neal, Hart, Roger, Lerner, Richard M., McEwen, Bruce, Meaney, Michael, Offord, Dan, Patrick, Donald, Peck, Magda, Trickett, Barbera, Weisner, Thomas and Zuckerman, Barry. *(Ecology Working Group) Ecology of Child Well-Being: Advancing the Science and the Science-Practice Link*. Georgia: Centre for Child Well-Being, 2002.

Clark, Helen, Marie Coll-Seck, Awa, Banjaree, Anshu, Peterson, Stefan, Dalglish, Sarah L., Ameratunga, Shanthi, Balabanova, Dina, Kishan Bhan, Maharaj, Bhutta, Zulfiqar A., Borrazzo, John, Claeson, Mariam, Doherty, Tanya, El-Jardali, Fadi, George, Asha S., Gichaga, Angela, Gram, Lu, Hipgrave, David B., Kwamie, Aku, Meng, Qingyue, Mercer, Raúl, Narain, Sunita, Nsungwa-Sabiiti, Jesca, Olumide, Adesola O., Osrin, David, Powell-Jackson, Timothy, Rasanathan, Kumanan, Rasul, Imran, Reid, Papaarangi, Requejo, Jennifer, Rohde, Sarah S., Rollins, Nigel, Romedenne, Magali, Singh Sachdev, Harshpal, Saleh, Rana, Shawar, Yusra R., Shiffman, Jeremy, Simon, Jonathon, Sly, Peter D., Stenberg, Karin, Tomlinson, Mark, Ved, Rajani R., and Costello, Anthony. A Future for the World's Children? A WHO–UNICEF–Lancet Commission. *The Lancet Commissions 395*(10224) (2020): 605–58.

Central Statistics Office. *Census of Population 2022: Summary Results,* 2023.

Department of Education and Skills. *Circular 0040/20: Arrangements for Inspection and School Self-Evaluation for the 2020/2021 School Year*. Dublin: Rialtas na hÉireann, 2020.

Department of Education and Skills. *Looking at our Schools 2016: A Quality Framework for Primary Schools*. Dublin: Rialtais na hÉireann, 2016.

Department of Education and Skills. *Statistical Bulletin- August 2024: Overview of Education: 2003/04–2023/24*. Dublin: Rialtas na hÉireann, 2024.

Department of Education and Skills. *Supporting the Wellbeing of School Communities as Schools Reopen: Guidance for Schools*. Dublin: Rialtas na hÉireann, 2020.

Department of Education and Skills. *Wellbeing Policy Statement and Framework for Practice 2018–2023 (Revised 2019)*. Dublin: Rialtas na hÉireann, 2019.

Dooley, Barbera, O' Connor, Clíodhna, Fitzgerald, Amanda and O' Reilly, Aileen. *My World Survey 2: The National Study of Youth Mental Health in Ireland*. Dublin: UCD and Jigsaw, 2019.

Ereaut, Gill and Whiting, Rebecca, Department for Children, Youth and Families. *What do We Mean by 'Wellbeing'?: And Why Might it Matter?* 2008.

Haynes, Laura, Service, Owain, Goldacre, Ben and Torgerson, David. *Test, Learn, Adapt: Developing Public Policy with Randomised Controlled Trials*. London: Cabinet Office, 2012.

Inchley, Jo, Currie, Dorothy, Budisavljevic, Sanja, Torsheim, Torbjørn, Jåstad, Atle, Cosma, Alina, Kelly, Colette, Már Arnarsson, Ársæll Már and Samdal, Oddrun. *Spotlight on Adolescent Health and Well-being: Findings from the 2017/2018 Health Behaviour in School-aged Children (HBSC) Survey in Europe and Canada. International Report. Volume 2. Key data*. Copenhagen: World Health Organisation Regional Office for Europe, 2020.

Islam, Nazrul and Winkel, John. Climate Change and Social Inequality. *UN Department of Economic and Social Affairs (DESA) Working Papers, No. 152*. NY: United Nations, 2017.

National Council for Curriculum and Assessment. *Guidelines for Wellbeing in Junior Cycle*. Dublin: NCCA, 2017.

National Council for Curriculum and Assessment. *Specification for Junior Cycle: Social, Personal and Health Education*. Dublin: NCCA, 2016.

National Council for Curriculum and Assessment. *The Framework for Junior Cycle*. Dublin: NCCA, 2015.

National Educational Psychological Service. *Wellbeing in Primary Schools: Guidelines for Mental Health Promotion*. Dublin: Rialtas na hÉireann, 2019.

Randles, Eileen. *Catholic Primary Schools Management Association Board of Management Handbook 2012*. Maynooth: CPSMA, 2012.

Report on Church of England Statistics for Mission 2017. <https://www.churchofengland.org/sites/default/files/2023-11/statisticsformission2022.pdf>. Accessed on 31 October 2024.

Suhrcke, Marc and de Paz Nieves, Carmen. *The Impact of Health and Health Behaviours on Educational Outcomes in High Income Countries: A Review of the Evidence*. Copenhagen: World Health Organisation Regional Office for Europe, 2011.

White, Janet. *Rapid Evidence Review: Reducing the Attainment Gap – The Role of Health and Wellbeing Interventions in Schools*. Edinburgh: NHS Health Scotland, 2017.

Websites

Abecina, Alex. Whose Virtues? Which Character Strengths? Positive Psychology in Christian Schools. Ethos Centre for Christianity and Society (2014). <http://www.ethos.org.au/online-resources/engage-mail/whose-virtues-which-character-strengths-positive-psychology>. Accessed on 17 September 2020.

American Psychological Association Database Webpage. Search Results for the term 'Mindfulness'. <https://psycnet.apa.org/search/results?type=direct&db=pi,pb,pa,pe,pt,pbc&fields=AnyField&term=mindfulness>. Accessed on 29 October 2024.

American Psychological Association Dictionary Webpage. Definition of Positive Psychology. <https://dictionary.apa.org/positive-psychology>. Accessed on 6 October 2020.

Batchelor, Stephen. A Secular Buddhist (2012). <https://gaiahouse.co.uk/wp-content/uploads/Stephen-Batchelor-A-Secular-Buddhist.pdf>. Accessed on 18 December 2019.

Beliefnet Web Page. Wendy Schuman Interview with Martin Seligman, The Psychology of Real Happiness: Psychologist Martin Seligman Helped Change His Profession's Focus from What's Wrong with People to What's Right with Them (2003). <https://www.beliefnet.com/wellness/health/2003/01/the-psychology-of-real-happiness.aspx>. Accessed on 1st October 2020.

Bodhi, Bhikku. A Look at the Kalama Sutta (1998). <https://www.accesstoinsight.org/lib/authors/bodhi/bps-essay_09.html>. Accessed on 31 December 2019.

Bodhi, Bhikku. The Noble Eightfold Path: The Way to the End of Suffering (2013). <http://www.accesstoinsight.org/lib/authors/bodhi/waytoend.html>. Accessed on 19 November 2019.

Burnett, Richard. Mindfulness in Schools: Learning Lessons from the Adults-Secular and Buddhist (2009) 1–48. <https://mindfulnessinschools.org/wp-content/uploads/2013/03/Mindfulness-in-schools-dissertation-Burnett.pdf>. Accessed on May 2021.

Catholic Education Service, About Us. <https://catholiceducation.ie/about-us/>. Accessed on 29 October 2024.

Catholic Schools Partnership, Catholic Schools – Looking to the Future (2012). <https://www.icatholic.ie/wp-content/uploads/2012/07/CSP-Future.pdf>. Accessed on 20 February 2022.

Catholic Schools Partnership. Understanding and Living the Ethos in a Catholic Primary School. <https://www.catholicschools.ie/understanding-and-living-the-ethos-in-a-catholic-primary-school/>. Accessed on 1 May 2021.

Chilcott, Lloyd. Academic Critique of Paws b, a Mindfulness Based Intervention for Children. University of Southampton Blog (2021). <https://blog.soton.ac.uk/edpsych/files/2021/07/PAWS-B-Jan-2021-Lloyd-Chilcott.pdf>. Accessed on 18 March 2024.

Christian Meditation Ireland, Meditation with Children. <http://www.christianmeditation.ie/?q=meditationwithchildren>. Accessed on 10 February 2021.

Department of Education Web Page on Extra Personal Vacation Days for Teachers. <https://www.education.ie/en/Education-Staff/Services/Breaks-Leave/Extra-Personal-Vacation-Days>. Accessed on 14 September 2020.

Department of Education Web Page on School Self Evaluation in Primary and Post-Primary Schools. <https://www.education.ie/en/Schools-Colleges/Services/Quality-Assurance/SSE-Primary-and-Post-Primary/School-Self Evaluation.html#:~:text=School%20self%2Devaluation%20(SSE),to%20improve%20outcomes%20for%20learners>. Accessed on 14 September 2020.

Forman, Fiona. An Introduction to Positive Psychology and the Weaving Well-Being Programme. CPD Presentation for Scoil an Spioraid Naoimh, Layton. (2018). <http://ssnlaytown.ie/wp-content/uploads/2018/08/Laytown-Weaving-Well-Being-002.pdf> Accessed on 7 September 2020.

Forman, Fiona. Summary of Findings of the Pilot Stage of the Weaving Wellbeing Programme. NUIG Health Promotion Conference (2019). <http://www.nuigalway.ie/media/healthpromotionresearchcentre/conference2019/Fiona-Forman.pdf>/>. Accessed on 8 September 2020.

Global Compact on Education Vademecum Home Page. <https://www.educationglobalcompact.org/resources/Risorse/vademecum-english.pdf>. Accessed on 29 October 2024.

Hawker Brownlow Education Publishers Home Page. <https://www.hbe.com.au/hb5343.html>. Accessed on 7 September 2020.

Home Page for Mindfulness-Based Cognitive Therapy. <http://www.mbct.com/>. Accessed on 4 August 2020.

Irish Catholic Bishops' Conference Web Page- Bishop Donal Murray, Catholic Primary Education in Contemporary Ireland: Facing New Horizons, 2009. <https://www.catholicbishops.ie/2009/05/22/address-by-bishop-donal-murray-bishop-of-limerick-and-chair-of-the-bishops-department-of-catholic-education-and-formation-at-the-mcauley-conference-series-catholic-primary-education-in-cont/>. Accessed on 16 February 2022.

Kabat-Zinn, Jon. Catalyzing Movement Towards a More Contemplative/Sacred-Appreciating/Non-Dualistic Society. The Contemplative Mind in Society Meeting of the Working Group, Sponsored by the Nathan Cummings Foundation & Fetzer Institute. 29 September–2 October 1994. <http://www.contemplative-mind.org/admin/wp-content/uploads/2012/09/kabat-zinn.pdf>. Accessed on 20 November 2019.

Lion's Roar Web Page. Interview by Danny Fisher with Jon Kabat-Zinn. Mindfulness and the Cessation of Suffering: An Exclusive New Interview with Mindfulness Pioneer Jon Kabat-Zinn. 2010. <http://www.lionsroar.com/mindfulness-and-the-cessation-of-suffering-an-exclusive-new-interview-with-mindfulness-pioneer-jon-kabat-zinn/>. Accessed on 18 November 2019.

Mindfulness in Schools Project Home Page. <https://mindfulnessinschools.org/about>. Accessed on 29 August 2020.

Mindfulness in Schools Page on Teaching the Paws b Curriculum. <https://mindfulnessinschools.org/teach-paws-b/> Accessed on 31 August 2020.

O'Toole, Catriona and O'Connor, Fiona. A Reprieve but not a Fix for Childhood Stresses: A Participatory Study of Schoolbased Mindfulness in an Irish Primary School. European Conference on Educational Research Presentation (2017). <https://www.maynoothuniversity.ie/sites/default/files/assets/document/ECER%202017%20Conference%20-%20Presentation%20by%20Dr.%20Catriona%20O%27Toole_0.pdf>. Accessed on 1 September 2020.

Podcast on McMindfulness with Dr Miles Neal. <https://innertruth.org/podcast/how-to-avoid-mcmindfulness-find-your-truth-with-dr-miles-neal>. Accessed on 24 November 2019.

Pew Forum: Believing without Belonging: Just How Secular is Europe? 5 December 2005. <https://www.pewforum.org/2005/12/05/believing-without-belonging-just-how-secular-is-europe/>. Accessed 8 August 2019.

Randles, Eileen: The Ethos of the Catholic Primary School' in Catholic Primary Schools Management Association Board of Management Handbook 2012. <https://www.cpsma.ie/wp-content/uploads/files/_Secure/Handbook/CPSMA_Handbook_2012.pdf>. Accessed on 15 February 2022.

Weaving Wellbeing Character Strengths Pupil Book Sample. <https://www.actnow.ie/wp-content/uploads/2018/04/Character-Strengths-Pupil-Book-Sample-Copy.pdf>. Accessed on 8 September 2020.

Weaving Wellbeing Concept Reinforcement and Progression Table. <https://weaving-wellbeing.com/wp-content/uploads/2015/07/WWB-Reinforcement-Progression-tableV4-for-WEB.jpg>. Accessed on 14 September 2020.

Weaving Wellbeing Home Page. <https://weavingwellbeing.com>. Accessed on 7 September 2020.

Weaving Wellbeing Mindmap. <https://weavingwellbeing.com/wp-content/uploads/2015/07/Mndmap-Weaving-Well-Being-Dec-2016-Low-Res.jpg>. Accessed on 8 September 2020.

Weaving Wellbeing Tools of Resilience Pupil Book Sample. <https://www.actnow.ie/wp-content/uploads/2018/04/Tools-of-Resilience-Pupil-Book-Sample-Copy.pdf>. Accessed on 8 September 2020.

Wellbeing Online Home Page for Washington State University. <https://wellbeingonline.wsu.edu/#:~:text=Wellbeing%20Online%20is%20dedicated%20to,holistic%20approach%20to%20healthy%20living>. Accessed on 4 August 2020.

Index

Religion, Education and Values

Debates about religion, education and values are more central to contemporary society than ever before. The challenges posed by the interaction between these different spheres will continue to increase as the effects of globalization and cultural pluralization impact on educational settings. Our radically changed and rapidly changing environment poses critical questions about how we should educate individuals to live in increasingly diverse societies.

Books in this series offer the most recent research, from a variety of disciplinary perspectives, on the interface between religion, education and values around the world. The series covers such themes as the history of religious education, the philosophies and psychologies of religious and values education, and the application of social science research methods to the study of young people's values and worldviews.

Books within the series are subject to peer review and include single and coauthored monographs and edited collections. Proposals should be sent to any or all of the series editors:

Professor Stephen G. Parker (s.parker@worc.ac.uk)
The Rev'd Canon Professor Leslie J. Francis (Leslie.Francis@warwick.ac.uk)
Professor Rob Freathy (r.j.k.freathy@ex.ac.uk)
Professor Mandy Robbins (mandy.robbins@glyndwr.ac.uk)

Vol. 1 Jeff Astley, Leslie J. Francis, Mandy Robbins and Mualla Selçuk (eds): Teaching Religion, Teaching Truth: Theoretical and Empirical Perspectives.
293 pages. 2012. ISBN 978-3-0343-0818-2

Vol. 2 Stephen Parker, Rob Freathy and Leslie J. Francis (eds):
Religious Education and Freedom of Religion and Belief.
286 pages. 2012. ISBN 978-3-0343-0754-3

Vol. 3 Ann Casson:
Fragmented Catholicity and Social Cohesion: Faith Schools in a Plural Society.
198 pages. 2013. ISBN 978-3-0343-0896-0

Vol. 4 Sylvia Baker:
Swimming Against the Tide: The New Independent Christian Schools and their Teenage Pupils.
259 pages. 2013. ISBN 978-3-0343-0942-4

Vol. 5 Nuraan Davids:
Women, Cosmopolitanism and Islamic Education: On the Virtues of Engagement and Belonging.
195 pages. 2013. ISBN 978-3-0343-1708-5

Vol. 6 Julian Stern:
Loneliness and Solitude in Education: How to Value Individuality and Create an Enstatic School.
224 pages. 2014. ISBN 978-3-0343-1733-7

Vol. 7 Stephen G. Parker, Rob Freathy and Leslie J. Francis (eds):
History, Remembrance and Religious Education.
423 pages. 2015. ISBN 978-3-0343-1720-7

Vol. 8 Trevor Cooling with Beth Green, Andrew Morris and Lynn Revell:
Christian Faith in English Church Schools: Research Conversations with Classroom Teachers.
205 pages. 2016. ISBN 978-3-0343-1938-6

Vol. 9 Julian Stern:
Virtuous Educational Research: Conversations on Ethical Practice.
258 pages. 2016. ISBN 978-3-0343-1880-8

Vol. 10 Jeff Astley and Leslie J. Francis (eds):
Diversity and Intersectionality: Studies in Religion, Education and Values.
264 pages. 2016. ISBN 978-3-0343-2252-2

Vol. 11 Robert A. Bowie:
Dignity and Human Rights Education: Exploring Ultimate Worth in a Post-Secular World.
314 pages. 2017. ISBN 978-3-0343-1940-9

Vol. 12 Olwyn E. Mark:
Educating for Sexual Virtue: A Moral Vision for Relationships and Sex Education.
254 pages. 2018. ISBN 978-1-78707-128-5

Vol. 13 Peter Cumper and Alison Mawhinney (eds):
Collective Worship and Religious Observance in Schools.
410 pages. 2018. ISBN 978-1-78707-655-6

Vol. 14 Jeff Astley, Leslie J. Francis and David W. Lankshear (eds):
Values, Human Rights and Religious Education: Contested Grounds.
350 pages. 2018. ISBN 978-1-78874-525-3

Vol. 15 Phra Nicholas Thanissaro:
The Intuitive Buddhist: Psychological Type as a New Hermeneutic of Buddhist Diversity in the West.
262 pages. 2020. ISBN 978-1-78997-185-9

Vol. 16 Youcef Sai:
Islamic Religious Education in Ireland: Insights and Perspectives.
218 pages. ISBN 978-1-78874-607-6

Vol. 17 Leslie J. Francis, David W. Lankshear and Stephen G. Parker (eds):
New Directions in Religious and Values Education: International Perspectives.
330 pages. 2021. ISBN 978-1-78997-876-6

Vol. 18 Antony Luby:
A Secular Principle: Dialogic RE from a Catholic Perspective
272 pages. 2021. ISBN 978-1-78997-643-4

Vol. 19 Thomas Carroll:
Mindfulness and Ethos: Compatibility, Challenges and Opportunities in the Irish Catholic Primary School.
328 pages. 2025. ISBN 978-1-80374-036-2

www.ingramcontent.com/pod-product-compliance
Ingram Content Group UK Ltd.
Pitfield, Milton Keynes, MK11 3LW, UK
UKHW021852100926
8556IPUK00020B/1192

9 781803 740362